Contributors

Audrey Knippa, MS, MPH, RN, CNE
Nursing Education Coordinator and
  Content Project Leader

Sheryl Sommer, PhD, MSN, RN, CNE
Director, Nursing Curriculum and
  Education Services

Brenda Ball, MEd, BSN, RN
Nursing Education Specialist

Lois Churchill, MN, RN
Nursing Education Specialist

Carrie B. Elkins, DHSc, MSN, PHCNS, BC
Nursing Education Specialist

Mary Jane Janowski, MA, BSN, RN
Nursing Resource Specialist

Sharon R. Redding, EdD, RN, CNE
Nursing Education Specialist

Karin Roberts, PhD, MSN, RN, CNE
Nursing Education Coordinator

Mendy G. Wright, DNP, MSN, RN
Nursing Education Specialist

Chris Crawford, BS Journalism
Product Developer and Editorial Project Leader

Derek Prater, MS Journalism
Lead Product Developer

Johanna Barnes, BA Journalism
Product Developer

Joey Berlin, BS Journalism
Product Developer

Hilary E. Groninger, BS Journalism
Product Developer

Megan E. Herre, BS Journalism
Product Developer

Amanda Lehman, BA English
Product Developer

Spring Lenox, BS Journalism
Product Developer

Robin Nelson, BA English
Product Developer

Joanna Shindler, BA Journalism
Product Developer

Morgan Smith, BS Journalism
Media Developer

Brant L. Stacy, BS Journalism, BA English
Product Developer

Mandy Tallmadge, BS Communication
Product Developer

Karen D. Wood, BS Journalism
Product Developer

Katherine Wood-Raclin, BA English, Mass
Communications
Product Developer

Consultants

Stephanie C. Butkus, MS, APRN, CPNP, CLC

Dr. Judy Drumm RN, DNS, CPN

P. Lea Monahan, PhD, RN

INTELLECTUAL PROPERTY NOTICE

IMPORTANT NOTICE TO THE READER

USER'S GUIDE

Welcome to the Assessment Technologies Institute® PN Nursing Care of Children Review Module Edition 8.0. The mission of ATI's Content Mastery Series® review modules is to provide user-friendly compendiums of nursing knowledge that will:

- Help you locate important information quickly.

- Assist in your remediation efforts.

- Provide exercises for applying your nursing knowledge.

- Facilitate your entry into the nursing profession as a newly licensed PN.

Organization

This review module is organized into units covering the foundations of nursing care of children, nursing care of children with system disorders, and nursing care of children with special needs. Chapters within these units conform to one of four organizing principles for presenting the content:

- Basic concepts

- Growth and development

- Procedures (diagnostic and therapeutic)

- Systems disorders

Basic concepts chapters begin with an overview describing the central concept and its relevance to nursing. Subordinate themes are in outline form to demonstrate relationships and present the information in a clear, succinct manner.

Growth and development chapters cover expected growth and development, including physical and psychosocial development and age-appropriate activities, and health promotion, including immunizations, health screenings, nutrition, and injury prevention.

Procedures chapters include an overview describing the procedure(s) covered in the chapter. These chapters will provide you with nursing knowledge relevant to each procedure, including indications, interpretations of findings, client outcomes, nursing actions, and complications.

Systems disorders chapters include an overview describing the disorder(s) and/or disease process. These chapters may provide information on health promotion and disease prevention before addressing data collection, including risk factors, subjective data, and objective data. Next, you will focus on collaborative care, including nursing care, medications, interdisciplinary care, therapeutic procedures, surgical interventions, care after discharge, and client outcomes. Finally, you will find complications related to the disorder, along with nursing actions in response to those complications.

Application Exercises

At the end of each chapter there are questions you can use to practice applying your knowledge. The Application Exercises include both NCLEX-style questions, such as multiple-choice and multiple-select items, and questions that ask you to apply your knowledge in other formats, such as short-answer and matching items. After completing the Application Exercises, go to the Application Exercise Answer Key to check your answers and rationales for correct and incorrect answers.

NCLEX® Connections

To prepare for the NCLEX-PN, it is important for you to understand how the content in this review module is connected to the NCLEX-PN test plan. You can find information on the detailed test plan at the National Council of State Boards of Nursing's Web site: https://www.ncsbn.org/. When reviewing content in this review module, regularly ask yourself, "How does this content fit into the test plan, and what types of questions related to this content should I expect?"

To help you in this process, we've included NCLEX Connections at the beginning of sections and units and with each question in the Application Exercises Answer Keys. The NCLEX Connections at the beginning of sections and units will point out areas of the detailed test plan that relate to the content within the section or unit. The NCLEX Connections attached to the Application Exercises Answer Keys will demonstrate how each exercise fits within the detailed content outline.

These NCLEX Connections will help you understand how the detailed content outline is organized, starting with major client needs categories and subcategories and followed by related content areas and tasks. The major client needs categories are:

- Safe and Effective Care Environment

  o Management of Care

  o Safety and Infection Control

- Health Promotion and Maintenance

- Psychosocial Integrity

- Physiological Integrity

  o Basic Care and Comfort

  o Pharmacological Therapies

  o Reduction of Risk Potential

  o Physiological Adaptation

An NCLEX Connection might, for example, alert you that content within a unit is related to:

- Physiological Adaptation

  o Potential for Alterations in Body Systems

    ▪ Compare current client clinical data to baseline information.

Icons

Throughout the review module you will see icons that will draw your attention to particular areas. Keep an eye out for these icons:

 This icon indicates an Overview, or introduction, to a particular subject matter. Descriptions and categories will typically be found in an Overview.

 This icon indicates Application Exercises and Application Exercises Answer Keys.

 This icon indicates NCLEX connections.

 This icon indicates content related to safety. When you see this icon, take note of safety concerns or steps that nurses can take to ensure client safety and a safe environment.

 This icon indicates that a media supplement, such as a graphic, an animation, or a video, is available. If you have an electronic copy of the review module, this icon will appear alongside clickable links to media supplements. If you have a hardcopy version of the review module, visit www.atitesting.com for details on how to access these features.

Feedback

ATI welcomes feedback regarding this review module. Please provide comments to: comments@atitesting.com.

Table of Contents

UNIT 1: FOUNDATIONS OF NURSING CARE OF CHILDREN

Section: Perspectives of Nursing Care of Children

- Family-Centered Nursing Care

- Physical Assessment Findings

- Health Promotion of the Infant (Birth to 1 year)

- Health Promotion of the Toddler (1 to 3 years)

- Health Promotion of the Preschooler (3 to 6 years)

- Health Promotion of the School-Age Child (6 to 12 years)

- Health Promotion of the Adolescent (12 to 20 years)

NCLEX® CONNECTIONS

When reviewing the chapters in this section, keep in mind the relevant sections of the NCLEX® outline, in particular:

CLIENT NEEDS: SAFETY AND INFECTION CONTROL

Relevant topics/tasks include:
- Accident/Error/Injury Prevention
  - Assist in or reinforce education to client about safety precautions.
- Home Safety
  - Reinforce client education on home safety precautions.

CLIENT NEEDS: HEALTH PROMOTION AND MAINTENANCE

Relevant topics/tasks include:
- Aging Process
  - Provide care that meets the special needs of infants or children aged 1 month to 12 years.
- Developmental Stages and Transitions
  - Compare client development to norms.
- Health Promotion/Disease Prevention
  - Identify and educate clients in need of immunizations.

UNIT 1	FOUNDATIONS OF NURSING CARE OF CHILDREN
Section:	Perspectives of Nursing Care of Children
Chapter 1	Family-Centered Nursing Care

Overview

- Families are groups of individuals that should remain constant in children's lives.

- Family is defined as what an individual considers it to be.

- Positive family relationships are characterized by parent-child interactions that show mutual warmth and respect.

- Family-centered nursing care includes:

  o Agreed upon partnerships between families of children, nurses, and health care providers, in which the families and children benefit.

  o Respecting cultural diversity and incorporating cultural views in the plan of care.

  o Understanding growth and developmental needs of children and their families.

  o Treating children and their families as clients.

  o Working with all types of families.

  o Collaborating with families regarding hospitalization, home, and community resources.

  o Allowing families to serve as experts regarding their children's health conditions, usual behaviors in different situations, and routine needs.

- Promoting family-centered care

  o Nurses should collect data to identify strengths and weaknesses of families.

  o Nurses should pay close attention when family members state that a child "isn't acting right" or has other concerns.

  o Nurses should consider children's opinions when providing care.

Family Composition

TYPE	MEMBERS
Nuclear family	Two parents and their children (biologic, adoptive, step, foster)
Traditional nuclear family	Married couple and their biologic children (only full brothers and sisters)
Single-parent family	One parent and one or more children
Blended family (also called reconstituted)	At least one stepparent, stepsibling, or half-sibling
Extended family	At least one parent, one or more children, and other individuals either related or not related
Gay/Lesbian family	Two members of the same sex that have a common-law tie and may or may not have children
Foster family	A child or children that have been placed in an approved living environment away from the family of origin – usually with one or two parents
Binuclear family	Parents that have terminated spousal roles but continue their parenting roles
Communal family	Individuals that share common ownership of property and goods and exchange services without monetary consideration

- Changes That Occur With the Birth (or Adoption) of the First Child

    o Parents' sense of self and how families work

    o Division of labor and roles within the relationships of couples

    o Relationships with grandparents

    o Work relationships

Parenting Styles

TYPE	DESCRIPTION	EXAMPLE
Dictatorial or authoritarian	• Parents try to control the child's behaviors and attitudes through unquestioned rules and expectations.	• The child may not watch television on school nights at all.
Permissive or laissez-faire	• Parents exert little or no control over the child's behaviors.	• The child may watch television whenever he wants to watch it.
Democratic or authoritative	• Parents direct the child's behavior by setting rules and explaining the reason for each rule setting. • Parents negatively reinforce deviations from the rules.	• The child may watch television for an hour if her homework is completed. • The privilege is taken away but may be reinstated based on new guidelines.

- Positive Parental Influences

    o   Parents have good mental health.

    o   Structure and routine is maintained in the household.

    o   Parents engage in activities with the child.

    o   There is communication that validates the child's feelings.

    o   The child is monitored for safety with special consideration for his developmental needs.

- Guidelines for Promoting Healthy Behavior in Children

    o   Set realistic limits and expectations based on the developmental level of the child.

    o   Validate the child's feelings.

    o   Provide reinforcement for appropriate behavior.

    o   Focus on the child's behavior when disciplining the child.

Data Collection

- Genogram – Medical history for parents, siblings, aunts, uncles, and grandparents

- Structure – Members in the family (mother, father, son)

- Developmental tasks – Tasks a family works on as the child grows (parents with a school-age child helping her to develop peer relations)

- Family functions/roles – Ways in which family members interact with each other (mother being the disciplinarian)

- Family stressors – Events that cause stress (illness of a child)

Client Outcomes

- The family will provide a safe environment for all family members.

Ⓐ APPLICATION EXERCISES

1. A 9-year-old child with sickle cell anemia lives with her father, stepmother, and half sibling. Which of the following describes this family's composition?

    A. Nuclear family

    B. Blended family

    C. Extended family

    D. Binuclear family

2. Which of the following is an example of parents maintaining structure and routine in the home environment?

    A. A mother purchasing a bicycle safety helmet for her son.

    B. A father monitoring a chart of the children assigned to set the table.

    C. The parents attending a parent-teacher meeting at their child's school.

    D. The parents discussing their vacation plans with the babysitter.

3. A nurse is collecting data from the parents of two school-age children. Which of the following data should be collected regarding the family? (Select all that apply.)

    _____ Health status of grandparents

    _____ Family members living in the home

    _____ Parents' involvement in children's school programs

    _____ Recent stressful family events

    _____ Heights and weights of children

(A) **APPLICATION EXERCISES ANSWER KEY**

1. A 9-year-old child with sickle cell anemia lives with her father, stepmother, and half sibling. Which of the following describes this family's composition?

   A. Nuclear family

   B. Blended family

   C. Extended family

   D. Binuclear family

   A blended family includes at least one stepparent, stepsibling, and/or half-sibling. A nuclear family includes two parents and their children. An extended family includes one or more parents, one or more children, and other family members such as a grandmother. A binuclear family includes parents that have terminated spousal roles but continue with parenting roles.

(N) NCLEX® Connection: Health Promotion and Maintenance, Developmental Stages and Transitions

2. Which of the following is an example of parents maintaining structure and routine in the home environment?

   A. A mother purchasing a bicycle safety helmet for her son.

   B. A father monitoring a chart of the children assigned to set the table.

   C. The parents attending a parent-teacher meeting at their child's school.

   D. The parents discussing their vacation plans with the babysitter.

   A father monitoring a chart of the children assigned to set the table is a way of maintaining structure and routine in the home environment. Purchasing a child's bicycle safety helmet focuses on monitoring safety based on the child's developmental needs. Parents' participation at their child's school and planning a family vacation are examples of family functions and roles.

(N) NCLEX® Connection: Health Promotion and Maintenance, Developmental Stages and Transitions

3. A nurse is collecting data from the parents of two school-age children. Which of the following data should be collected regarding the family? (Select all that apply.)

   __X__   **Health status of grandparents**

   __X__   **Family members living in the home**

   __X__   **Parents' involvement in children's school programs**

   __X__   **Recent stressful family events**

   _____   Heights and weights of children

Medical history of the grandparents, identifying family members, developmental tasks of the family such as involvement in their child's education, disciplinary activities and family stressors are all data to be collected regarding the family. The height and weight of the children is data related to physical assessment findings of the children.

NCLEX® Connection: Health Promotion and Maintenance, Developmental Stages and Transitions

UNIT 1	FOUNDATIONS OF NURSING CARE OF CHILDREN
Section:	Perspectives of Nursing Care of Children
Chapter 2	Physical Assessment Findings

Overview

- Perform examinations in nonthreatening environments.

- Modify exam techniques to accommodate children's developmental needs.

- Observe behaviors that signal children's readiness to cooperate.

- Involve children and family members in examinations. Adolescents may prefer to be examined without family members present.

- Praise children for cooperation during exams.

Nursing Considerations

- Keep the room warm and well lit.

- Distract children when bringing into the room equipment that can be perceived as threatening.

- Provide privacy.

- Tell children, using age-appropriate language, what to expect as the physical exam is being performed.

- Examine children while they are positioned securely and comfortably. For example, a toddler may sit on a parent's lap if desired.

- Examine children in an organized sequence when possible.

- Encourage children and/or families to ask questions during physical exams.

Expected Vital Signs

- Temperature

    o Birth to 1 year (axillary) – 36.5 to 37.2 ° C (97.7 to 98.9° F)

    o 1 to 12 years (oral) – 36.7 to 37.7° C (98.1 to 99.9° F)

    o 12 years and older (oral) – 36.6 to 36.7° C (97.8 to 98.0° F)

- Pulse
  - Birth to 1 week – 100 to 160/min with brief fluctuations above and below this range, depending on activity level (crying, sleeping)
  - 1 week to 3 months – 100 to 220/min
  - 3 months to 2 years – 80 to 150/min
  - 2 to 12 years – 70 to 110/min
  - 12 years and older – 50 to 90/min
- Respirations
  - Newborn – 30 to 60/min with short periods of apnea (less than 15 seconds)
  - Newborn to 1 year – 30/min
  - 1 to 2 years – 25 to 30/min
  - 2 to 6 years – 21 to 24/min
  - 6 to 12 years – 19 to 21/min
  - 12 years and older – 16 to 18/min
- Blood Pressure
  - Age, height, and gender all influence blood pressure readings. Readings should be compared with standard measurements (The National High Blood Pressure Program tables).
  - Infants – 60 to 80 mm Hg systolic and 40 to 50 mm Hg diastolic
  - The following chart provides examples of expected ranges of blood pressure by age and gender.

AGE	GIRLS		BOYS	
	SYSTOLIC (MM HG)	DIASTOLIC (MM HG)	SYSTOLIC (MM HG)	DIASTOLIC (MM HG)
1 year	97 to 107	53 to 60	94 to 106	50 to 59
3 years	100 to 110	61 to 68	100 to 113	59 to 67
6 years	104 to 114	67 to 75	105 to 117	67 to 76
10 years	112 to 122	73 to 80	110 to 123	73 to 82
16 years	122 to 132	79 to 86	125 to 138	79 to 87

Expected Physical Assessment Findings

- General Appearance
  - Appears undistressed
  - Appears clean and well-kept
  - Muscle tone
    - When supine, limp posture with extension of the extremities is expected.
    - Erect head posture is expected in infants after 4 months of age.
  - Has no body odors
  - Makes eye contact when addressed (except infants)
  - Follows simple commands as age appropriate
  - Uses speech, language, and motor skills spontaneously
  - Growth – Growth can be measured using weight, height, body mass index (BMI), and head circumference. Growth charts are tools that can be used to assess the overall health of a child. To see growth charts by age and gender, visit the Web site for the Centers for Disease Control and Prevention (http://www.cdc.gov).
- Skin, Hair, and Nails
  - Skin
    - Skin color may show normal variations based on race and ethnicity.
    - Temperature should be warm or slightly cool to the touch.
    - Skin turgor should demonstrate brisk elasticity with adequate hydration.
    - Skin texture should be smooth and slightly dry.
    - Lesions are not expected findings.
    - Skin folds should be symmetric.
  - Hair
    - Hair should be evenly distributed and smooth.
    - Children approaching adolescence should be assessed for the presence of secondary hair growth.
  - Nails
    - Pink over the nail bed and white at the tips
    - Smooth and firm (but slightly flexible in infants)
    - No clubbing
- Lymph nodes should be nonpalpable, but lymph nodes that are small, palpable, nontender, and mobile in children may still be considered normal.

- Head and Neck
  - Head
    - The shape of the head should be symmetric.
    - Fontanels should be flat. The posterior fontanel usually closes between 2 and 3 months of age, and the anterior fontanel usually closes between 12 and 18 months of age.
  - Face
    - Symmetric appearance and movement
    - Proportional features
  - Neck
    - Short in infants
    - No palpable masses
    - Midline trachea
    - Full range of motion present whether assessed actively or passively
- Eyes
  - Visual acuity – May be difficult to check in children under 3 years of age
    - Visual acuity in infants can be checked by holding an object in front of the eyes and checking to see if they are able to fix on the object and follow it.
    - Older children should be tested using a Snellen chart or symbol chart.
  - Color vision should be checked using the Ishihara color test. Children should be able to correctly identify shapes.
  - Peripheral visual fields should be:
    - Upward 50°
    - Downward 70°
    - Nasally 60°
    - Temporally 90°
  - Extraocular movements may not be symmetric in newborns.
    - Corneal light reflex should be symmetric.
    - Cover/uncover test should demonstrate equal movement of the eyes. The presence of strabismus should be further evaluated in children between 4 and 6 years of age.
    - Six cardinal fields of gaze should demonstrate no nystagmus.
  - Eyebrows should be symmetric and evenly distributed from the inner to the outer canthus.
  - Eyelids should close completely and open to allow the lower border and most of the upper portion of the iris to be seen.

- o Eyelashes should curve outward and be evenly distributed with no inflammation around any of the hair follicles.
- o Conjunctiva
  - Palpebral is pink.
  - Bulbar is transparent.
- o Lacrimal apparatus is without excessive tearing, redness, or discharge.
- o Sclera should be white.
- o Corneas should be clear.
- o Pupils should be:
  - Round
  - Equal in size
  - Reactive to light
  - Accommodating (can be tested in older children)
- o Irises should be round with the permanent color manifesting around 6 to 12 months of age.

- Internal Exam
  - o Red reflex should be present in infants.
  - o Arteries, veins, optic discs, and maculas may be visualized in older children and adolescents.

- Ears
  - o Alignment
    - The top of the auricles should meet in an imaginary horizontal line that extends from the outer canthus of the eye.
  - o External ear
    - The external ear should be free of lesions and nontender.
    - The ear canal should be free of foreign bodies or discharge.
    - Cerumen is an expected finding.
  - o Internal ear
    - In infants and children under 3 years of age, pull the pinna down and back to visualize the tympanic membrane.
    - In children older than 3 years of age, pull the pinna up and back to visualize.
    - The tympanic membrane should be pearly gray.
    - The light reflex should be visible.

- Umbo (tip of the malleolus) and manubrium (long process or handle) are the bony landmarks that should be visible.

- The ear canal should be pink with fine hairs.

  o Hearing

- Newborns should have intact acoustic blink reflexes to sudden sounds.

- Infants should turn toward sounds.

- Screen older children by whispering a word from behind to see if they can identify the word.

- Nose

  o The position should be midline.

  o Patency should be present for each nostril without excessive flaring.

  o Internal structures

- The septum is midline and intact.

- The mucosa is deep pink and moist with no discharge.

  o Assess smell in older children.

- Mouth and Throat

  o Lips

- Darker pigmented than facial skin

- Smooth, soft, and moist

  o Gums

- Coral pink

- Tight against the teeth

  o Mucous membranes

- Without lesions

- Moist and pink

  o Tongue

- Infants may have white coatings on their tongues from milk that can be easily removed. Oral candidiasis coating is not easily removed.

- Children and adolescents should have pink, symmetric tongues that they are able to move beyond their lips.

  o Teeth

- Infants should have six to eight teeth by 1 year of age.

- Children and adolescents should have teeth that are white and smooth, with 20 deciduous and 32 permanent teeth.

- o Hard and soft palates – Intact, firm, and concave
- o Uvula – Intact and moves with vocalization
- o Tonsils
  - Infants – May not be able to visualize
  - Children – Barely visible to prominent, same color as surrounding mucosa, deep crevices that hold food particles
- o Speech
  - Infants – Strong cry
  - Children and adolescents – Clear and articulate
- Thorax and Lungs
  - o Chest shape
    - Infants – Shape is almost circular with anteroposterior diameter equaling the transverse or lateral diameter
    - Children and adolescents – The transverse diameter to anteroposterior diameter changes to 2:1.
  - o Ribs and sternum – More soft and flexible in infants, symmetric, and smooth with no protrusions or bulges
  - o Movement – Symmetric, no retractions
    - Infants – Irregular rhythms are common.
    - Children younger than 7 – More abdominal movement is seen during respirations.
  - o Breath sounds
    - Infants – Harsher and easier to hear than in adults; harder to differentiate between upper versus lower respiratory sounds
    - Children and adolescents – Vesicular sounds heard over the lung fields
  - o Breasts
    - Newborns – Breasts may be enlarged during the first several months.
    - Children and adolescents – Nipples and areolas are darker pigmented and symmetric.
    - Females – Breasts typically develop between 10 to 14 years of age. The breasts should appear asymmetric, have no masses, and be palpable.
    - Males may develop a firm, approximately 2-cm area of breast tissue or gynecomastia.

- Circulatory System

  - Heart sounds – S1 and S2 heart sounds should be clear and crisp. S1 is louder at the apex of the heart. S2 is louder near the base of the heart. Sinus arrhythmias that are associated with respirations are common. Physiologic splitting of S2 and S3 heart sounds are expected findings in children.

  - Pulses

    - Infants – Brachial, temporal, and femoral pulses should be palpable, full, and localized.

    - Children and adolescents – Pulse locations and expected findings are the same as those in adults.

- Abdomen – Without tenderness, no guarding. Peristaltic waves may be visible in thinner children.

  - Shape – Symmetric and without protrusions around the umbilicus

    - Infants and toddlers have rounded abdomens.

    - Children and adolescents should have flat abdomens.

  - Bowel sounds should be heard every 5 to 30 seconds.

  - Descending colon – Cylindric mass that is possibly palpable in the lower left quadrant due to the presence of stool

- Musculoskeletal System

  - Length, position, and size are symmetric.

  - Joints – Stable and symmetric with full range of motion and no crepitus or redness

  - Spine

    - Infants – Spines should be without dimples or tufts of hair. They should be midline with an overall C-shaped lateral curve.

    - Toddlers appear squat with short legs and protuberant abdomens.

    - Preschoolers appear more erect than toddlers.

    - Children should develop the cervical, thoracic, and lumbar curvatures like that of adults.

    - Adolescents' spines should remain midline (no scoliosis noted).

  - Gait

    - Toddlers and young children – A bowlegged or knock-knee appearance is a common finding. Feet should face forward while walking.

    - Older children and adolescents – A steady gait should be noted with even wear on the soles of shoes.

- Neurologic System

REFLEX	EXPECTED FINDING	EXPECTED AGE
Sucking and rooting reflexes	• Stroke an infant's cheek or the edge of an infant's mouth. ○ The infant turns her head toward the side that is touched and starts to suck.	Birth to 4 months
Palmar grasp	• Place an object in an infant's palm. ○ The infant grasps the object.	Birth to 6 months
Plantar grasp	• Touch the sole of an infant's foot. ○ The infant's toes curl downward.	Birth to 8 months
Moro reflex (startle)	• Strike a flat surface an infant is lying on, or allow the head and trunk of an infant in a semi-sitting position to fall backward to an angle of at least 30°. ○ The infant's arms and legs symmetrically extend and then abduct while her fingers spread to form a C shape.	Birth to 4 months
Tonic neck reflex (fencer position)	• Turn an infant's head to one side. ○ The infant extends the arm and leg on that side and flexes the arm and leg on the opposite side.	Birth to 3 to 4 months
Babinski reflex	• Stroke the outer edge of the sole of an infant's foot up toward the toes. ○ The infant's toes fan upward and out.	Birth to 1 year
Stepping	• Hold an infant upright with his feet touching a flat surface. ○ The infant makes stepping movements.	Birth to 4 weeks

	CRANIAL NERVES	
CRANIAL NERVE	**EXPECTED FINDINGS INFANT**	**EXPECTED FINDINGS CHILD/ADOLESCENT**
I Olfactory	• Difficult to test	• Identifies smells through each nostril individually
II Optic	• Looks at face and tracks with eyes	• Has intact visual acuity, peripheral vision, and color vision
III Oculomotor	• Blinks in response to light • Has pupils that are reactive to light	• Has no nystagmus and PERRLA are intact
IV Trochlear	• Looks at face and tracks with eyes	• Has the ability to look down and in with eyes
V Trigeminal	• Has rooting and sucking reflexes	• Is able to clench teeth together • Detects touch on face with eyes closed
VI Abducens	• Looks at face and tracks with eyes	• Is able to see laterally with eyes
VII Facial	• Has symmetric facial movements	• Has the ability to differentiate between salty and sweet on tongue • Has symmetric facial movements
VIII Acoustic	• Tracks a sound • Blinks in response to a loud noise	• Does not experience vertigo • Has intact hearing
IX Glossopharyngeal	• Has an intact gag reflex	• Has an intact gag reflex • Is able to taste sour sensations on back of tongue
X Vagus	• Has no difficulties swallowing	• Speech clear, no difficulties swallowing
XI Spinal Accessory	• Moves shoulders symmetrically	• Has equal strength of shoulder shrug against examiner's hands
XII Hypoglossal	• Has no difficulties swallowing • Opens mouth when nares are occluded	• Has a tongue that is midline • Is able to move tongue in all directions with equal strength against tongue blade resistance

- o Deep tendon reflexes should demonstrate the following:
  - Partial flexion of the lower arm at the biceps tendon
  - Partial extension of the lower arm at the triceps tendon
  - Partial extension of the lower leg at the patellar tendon
  - Plantar flexion of the foot at the Achilles tendon
- o Cerebellar function (children and adolescents)
  - Finger to nose test – Rapid coordinated movements
  - Heel to shin test – Able to run the heel of one foot down the shin of the other leg while standing
  - Romberg test – Able to stand with slight swaying while eyes are closed
- o Language, cognition, and fine and gross motor development can be screened using a standardized tool such as the Denver Developmental Screening Test – Revised (Denver II). Referrals for further evaluation should not be based solely on results of one tool, but on a combination of data collected from psychosocial and medical histories and a physical examination.

- Genitalia
  - o Male
    - Hair distribution is diamond shaped after puberty in adolescent males. No pubic hair is noted in infants and small children.
    - Penis
      - □ Penis should appear straight.
      - □ Urethral meatus should be at the tip of the penis.
      - □ Foreskin may not be retractable in infants and small children who are uncircumcised.
      - □ Enlargement of the penis occurs during adolescence.
    - Scrotum
      - □ The scrotum hangs separately from the penis.
      - □ The skin on the scrotum has a rugated appearance and is loose.
      - □ The left testicle hangs slighter lower than the right.
      - □ The inguinal canal should be absent of swelling.
      - □ During puberty, the testes and scrotum enlarge with darker scrotal skin.

- ○ Female
  - ■ Hair distribution over the mons pubis should be documented in terms of amount and location during puberty. Hair should appear in an inverted triangle. No pubic hair should be noted in infants or small children.
  - ■ Labia – Symmetric, without lesions, moist on the inner aspects
  - ■ Clitoris – Small, without bruising or edema
  - ■ Urethral meatus – Slit-like in appearance with no discharge
  - ■ Vaginal orifice – The hymen may be absent, or it may completely or partially cover the vaginal opening prior to sexual intercourse.
- ○ Anus – Surrounding skin should be intact with sphincter tightening noted if the anus is touched. Routine rectal exams are not done with the pediatric population.

(A) APPLICATION EXERCISES

1. List five basic assessments that should be included in the physical assessment of a child over 3 years of age.

2. When assessing blood pressure in children, the nurse should be aware that

    A. systolic and diastolic ranges will gradually increase with age.

    B. systolic and diastolic ranges will gradually decrease with age.

    C. there is no difference in the expected range between boys and girls.

    D. girls will have a slightly higher reading in the expected range.

3. When collecting data from a toddler, which of the following characteristics should the nurse expect to find? (Select all that apply.)

    _____ Bowlegged gait

    _____ Abdominal breathing

    _____ Established eye color

    _____ Absent red reflex

    _____ Bowel sounds heard every 2 to 3 min on auscultation

4. When collecting data from an infant, which of the following techniques should the nurse use to elicit the stepping reflex?

    A. Hold the infant upright with his feet touching a flat surface.

    B. Strike a flat surface on which the infant is lying.

    C. Place an object in the infant's palm.

    D. Stroke the outer edge of the sole of the infant's foot up toward the toes.

(A) APPLICATION EXERCISES ANSWER KEY

1. List five basic assessments that should be included in the physical assessment of a child over 3 years of age.

    Height, weight, temperature, respiratory rate, heart rate, and blood pressure

(N) NCLEX® Connection: Health Promotion and Maintenance, Data Collection Techniques

2. When assessing blood pressure in children, the nurse should be aware that

    A. systolic and diastolic ranges will gradually increase with age.
    B. systolic and diastolic ranges will gradually decrease with age.
    C. there is no difference in the expected range between boys and girls.
    D. girls will have a slightly higher reading in the expected range.

    The expected range of diastolic and systolic blood pressure in children will gradually increase with age. Boys will have slightly higher readings than girls in the expected range.

(N) NCLEX® Connection: Health Promotion and Maintenance, Data Collection Techniques

3. When collecting data from a toddler, which of the following characteristics should the nurse expect to find? (Select all that apply.)

__X__	**Bowlegged gait**
__X__	**Abdominal breathing**
__X__	**Established eye color**
_____	Absent red reflex
_____	Bowel sounds heard every 2 to 3 min on auscultation

    Physical characteristics of the toddler include bowlegged or knock-knee appearance and feet facing forward while walking, more abdominal movements seen during respirations, and permanent eye color established by 6 to 12 months of age. The red reflex is present and bowel sounds should be heard on auscultation every 5-30 seconds.

(N) NCLEX® Connection: Health Promotion and Maintenance, Data Collection Techniques

4. When collecting data from an infant, which of the following techniques should the nurse use to elicit the stepping reflex?

   A. Hold the infant upright with his feet touching a flat surface.

   B. Strike a flat surface on which the infant is lying.

   C. Place an object in the infant's palm.

   D. Stroke the outer edge of the sole of the infant's foot up toward the toes.

   The stepping reflex can be elicited when the infant is held upright with the feet touching a flat surface. The infant will make stepping movements. Striking a flat surface on which the infant is lying will elicit the Moro reflex. The infant's arms and legs extend symmetrically and then abduct while her fingers spread to form a C shape. Placing an object in the infant's palm will elicit the grasp reflex. The infant will grasp the object. Lightly stroking the outer edge of the infant's sole up toward the toes will elicit the Babinski reflex. The infant's toes should fan upward and out.

   NCLEX® Connection: Health Promotion and Maintenance, Data Collection Techniques

UNIT 1	FOUNDATIONS OF NURSING CARE OF CHILDREN
Section:	Perspectives of Nursing Care of Children
Chapter 3	Health Promotion of the Infant (Birth to 1 Year)

Overview

- Infants are clients up to 1 year of age. Safe, client-centered care includes demonstrated knowledge of:

  ○ Expected growth and development, including physical, cognitive, and psychosocial development

  ○ Age-appropriate activities

  ○ Health promotion activities including immunizations, nutrition, and injury prevention.

Expected Growth and Development

- Physical Development

  ○ The infant's posterior fontanel closes by 2 to 3 months of age.

  ○ The infant's anterior fontanel closes by 12 to 18 months of age.

  ○ Weight, height, and head circumference measurements are used to track the size of infants.

    ■ Weight – Infants gain approximately 150 to 210 g (about 5 to 7 oz) weekly during the first 6 months of age. Infants should double their birth weight by 4 to 7 months and triple their birth weight by the end of the first year of life.

    ■ Height – Infants grow approximately 2.5 cm (1 in) per month the first 6 months of age, and then approximately 1.25 cm (0.5 in) per month for the next 6 months.

    ■ Head circumference – The circumference of infants' heads increases approximately 1.5 cm (0.6 in) per month for the first 6 months of life, and then approximately 0.5 cm (0.2 in) between 6 and 12 months of age.

  ○ Dentition – Six to eight teeth should erupt in infants' mouths by the end of the first year of age.

    ■ Teething pain can be eased using cold teething rings, over-the-counter teething gels, or acetaminophen (Tylenol) and/or ibuprofen (Advil). Ibuprofen should be used only in infants over the age of 6 months.

    ■ Clean infants' teeth using cool, wet washcloths.

    ■ Bottles should not be given to infants when they are falling asleep. This will help to avoid prolonged exposure to milk or juice that can cause dental caries (bottle mouth syndrome).

AGE	GROSS MOTOR SKILLS	FINE MOTOR SKILLS
1 month	Demonstrates head lag	• Has a grasp reflex
2 months	Lifts head off mattress	• Holds hands in an open position
3 months	Raises head and shoulders off mattress	• No longer has a grasp reflex • Keeps hands loosely open
4 months	Rolls from back to side	• Places objects in mouth
5 months	Rolls from front to back	• Uses palmar grasp dominantly
6 months	Rolls from back to front	• Holds bottle
7 months	Bears full weight on feet	• Moves objects from hand to hand
8 months	Sits unsupported	• Begins using pincer grasp
9 months	Pulls to a standing position	• Has a crude pincer grasp
10 months	Changes from a prone to a sitting position	• Grasps rattle by its handle
11 months	Walks while holding on to something	• Places objects into a container
12 months	Sits down from a standing position without assistance	• Tries to build a two-block tower without success

 View Media Supplement: Fine and Gross Motor Development (Video)

- Cognitive Development
  - Piaget – Sensorimotor Stage (birth to 24 months)
    - There are three things that occur during this time: separation, object permanence, and mental representation.
      - Separation is when infants learn to separate themselves from other objects in the environment.
      - Object permanence is the process by which infants know that an object still exists when it is hidden from view. This occurs at approximately 9 months of age.
      - Mental representation is the recognition of symbols.
  - Language
    - Vocalizes with cooing noises
    - Responds to noises
    - Turns head to the sound of a rattle
    - Laughs and squeals 6 m.
    - Pronounces single-syllable words
    - Begins speaking two-word phrases and progresses to speaking three-word phrases

- Psychosocial Development

  - The stage of psychosocial development for infants, according to Erikson, is trust versus mistrust.

  - Infants trust that their feeding, comfort, stimulation, and caring needs will be met.

  - Social development is initially influenced by infants' reflexive behaviors and includes attachment, separation, recognition/anxiety, and stranger fear.

    - Attachment is seen when infants begin to bond with their parents. This development is seen within the first month, but it actually begins before birth. The process is enhanced when infants and parents are in good health, have positive feeding experiences, and receive adequate rest.

    - Separation recognition occurs during the first year as infants learn physical boundaries from other people. Learning how to respond to people in their environments is the next phase of development. Positive interactions with parents, siblings, and other caregivers help to establish trust.

    - Separation anxiety develops between 4 and 8 months of age. Infants will protest loudly when separated from parents, which can cause considerable anxiety for parents.

    - Stranger fear becomes evident between 6 and 8 months of age, when infants are less likely to accept strangers.

  - Self-Concept Development

    - By the end of the first year, infants will be able to distinguish themselves as being separate from their parents.

  - Body-Image Changes

    - Infants will discover that their mouths are pleasure producers (Freud – Oral stage).

    - Hands and feet are seen as objects of play.

    - Infants discover that smiling causes others to react.

- Age-Appropriate Activities

  - Infants will have short attention spans and will not interact with other children during play (solitary play). Appropriate toys and activities that stimulate the senses and encourage development include:

    - Rattles

    - Mobiles

    - Teething toys

    - Nesting toys

    - Playing pat-a-cake

    - Playing with balls

    - Reading books

Health Promotion

- Immunizations

  o 2010 Centers for Disease Control and Prevention (CDC) immunization recommendations for healthy infants less than 12 months of age (http://www.cdc.gov) include:

    - Birth – Hepatitis B (Hep B)

    - 2 months – Diphtheria and tetanus toxoids and pertussis (DTaP), rotavirus vaccine (RV), inactivated poliovirus (IPV), Haemophilus influenzae type B (Hib), pneumococcal vaccine (PCV), and Hep B

    - 4 months – DTaP, RV, IPV, Hib, PVC

    - 6 months – DTaP, IPV (6 to 18 months), PVC, and Hep B (6 to 12 months); RotaTeq, an alternative formulation for RV, requires 3 doses that must be completed by 32 weeks of age.

    - 6 to 12 months – Seasonal influenza vaccination yearly; the trivalent inactivated influenza vaccine (TIV) is available as an intramuscular injection.

- Nutrition

  o Tell parents about feeding alternatives.

    - Breastfeeding provides a complete diet for infants during the first 6 months of life and is recommended by health care providers.

    - Iron-fortified formula is an acceptable alternative to breast milk. Cows' milk is not recommended.

  o Instruct parents to introduce solid food between 4 and 6 months of age. Parents should:

    - Recognize readiness such as interest in solid foods, voluntary control of the head and trunk, and hunger less than 4 hr after vigorous nursing or intake of 8 oz of formula.

    - Offer iron-fortified rice cereal first.

    - Introduce new foods one at a time, over a 5- to 7-day period to observe for signs of allergy or intolerance, which may include fussiness, rash, vomiting, diarrhea, and constipation. Start first with vegetables or fruits between 6 and 8 months of age. Add meats after both have been introduced.

    - Delay milk, eggs, wheat, citrus fruits, peanuts, peanut butter, and honey until after the first year of life. Use caution if there is a family history of allergies.

    - Decrease breast milk/formula as intake of solid foods increases.

    - Offer table foods that are cooked, chopped, and unseasoned by 9 months of age.

    - Appropriate finger foods include ripe bananas; toast strips; graham crackers; cheese cubes; noodles; and peeled chunks of apples, pears, or peaches.

    - Encourage parents to use iron-enriched foods after infants are 6 months of age.

- ○ Instruct parents to wean infants when they are able to drink from cups with handles (sometime after 6 months). Parents should:
  - Replace one feeding with breast milk or formula in a cup with handles.
  - Replace bedtime feedings.
- • Injury Prevention
  - ○ Aspiration of foreign objects
    - Instruct parents to:
      - □ Avoid small objects that can become lodged in the throat (grapes, coins, candy).
      - □ Provide age-appropriate toys.
      - □ Check clothing for safety hazards (loose buttons).
  - ○ Bodily harm
    - Remind parents to:
      - □ Keep sharp objects out of reach.
      - □ Keep infants away from heavy objects that can be pulled down onto them.
      - □ Do not leave infants unattended with any animals present.
      - □ Monitor infants for shaken baby syndrome.
  - ○ Burns
    - Instruct parents to:
      - □ Check the temperature of bathwater.
      - □ Turn down thermostats on hot water heaters.
      - □ Keep working smoke detectors in the home.
      - □ Keep handles of pots and pans turned to the back of stoves.
      - □ Use sunscreen when infants will be exposed to the sun.
      - □ Cover electrical outlets.
  - ○ Drowning
    - Remind parents to not leave infants unattended in bathtubs.
  - ○ Falls
    - Instruct parents to:
      - □ Keep crib mattresses in the lowest position possible with the rails all the way up.
      - □ Use restraints in infant seats.
      - □ Place infant seats on the ground or floor if used outside of the car, and do not leave unattended or on elevated surfaces.
      - □ Use safety gates across stairs.

- o Poisoning
  - Tell parents to:
    - □ Avoid exposure to lead paint.
    - □ Keep toxins and plants out of reach.
    - □ Keep safety locks on cabinets with cleaners and other household chemicals.
    - □ Keep the phone number for a poison control center near the phone.
    - □ Keep medications in childproof containers, away from the reach of infants.
    - □ Keep a working carbon monoxide detector in the home.
- o Motor-vehicle injuries
  - Instruct parents to place infants in approved rear-facing car seats in the back seat, preferably in the middle, (away from air bags and side impact). Place infants in rear-facing car seats for the first year of life and until they weigh 9.1 kg (20 lb). It is recommended to have infants ride rear-facing until they have reached the weight limit allowed for the car seat (as long as the top of the infant's head does not extend above the top of the seat back). In addition, a five-point harness or T-shield should be part of a convertible restraint.
- o Suffocation
  - Instruct parents to:
    - □ Avoid plastic bags.
    - □ Keep balloons away from infants.
    - □ Ensure crib mattresses fit snugly.
    - □ Avoid use of drop-side cribs due to the risk of suffocation and strangulation. Many manufacturers no longer sell drop-side cribs. Information about crib safety may be found on the U.S. Consumer Product Safety Commission Web site (http://www.cpsc.gov).
  - Ensure crib slats are no farther apart than 6 cm (2.4 in).
  - Remove crib mobiles or crib gyms by 4 to 5 months of age.
  - Keep pillows out of the crib.
  - Place infants on their backs for sleep.
  - Keep toys with small parts out of reach.
  - Remove drawstrings from jackets and other clothing.

(A) APPLICATION EXERCISES

1. Which of the following foods should be introduced into the diet <u>after</u> the first year of life?

   A. Cow's milk
   B. Baked squash
   C. Fresh nectarines
   D. Toast with jelly

2. The mother of an 11-month-old infant reveals that her infant has started walking. What poison prevention activities should the nurse discuss with the mother?

3. Which of the following is the correct position for the car seat of an infant who weighs less than 20 lb?

   A. Rear-facing in the middle of the back seat
   B. Forward-facing in the middle of the back seat
   C. Forward-facing on the passenger side of the back seat
   D. Rear-facing on the passenger side of the back seat

4. A woman calls the clinic saying she is a first-time grandmother and her daughter and grandchild are coming for a visit. She asks the nurse what type of toys and activities she could plan for her 6-month-old grandchild. (Select all that apply.)

   _____ Large nesting cups
   _____ Teething toy
   _____ Playing pat-a-cake
   _____ Pretend play
   _____ Playing dress-up

APPLICATION EXERCISES ANSWER KEY

1. Which of the following foods should be introduced into the diet after the first year of life?

   A. Cow's milk
   B. Baked squash
   C. Fresh nectarines
   D. Toast with jelly

   Delay milk, eggs, wheat, citrus fruits, peanuts, peanut butter, and honey until after the first year of life. Use caution if there is a family history of allergies. Baked squash, fresh nectarines, and toast with jelly are table foods that are can be chopped, cooked, and unseasoned and are appropriate by 9 months of age.

    NCLEX® Connection: Basic Care and Comfort, Nutrition and Oral Hydration

2. The mother of an 11-month-old infant reveals that her infant has started walking. What poison prevention activities should the nurse discuss with the mother?

   Poison prevention activities include placing any poisonous houseplants or toxic substances out of reach, installing safety locks on cabinets where household cleaning agents and chemicals are stored, and keeping all medications in childproof bottles.

    NCLEX® Connection: Health Promotion and Maintenance, Developmental Stages and Transitions

3. Which of the following is the correct position for the car seat of an infant who weighs less than 20 lb?

   A. Rear-facing in the middle of the back seat
   B. Forward-facing in the middle of the back seat
   C. Forward-facing on the passenger side of the back seat
   D. Rear-facing on the passenger side of the back seat

   Place infants in approved rear-facing car seats in the back seat, preferably in the middle, for the first year of life and until weighing 20 lb. The car seat should be away from air bags and side impact. Facing forward in the middle of the back seat or on the passenger side of the back seat are incorrect positions. Rear-facing on the passenger side of the back seat is in a side impact area.

    NCLEX® Connection: Safety and Infection Control, Accident/Error/Injury Prevention

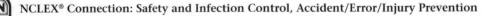

4. A woman calls the clinic saying she is a first-time grandmother and her daughter and grandchild are coming for a visit. She asks the nurse what type of toys and activities she could plan for her 6-month-old grandchild. (Select all that apply.)

    | X | **Large nesting cups** |
    | X | **Teething toy** |
    | X | **Playing pat-a-cake** |
    | _____ | Pretend play |
    | _____ | Playing dress-up |

    Age-appropriate toys and activities for infants include large nesting cups, teething toys, and playing pat-a-cake. Playing dress up-or pretend play are appropriate activities for the preschool-age child.

    (N) NCLEX® Connection: Health Promotion and Maintenance, Developmental Stages and Transitions

UNIT 1	FOUNDATIONS OF NURSING CARE OF CHILDREN
Section:	Perspectives of Nursing Care of Children
Chapter 4	Health Promotion of the Toddler (1 to 3 Years)

Overview

- Toddlers are clients 1 to 3 yr of age. Safe, client centered care includes demonstrating knowledge of:

  - Expected growth and development, including physical, cognitive, and psychosocial development.

  - Age-appropriate activities.

  - Health promotion activities, including immunizations, nutrition, and injury prevention.

Expected Growth and Development

- Physical Development

  - Anterior fontanels close by 18 months of age.

  - Weight – At 30 months of age, toddlers should weigh four times their birth weights.

  - Height – Toddlers grow about 7.5 cm (3 in) per year.

AGE	GROSS MOTOR SKILLS	FINE MOTOR SKILLS
15 months	• Walks without help • Creeps up stairs	• Uses a cup well • Builds a tower of two blocks
18 months	• Assumes a standing position	• Manages a spoon without rotation • Turns pages in a book, two or three at a time
2 years	• Walks up and down stairs	• Builds a tower of six or seven blocks
2.5 years	• Jumps in place with both feet • Stands on one foot momentarily	• Draws circles • Has good hand-finger coordination

- Cognitive Development

  - Piaget – The sensorimotor stage transitions to the preoperational stage.

    - The concept of object permanence is fully developed.

    - Toddlers have memories of events that relate to them.

- Domestic mimicry (playing house) is evident.
- Preoperational thought does not allow for toddlers to understand other viewpoints, but it does allow them to symbolize objects and people to imitate previously seen activities.
  - Language
    - Language increases to about 400 words with toddlers speaking in two- to three-word phrases.
- Psychosocial Development
  - The stage of psychosocial development for toddlers, according to Erikson, is autonomy versus shame and doubt.
    - Independence is paramount for toddlers, who are attempting to do everything for themselves.
    - Separation anxiety continues to occur when parents leave toddlers.
  - Moral Development
    - Moral development is closely associated with cognitive development.
    - Egocentric – Toddlers are unable to see things from the perspectives of others; they can only view things from their personal points of view.
    - Punishment and obedience orientation begin with a sense that good behavior is rewarded and bad behavior is punished.
  - Self-Concept Development
    - Toddlers progressively see themselves as separate from their parents and increase their explorations away from them.
  - Body-Image Changes
    - Toddlers appreciate the usefulness of various body parts.
    - Toddlers will develop gender identity by 3 years of age.
- Age-Appropriate Activities
  - Solitary play evolves into parallel play, in which toddlers observe other children and then may engage in activities nearby.
  - Appropriate activities
    - Filling and emptying containers
    - Playing with blocks
    - Looking at books
    - Playing with toys that can be pushed and pulled
    - Tossing balls
  - Temper tantrums result when toddlers are frustrated with restrictions on independence. Providing consistent, age-appropriate expectations helps toddlers to work through frustration.

     o   Begin toilet training when it is recognized that toddlers have the sensation of needing to urinate or defecate. Parents should demonstrate patience and consistency in toilet training. Nighttime control may develop last of all.

     o   Impose consistent discipline with well-defined boundaries that are established to develop appropriate social behavior.

Health Promotion

- Immunizations

  - 2010 Centers for Disease Control and Prevention (CDC) immunization recommendations for healthy toddlers 12 months to 3 years of age (http://www.cdc.gov) include:

    - 12 to 15 months – Inactivated poliovirus (IPV) (6 to 18 months); Haemophilus influenzae type B (Hib); pneumococcal vaccine (PCV); measles, mumps, and rubella (MMR); and varicella

    - 12 to 23 months – Hepatitis A (Hep A), given in two doses at least 6 months apart

    - 15 to 18 months – Diphtheria and tetanus toxoids and pertussis (DTaP)

    - 12 to 36 months – Yearly seasonal trivalent inactivated influenza vaccine (TIV); the live, attenuated influenza vaccine (LAIV) by nasal spray (at 2 years of age)

- Nutrition

  - Tell parents that:

    - Toddlers are generally picky eaters who will repeatedly request their favorite foods.

    - Toddlers generally prefer finger foods because of increasing autonomy.

    - Regular meal times and nutritious snacks best meet nutrient needs.

    - Dietary recommendations outlined by the United States Department of Agriculture can be found at http://www.mypyramid.gov.

  - Instruct parents to:

    - Expect that exposure to a new food may need to occur 8 to 15 times before toddlers develop an acceptance of it.

    - If there is a family history of allergy, introduce cow's milk, chocolate, citrus fruits, egg whites, seafood, and nut butters gradually while monitoring for reactions.

    - Have toddlers consume 24 to 30 oz of milk per day, and they may switch from drinking whole milk to drinking low-fat milk (2% fat) at 2 years of age.

    - Limit juice consumption to 4 to 6 oz per day.

    - Provide food serving size of 1 tbsp for each year of age.

    - Avoid snacks or desserts that are high in sugar, fat, or sodium.

    - Avoid foods that are potential choking hazards (nuts, grapes, hot dogs, peanut butter, raw carrots, tough meats, popcorn).

- Provide adult supervision during snack and mealtimes.
- Cut foods into small, bite-size pieces to make them easier to swallow and to prevent choking.
- Do not let toddlers engage in drinking or eating during play activities or while lying down.

- Dental health
  - Have toddlers:
    - Brush daily.
    - Floss daily.
    - Have regular checkups.
    - Have regular fluoride treatments.
- Injury Prevention
  - Aspiration of foreign objects
    - Avoid small objects (grapes, coins, candy) that can become lodged in the throat.
    - Keep toys that have small parts out of reach.
    - Provide age-appropriate toys.
    - Check clothing for safety hazards (loose buttons).
    - Keep balloons away from toddlers.
  - Bodily harm
    - Remind parents to:
      - Keep sharp objects out of reach.
      - Keep firearms in locked boxes or cabinets.
      - Do not leave toddlers unattended with any animals present.
      - Reinforce stranger safety to toddlers.
  - Burns
    - Have parents:
      - Check the temperature of bath water.
      - Turn down thermostats on hot water heaters.
      - Keep working smoke detectors in the home.
      - Turn pot handles toward the back of the stove.
      - Cover electrical outlets.
      - Have toddlers wear sunscreen when outside.

- o Drowning
  - ▪ Instruct parents to:
    - □ Not leave toddlers unattended in bathtubs.
    - □ Keep toilet lids closed.
    - □ Closely supervise toddlers when near pools or any other body of water.
    - □ Begin swimming instruction for toddlers.
- o Falls
  - ▪ Remind parents to:
    - □ Keep doors and windows locked.
    - □ Keep crib mattresses in the lowest position with the rails all the way up.
    - □ Use safety gates across stairs.
- o Motor vehicle injuries
- o Instruct parents to:
  - □ Use approved car seats in the backseats of cars (away from air bags).
  - □ Place toddlers in approved rear-facing car seats in the backseat until they weigh 9.1 kg (20 lb). Toddlers may then sit in approved forward-facing car seats in the back seat. Toddlers may usually remain in car seats until 4 years of age and/or 40 lb.
- o Poisoning
  - ▪ Encourage parents to:
    - □ Avoid exposure to lead paint.
    - □ Place safety locks on cabinets that contain cleaners and other chemicals.
    - □ Place the phone number for a poison control center near the phone.
    - □ Keep medications in childproof containers, away from the reach of toddlers.
    - □ Place a working carbon monoxide detector in the home.
- o Suffocation
  - ▪ Instruct parents to:
    - □ Avoid plastic bags.
    - □ Ensure crib mattresses fit tightly.
    - □ Avoid drop-side cribs due to the risk of suffocation and strangulation. Many manufacturers no longer sell drop-side cribs. Information about crib safety may be found on the U.S. Consumer Product Safety Commission Web site (http://www.cpsc.gov).
    - □ Ensure crib slats are no farther apart than 6 cm (2.4 in).
    - □ Keep pillows out of cribs.
    - □ Remove drawstrings from jackets and other clothing.

Ⓐ APPLICATION EXERCISES

1. List the immunizations recommended for each of the following age groups listed below.

   12 to 15 months

   12 to 23 months

   15 to 18 months

   12 to 36 months

2. The parent of an 18-month-old toddler asks about toilet training. What response by the nurse is appropriate?

3. A nurse is admitting a 20-month-old toddler to the pediatric unit. Based on the child's developmental stage, which of the following toys should the nurse place in the hospital room?

   A. Small car with wheels
   B. 100-piece puzzle
   C. Water colors and paint book
   D. Comic books

4. A toddler who swallowed beads and was taken to the emergency department is being seen at the clinic for a follow-up visit. Which of the following safety instructions related to the risk of aspiration should the nurse review with the mother? (Select all that apply.)

   _____ Cut foods such as grapes and hot dogs into small pieces.
   _____ Avoid toys that have small parts.
   _____ Check clothing for loose buttons.
   _____ Verify that bath water is warm before bathing.
   _____ Turn pot handles to the back of the stove.

APPLICATION EXERCISES ANSWER KEY

1. List the immunizations recommended for each of the following age groups listed below.

    12 to 15 months – **IPV (6 to 18 months), Hib, PCV, MMR, and varicella**

    12 to 23 months – **Hep A, given in two doses, at least 6 months apart**

    15 to 18 months – **DTaP**

    12 to 36 months – **Yearly Influenza (TIV)**

 NCLEX® Connection: Health Promotion and Maintenance, Health Promotion/Disease Prevention

2. The parent of an 18-month-old toddler asks about toilet training. What response by the nurse is appropriate?

    Toilet training can begin when the parent recognizes that the toddler is aware of the need to urinate or defecate. The parent can observe cues such as a change in the toddler's facial expressions or body movements. Parents should be patient and consistent in their toilet training techniques, knowing that nighttime control is the last to develop.

 NCLEX® Connection: Health Promotion and Maintenance, Developmental Stages and Transitions

3. A nurse is admitting a 20-month-old toddler to the pediatric unit. Based on the child's developmental stage, which of the following toys should the nurse place in the hospital room?

    A. Small car with wheels
    B. 100-piece puzzle
    C. Water colors and paint book
    D. Comic books

    Appropriate toys for toddlers include push-pull toys, balls, blocks, large picture books, puzzles with few and large pieces, and containers that can be emptied and filled, such as with bath water. Puzzles with more pieces and water colors and paint books are appropriate to the preschool-age child. Large puzzles with many pieces and comic books are appropriate to the school-age child.

 NCLEX® Connection: Health Promotion and Maintenance, Developmental Stages and Transitions

4. A toddler who swallowed beads and was taken to the emergency department is being seen at the clinic for a follow-up visit. Which of the following safety instructions related to the risk of aspiration should the nurse review with the mother? (Select all that apply.)

   __X__ **Cut foods such as grapes and hot dogs into small pieces.**

   __X__ **Avoid toys that have small parts.**

   __X__ **Check clothing for loose buttons.**

   _____ Verify that bath water is warm before bathing.

   _____ Turn pot handles to the back of the stove.

   Safety concerns related to aspiration include avoiding small food items which can easily become lodged in a child's throat, avoiding toys that have small parts, and checking clothing for loose objects such as buttons, which can be swallowed and are hazardous. Verifying that the temperature of bath water is warm and keeping pot handles turned to the back of the stove are not related to the risk of aspiration. They are safety measures implemented to prevent burns.

   Ⓝ **NCLEX® Connection: Safety and Infection Control, Accident/Error/Injury Prevention**

UNIT 1	FOUNDATIONS OF NURSING CARE OF CHILDREN
Section:	Perspectives of Nursing Care of Children
Chapter 5	Health Promotion of the Preschooler (3 to 6 Years)

Expected Growth and Development

- Physical Development

    o Weight – Preschoolers should gain about 2 to 3 kg (4.5 to 6.5 lb) per year.

    o Height – Preschoolers should grow about 6.2 to 7.5 cm (2.5 to 3 inches) per year.

    o Preschoolers' bodies evolve away from the characteristically unsteady wide stances and protruding abdomens of toddlers, into a more graceful, posturally erect, and sturdy physicality.

    o Fine and gross motor skills

        ▪ Preschoolers should show improvement in fine motor skills, which will be displayed by activities like copying figures on paper and dressing independently.

AGE	GROSS MOTOR SKILLS
3 years	• Rides a tricycle • Jumps off bottom step • Stands on one foot for a few seconds
4 years	• Skips and hops on one foot • Throws a ball overhead
5 years	• Jumps rope • Walks backward with heel to toe • Moves up and down stairs easily

- Cognitive Development

    o Piaget – Preschoolers are still in the preoperational phase of cognitive development. They participate in preconceptual thought (from 2 to 4 years of age) and intuitive thought (from 4 to 7 years of age).

        ▪ Preconceptual thought – Preschoolers make judgments based on visual appearances. Misconceptions in thinking during this stage include:

            □ Artificialism – Everything is made by humans.

            □ Animism – Inanimate objects are alive.

            □ Imminent justice – A universal code exists that determines law and order.

- Intuitive thought – Preschoolers can classify information, and they become aware of cause-and-effect relationships.
  - Time – Preschoolers begin to understand the concepts of the past, present, and future. By the end of the preschool years, children may comprehend days of the week.
  - Language – The vocabulary of preschoolers continues to increase. Preschoolers can speak in sentences and identify colors, and they enjoy talking.
- Psychosocial Development
  - The stage of psychosocial development for preschoolers, according to Erikson, is initiative versus guilt.
    - Preschoolers may take on many new experiences, despite not having all of the physical abilities necessary to be successful at everything. Guilt may occur when preschoolers are unable to accomplish a task and believe they have misbehaved. Guiding preschoolers to attempt activities within their capabilities while setting limits is appropriate.
  - Moral Development
    - Preschoolers continue in the good-bad orientation of the toddler years, but they begin to understand behaviors in terms of what is socially acceptable.
  - Self-Concept Development
    - Preschooler feels good about themselves with regard to mastering skills that allow independence (dressing, feeding). During stress, insecurity, or illness, preschoolers may regress to previous immature behaviors or develop habits (nose-picking, bedwetting, thumb-sucking).
  - Body-Image Changes
    - Mistaken perceptions of reality coupled with misconceptions in thinking lead to active fantasies and fears. The greatest fear is that of bodily harm, resulting in fear of the dark or animals.
    - Sex-role identification is occurring.
  - Social Development
    - Preschoolers generally do not exhibit stranger anxiety and have less separation anxiety. However, prolonged separation, such as during hospitalization, can provoke anxiety. Favorite toys and appropriate play should be used to help ease preschoolers' fears.
    - Pretend play is healthy and allows preschoolers to determine the difference between reality and fantasy.
  - Sleep disturbances frequently occur during early childhood, and problems range from difficulties going to bed to night tremors. Advise parents to:
    - Assess whether or not the bedtime is too early if preschoolers are still taking naps. On average, preschoolers need about 12 hr of sleep per day. Some still require a daytime nap.
    - Keep a consistent bedtime routine.

- Use a night-light.
- Reassure preschoolers who have been frightened, but avoid allowing preschoolers to sleep with their parents.

- Age-Appropriate Activities

  o Parallel play shifts to associative play during the preschool years. Play is not highly organized, but cooperation does exist between children. Appropriate activities include:

    - Playing ball
    - Putting puzzles together
    - Riding tricycles
    - Playing pretend and dress-up activities
    - Role playing
    - Painting
    - Sewing cards and beads
    - Reading books

Health Promotion

- Immunizations

  o The 2010 Centers for Disease Control and Prevention (CDC) immunization recommendations for healthy preschoolers 3 to 6 years of age (http://www.cdc.gov) include:

    - 4 to 6 years – Diphtheria and tetanus toxoids and pertussis (DTaP); measles, mumps, and rubella (MMR); varicella; and inactivated poliovirus (IPV)
    - 36 to 59 months – Yearly seasonal influenza vaccine; trivalent inactivated influenza vaccine (TIV); or live, attenuated influenza vaccine (LAIV) by nasal spray

- Health Screenings

  o Vision screening is routinely done in the preschool population as part of the prekindergarten physical exam. Visual impairments such as myopia and amblyopia can be detected and treated before poor visual acuity impairs learning.

(M) **View Media Supplement:** Pediatric Eye Chart (Image)

- Nutrition

- Inform parents that:

  - Preschoolers consume about 1,800 calories per day.

  - Picky eating may remain a behavior in preschoolers, but often by 5 years of age they become more willing to sample different foods.

  - Preschoolers need 13 to 19 g/day of complete protein in addition to adequate calcium, iron, folate, and vitamins A and C.

- Injury Prevention

  o Bodily harm

  - Tell parents to:

    □ Keep firearms in locked cabinets or containers.

    □ Reinforce stranger safety.

    □ Ensure preschoolers wear protective equipment (helmet, pads).

  o Burns

  - Instruct parents to:

    □ Turn thermostats down on hot water heaters.

    □ Keep working smoke detectors in the home.

    □ Ensure preschoolers have sunscreen applied when outside.

  o Drowning

  - Tell parents to:

    □ Not leave preschoolers unattended in bathtubs.

    □ Closely supervise preschoolers when near the pool or any other body of water.

    □ Reinforce to preschoolers how to swim.

  o Motor vehicle injuries

  - Instruct parents to:

    □ Place preschoolers in approved forward-facing car seats in the backseat away from airbags. Usually preschoolers may remain in car seats until 4 years of age and/or 40 lb. Use booster seats in the backseat when preschoolers have outgrown car seats. Restrain children in car seats or booster chairs until adult seat belts fit correctly. Laws may vary from state to state and requirements may be up to a weight of 80 lb and a height of 4 feet 9 inches, which is when adult seat belts will most likely fit correctly.

- o Poisoning
  - ▪ Instruct parents to:
    - □ Avoid exposure to lead paint.
    - □ Keep plants out of reach.
    - □ Place safety locks on cabinets with cleaners and other chemicals.
    - □ Keep the phone number for a poison control center near the phone.
    - □ Keep medications in childproof containers, out of reach of preschoolers.
    - □ Keep a working carbon monoxide detector in the home.

Ⓐ APPLICATION EXERCISES

1. A nurse is reinforcing nutrition education to a group of parents whose children attend a local day-care center. Which of the following is an effective way to encourage good nutrition habits in preschool children?

    A. Introduce different foods along with foods the child enjoys.

    B. Allow the child to choose other foods if he doesn't like what is being served.

    C. Place adult-size portions on the child's plate.

    D. Insist the child finish all the food given at a meal.

2. What immunizations should a pre-school age child receive if all immunizations have been kept up to date?

3. The parents of a preschooler are worried because their son is having difficulty sleeping through the night after spending 2 weeks at his grandparents' house. How should the nurse respond to the parents' concern?

4. A nurse is leading a health promotion class about the preschool-age child for employees of a local day-care center. Which of the following should be included in this presentation? (Select all that apply.)

    _____ Teach preschoolers to swim.

    _____ Daily dietary needs include complete proteins such as meats and eggs.

    _____ Fear of the dark or animals is a common concern.

    _____ Use adult seat belts when in the car.

    _____ Vision screening does not begin until the child starts school.

5. Play activities of the preschool-age child include

    A. having imaginary playmates.

    B. complex board games.

    C. parallel play.

    D. selective collection of objects.

APPLICATION EXERCISES ANSWER KEY

1. A nurse is reinforcing nutrition education to a group of parents whose children attend a local day-care center. Which of the following is an effective way to encourage good nutrition habits in preschool children?

   A. Introduce different foods along with foods the child enjoys.

   B. Allow the child to choose other foods if he doesn't like what is being served.

   C. Place adult-size portions on the child's plate.

   D. Insist the child finish all the food given at a meal.

   Preschoolers learn by example. Serving foods children enjoy and introducing new and different foods encourages good nutrition habits. Picky eating habits may continue but by age 5, children are more willing to try different foods. Allowing children to choose other foods if they don't like what is being served reinforces the picky-eating habit. Children need about half the amount of kilo-calories of an adult, so portion size should be appropriate. Children need to learn how to self-regulate their hunger and satisfaction. Insisting children eat when they are no longer hungry can lead to unnecessary weight gain

 NCLEX® Connection: Basic Care and Comfort, Nutrition and Oral Hydration

2. What immunizations should a pre-school age child receive if all immunizations have been kept up to date?

   Diphtheria and tetanus toxoids and pertussis (DTaP); inactivated poliovirus (IPV); measles, mumps, and rubella (MMR); and varicella. In addition, preschoolers who are 36 to 59 months should receive yearly seasonal influenza vaccine; trivalent inactivated influenza vaccine (TIV); or live, attenuated influenza vaccine (LAIV) by nasal spray.

 NCLEX® Connection: Health Promotion and Maintenance, Health Promotion/Disease Prevention

3. The parents of a preschooler are worried because their son is having difficulty sleeping through the night after spending 2 weeks at his grandparents' house. How should the nurse respond to the parents' concern?

   Sleep disturbances are common during early childhood. Ask the parents to review their child's bedtime routine with the grandparents as it may have been different. Children need consistency in their bedtime routine. The child may have napped and gone to bed later than at home. Having a night-light at home, but not one while away, could upset the child's routine. Other routines that the parents had at home, such as reading at bedtime, telling a story, or quiet play, may have been different.

 NCLEX® Connection: Health Promotion and Maintenance, Developmental Stages and Transitions

4. A nurse is leading a health promotion class about the preschool-age child for employees of a local day-care center. Which of the following should be included in this presentation? (Select all that apply.)

   X   **Teach preschoolers to swim.**

   X   **Daily dietary needs include complete proteins such as meats and eggs.**

   X   **Fear of the dark or animals is a common concern.**

   _____   Use adult seat belts when in the car.

   _____   Vision screening does not begin until the child starts school.

   Include the need for preschoolers to be taught to swim, dietary needs including complete proteins such as meat and eggs, and that the fear of the dark or animals is a common concern. Use car seats until 4 years of age and/or 40 lb. Place the child in a booster seat until adult seat belts fit properly. Vision screening should be part of the routine prekindergarten physical exam.

   (N) **NCLEX® Connection: Health Promotion and Maintenance, Developmental Stages and Transitions**

5. Play activities of the preschool-age child include

   A. having imaginary playmates.

   B. complex board games.

   C. parallel play.

   D. selective collection of objects.

   Play activities involve having imaginary playmates and pretend play. Preschool children ride tricycles and like creative activities such as painting, sewing sets, illustrated books, and playing ball. Parallel play is characteristic of toddlers. Organized and selective collections of similar objects and complex board games are activities of the school-age child.

   (N) **NCLEX® Connection: Health Promotion and Maintenance, Developmental Stages and Transitions**

UNIT 1	FOUNDATIONS OF NURSING CARE OF CHILDREN
Section:	Perspectives of Nursing Care of Children
Chapter 6	Health Promotion of the School-Age Child (6 to 12 Years)

Overview

- School-age children are clients 6 to 12 yr of age. Safe, client-centered care includes demonstrating knowledge of:

    o Expected growth and development including physical, cognitive, and psychosocial development.

    o Age-appropriate activities.

    o Health promotion activities including immunizations, health screening, nutrition, and injury prevention.

Expected Growth and Development

- Physical Development

    o Weight – School-age children will gain about 2 to 4 kg (4.4 to 8.8 lb) per year.

    ▪ Weight gain typically occurs between 9 and 12 years of age (girls from 9 to 12 and boys from 10 to 12 years of age).

    o Height – School-age children will grow about 5 cm (2 inches) per year.

    ▪ Changes in height usually occur after 10 to 12 years of age for girls and 12 to 14 years of age for boys (after the period of weight gain).

    o Changes related to puberty begin to appear in females.

    ▪ Budding of breasts

    ▪ Appearance of pubic hair

    ▪ Onset of menarche

    o Changes related to puberty begin to appear in males.

    ▪ Enlargement of testicles with changes in the scrotum (increased looseness)

    ▪ Appearance of pubic hair

    o Permanent teeth erupt.

    o Visual acuity improves to 20/20.

    o Auditory acuity and sense of touch is fully developed.

- ○ Fine and gross motor development
  - ■ During the school-age years, coordination continues to improve.
- Cognitive Development
  - ○ Piaget – Concrete operations
    - ■ Sees weight and volume as unchanging
    - ■ Understands simple analogies
    - ■ Understands time (days, seasons)
    - ■ Classifies more complex information
    - ■ Understands various emotions
    - ■ Becomes self-motivated
    - ■ Is able to solve problems
  - ○ Language
    - ■ Defines many words and understands rules of grammar
    - ■ Understands that a word may have multiple meanings
- Psychosocial Development *Erickson (Industry vs. Inferiority)*
  - ○ The stage of psychosocial development for school-age children, according to Erikson, is industry versus inferiority.
    - ■ A sense of industry is achieved through advancements in learning.
    - ■ School-age children are motivated by tasks that increase self-worth.
    - ■ Fears of ridicule by peers and teachers over school-related issues are common. Some children manifest nervous behaviors (nail-biting) to deal with the stress.
  - ○ Moral Development
    - ■ Early on, school-age children may not understand the reasoning behind many rules and may try to find ways around them. Instrumental exchange ("I'll help you if you help me") is in place. Children want to make the best deal, and they do not really consider elements of loyalty, gratitude, or justice as they make decisions.
    - ■ In the latter part of the school-age years, children move into a law-and-order orientation with more emphasis placed on justice being administered.
  - ○ Self-Concept Development
    - ■ School-age children strive to develop a healthy self-respect by finding out in what areas they excel.
    - ■ School-age children need parents to encourage them regarding educational or extracurricular successes.

- o Body-Image Changes
  - Address curiosity about sexuality with education regarding sexual development and the reproductive process.
  - School-age children are more modest than preschoolers and place more emphasis on privacy issues.
- o Social Development
  - Peer groups play an important part in social development. Peer pressure begins to take effect.
  - Friendships begin to form between same-gender peers. This is the time period when clubs and best friends are popular.
  - Children prefer the company of same-gender companions.
  - Most relationships come from school associations.
  - Children may rival same-gender parents.
  - Conformity becomes evident.

- Age-Appropriate Activities
  - o Competitive and cooperative play is predominant.
  - o Children from 6 to 9 years of age
    - Play simple board and number games.
    - Play hopscotch.
    - Jump rope.
    - Collect rocks, stamps, cards, coins, or stuffed animals.
    - Ride bicycles.
    - Build simple models.
    - Join organized sports (for skill building).
  - o Children from 9 to 12 years of age
    - Make crafts.
    - Build models.
    - Collect things/engage in hobbies.
    - Solve jigsaw puzzles.
    - Play board and card games.
    - Join organized competitive sports.

Health Promotion

- Immunizations

  o 2010 Centers for Disease Control and Prevention (CDC) immunization recommendations for healthy school-age children 6 to 12 years of age (http://www.cdc.gov) include:

  - If not given between 4 and 5 years of age, children should receive the following vaccines by 6 years of age – Diphtheria and tetanus toxoids and pertussis (DTaP); inactivated poliovirus (IPV); measles, mumps, and rubella (MMR); and varicella

  - Yearly seasonal influenza vaccine – Trivalent inactivated influenza vaccine (TIV) or live, attenuated influenza vaccine (LAIV) by nasal spray

  - 11 to 12 years – Tetanus and diphtheria toxoids and pertussis vaccine (Tdap), meningococcal vaccine (MCV4), human papillomavirus vaccine (HPV2) in three doses (for females), and HPV4 (for males)

- Health Screenings

  o Scoliosis – School-age children should be screened for scoliosis by examining for a lateral curvature of the spine before and during growth spurts. Screening may take place at schools or health care facilities.

- Nutrition

  o Inform parents that:

  - By the end of the school-age years, children should be eating adult proportions of food. They need quality nutritious snacks.

  - Obesity is an increasing concern of this age group that predisposes children to low self-esteem, diabetes, heart disease, and high blood pressure.

  o Advise parents to:

  - Avoid using food as a reward.

  - Emphasize physical activity.

  - Ensure that a balanced diet is consumed. Recommendations posted by the United States Department of Agriculture may be found on the Web (http://www.mypyramid.gov).

  - Teach children to make healthy food selections for meals and snacks.

  - Avoid eating fast-food frequently.

  - Avoid skipping meals.

  o Dental health

  - Encourage parents to ensure that children:

    □ Brush daily.

    □ Floss daily.

    □ Have regular checkups.

    □ Have regular fluoride treatments.

- Injury Prevention
  - Bodily harm
    - Instruct parents to:
      - Keep firearms in locked cabinets or boxes.
      - Discourage play on trampolines.
      - Identify safe play areas.
      - Reinforce stranger safety.
      - Ensure children wear helmets and/or pads when rollerblading, skateboarding, bicycling, riding scooters, skiing, and snowboarding.
  - Burns
    - Remind parents to:
      - Reinforce fire safety and potential burn hazards.
      - Keep working smoke detectors in the home.
      - Ensure children use sunscreen when outside.
  - Drowning
    - Instruct parents to:
      - Supervise children when swimming or when near a body of water.
      - Reinforce to children how to swim.
  - Motor vehicle injuries
    - Remind parents to:
      - Restrain children in car seats or booster chairs until adult seat belts fit correctly. Laws may vary from state to state and requirements may be up to a weight of 36.3 kg (80 lb) and a height of 4 feet 9 inches, which is when adult seat belts will most likely fit correctly. Properly fitting adult seat belts should have the lap belt lying across the upper thighs and the shoulder belt fitting across the chest.
      - Children less than 13 years of age are safest in the back seat.
  - Poisoning/Substance abuse
    - Have parents:
      - Keep cleaners or chemicals in locked cabinets or out of reach of younger children.
      - Reinforce to children to say "no" to illegal drugs and alcohol.

Ⓐ APPLICATION EXERCISES

1. When teaching a class about puberty to school-age children, a question is asked about what changes occur. What is an appropriate response by the nurse?

2. Which of the following health screenings of the school-age child is often done by the school nurse?

    A. Scoliosis

    B. Diabetes mellitus

    C. Fine motor skills

    D. Gross muscle coordination

3. What immunizations should a school-age child receive between the ages of 11 and 12?

4. The director of a summer camp for school-age children asks a nurse to review a list of planned activities. Which of the following should be avoided due to safety concerns? (Select all that apply.)

    _____ Jumping on a trampoline

    _____ Building a campfire

    _____ Riding scooters

    _____ Same-gender team games

    _____ Jump rope competitions

APPLICATION EXERCISES ANSWER KEY

1. When teaching a class about puberty to school-age children, a question is asked about what changes occur. What is an appropriate response by the nurse?

    Pubertal changes in girls include the development of breast buds, the appearance of pubic hair, and the onset of menarche. In boys, pubic hair appears, the testicles enlarge, and the scrotal sac becomes loose.

 NCLEX® Connection: Health Promotion and Maintenance, Developmental Stages and Transitions

2. Which of the following health screenings of the school-age child is often done by the school nurse?

    A. Scoliosis

    B. Diabetes mellitus

    C. Fine motor skills

    D. Gross muscle coordination

    A scoliosis screening may take place at the school or a health care facility. The school nurse does not routinely screen for diabetes, fine motor skills, and gross motor coordination.

 NCLEX® Connection: Health Promotion and Maintenance, Health Promotion/Disease Prevention

3. What immunizations should a school-age child receive between the ages of 11 and 12?

    Tetanus and diphtheria toxoids and pertussis vaccine (Tdap); human papillomavirus vaccine (HPV2) in 3 doses (for females) and HPV4 (for males); yearly seasonal influenza vaccine: trivalent inactivated influenza vaccine (TIV) or live, attenuated influenza vaccine (LAIV) by nasal spray.

 NCLEX® Connection: Health Promotion and Maintenance, Health Promotion/Disease Prevention

4. The director of a summer camp for school-age children asks a nurse to review a list of planned activities. Which of the following should be avoided due to safety concerns? (Select all that apply.)

___X___ **Jumping on a trampoline**

_____ Building a campfire

_____ Riding scooters

_____ Same-gender team games

_____ Jump rope competitions

Avoid play on trampolines. School-age children should be taught fire safety and building a campfire is an appropriate activity. Riding scooters while wearing pads and jump rope competitions are appropriate activities. Same-gender team games do not pose a safety concern and are often preferred by school-age children.

NCLEX® Connection: Health Promotion and Maintenance, Developmental Stages and Transitions

UNIT 1	FOUNDATIONS OF NURSING CARE OF CHILDREN
Section:	Perspectives of Nursing Care of Children
Chapter 7	Health Promotion of the Adolescent (12 to 20 Years)

Overview

- Adolescents are clients between the ages of 12 and 20 yr. Safe, client-centered care includes demonstrating knowledge of:

  o Expected growth and development including physical, cognitive, and psychosocial development.

  o Age-appropriate activities.

  o Health promotion activities, including immunizations, health screening, nutrition, and injury prevention

Expected Growth and Development

- Physical Development

  o The final 20% to 25% of height is achieved during puberty.

  o Acne may appear during adolescence.

  o Girls may cease to grow at about 2 to 2.5 years after the onset of menarche. They will grow 5 to 20 cm (2 to 8 in) and gain 7 to 25 kg (15.5 to 55 lb).

  o Boys tend to stop growing at around 18 to 20 years of age. They will grow 10 to 30 cm (4 to 12 inches) and gain 7 to 30 kg (15.5 to 66 lb).

  o Sexual maturation and puberty last for approximately 2 years from Tanner stage 1 to stage 4.

  o In girls, sexual maturation occurs in the following order:

    ▪ Appearance of breast buds

    ▪ Growth of pubic hair (although some girls may have hair growth prior to breast bud development)

    ▪ Onset of menstruation

  o In males, sexual maturation occurs in the following order:

    ▪ Increase in the size of the testes and scrotum

    ▪ Appearance of pubic hair

    ▪ Rapid growth of genitalia

- - Growth of axillary hair
  - Appearance of downy hair on upper lip
  - Change in voice
  - Sleep habits change with puberty due to increased metabolism and rapid growth during the adolescent years. Changes are characterized by staying up late, sleeping in later in the morning, and perhaps sleeping longer than was done during the school-age years.
- Cognitive Development
  - Piaget – Formal operations
    - Capable of thinking at an adult level
    - Able to think abstractly and deal with principles
    - Capable of evaluating the quality of their own thinking
    - Able to maintain attention for longer periods of time
    - Highly imaginative and idealistic
    - Capable of making decisions through logical operations
    - Future oriented
    - Capable of using deductive reasoning
    - Able to understand how the actions of an individual influence others
  - Language
    - Adolescents develop jargon within their peer groups. They are able to communicate one way with peer groups and another way with adults or teachers. Development of communication skills is essential for adolescents.
- Psychosocial Development
  - The psychosocial development stage of adolescents, according to Erikson, is identity versus role confusion.
    - Adolescents develop a sense of personal identity that is influenced by expectations of their families.
      - □ Group identity – Adolescents may become part of a peer group that greatly influences behavior.
  - Vocationally – Adolescents solidify work habits and plan for future college and careers.
  - Sexually – There is increased interest in the opposite gender.
  - Health perceptions – Adolescents may view themselves as invincible to bad outcomes of risky behaviors.

- o Moral Development

  - ▪ Conventional law and order – Rules are not seen as absolutes. Each situation needs to be looked at, and perhaps the rules will need to be adjusted. Not all adolescents attain this level of moral development during these years.

- o Self-Concept Development

  - ▪ A healthy self-concept is developed by having healthy relationships with peers, family, and teachers. Identifying a skill or talent helps maintain a healthy self-concept. Participation in sports, hobbies, or the community can have a positive outcome.

- o Body-Image Changes

  - ▪ Adolescents seem particularly concerned with the body images portrayed by the media. Changes that occur during puberty result in comparisons between individual adolescents and their surrounding peer groups. Parents also give their input as to hair styles, dress, and activities. Adolescents may require help if depression or eating disorders result due to poor body image.

- o Social Development

  - ▪ Peer relationships develop. These relationships act as a support system for adolescents.

  - ▪ Best-friend relationships are more stable and longer lasting than they were in previous years.

  - ▪ Parent-child relationships change to allow a greater sense of independence.

- • Age-Appropriate Activities

  - o Nonviolent video games

  - o Nonviolent music

  - o Sports

  - o Caring for a pet

  - o Career-training programs

  - o Reading

  - o Social events (going to the movies, school dances)

Health Promotion

- • Immunizations

  - o 2010 Centers for Disease Control and Prevention (CDC) recommendations for healthy adolescents 12 to 20 years of age (http://cdc.gov) include the following vaccines if not given at age 11 to 12 – Tetanus and diphtheria toxoids and pertussis vaccine (Tdap); meningococcal (MCV4); human papillomavirus vaccine (HPV2 series for females and HPV4 series for males); and yearly influenza vaccine (trivalent inactivated influenza vaccine [TIV] or live, attenuated influenza vaccine [LAIV] by nasal spray)

- Health Screenings

  o Scoliosis – Continue scoliosis screenings during the adolescent years. These screenings should include an examination for a lateral curvature of the spine before and during growth spurts. Screenings may take place at school or at a health care facility.

- Nutrition

  o Tell parents that:

    ▪ Rapid growth and high metabolism require increases in quality nutrients. Nutrients that tend to be deficient during this stage of life are iron, calcium, and vitamins A and C.

    ▪ Eating disorders commonly develop during adolescence (more prevalent in girls than in boys) due to a fear of being overweight, fad diets, and/or the desire to maintain control over some aspect of life. Eating disorders include anorexia nervosa, bulimia nervosa, and obesity.

  o Advise parents to:

    ▪ Avoid using food as a reward.

    ▪ Emphasize physical activity.

    ▪ Ensure that a balanced diet is consumed. Healthy food recommendations are posted by the United States Department of Agriculture (http://www.mypyramid.gov).

    ▪ Teach children to make healthy food selections for meals and snacks.

  o Dental health

    ▪ Encourage parents to ensure that adolescents:

      ☐ Brush daily.

      ☐ Floss daily.

      ☐ Have regular checkups.

      ☐ Have regular fluoride treatments.

- Injury Prevention

  o Bodily harm

    ▪ Remind parents to:

      ☐ Keep firearms in a locked cabinet or box.

      ☐ Teach proper use of sporting equipment prior to use.

      ☐ Insist on helmet use and/or pads when rollerblading, skateboarding, bicycling, riding scooters, skiing, and snowboarding.

      ☐ Avoid trampolines.

- ☐ Be aware of changes in mood. Monitor for self-harm in adolescents who are at risk. Watch for:
  - ▸ Poor school performance
  - ▸ Lack of interest in things that were of interest to the adolescent in the past
  - ▸ Social isolation
  - ▸ Disturbances in sleep or appetite
  - ▸ Expression of suicidal thoughts

- ○ Burns
  - ■ Instruct parents to:
    - ☐ Teach fire safety.
    - ☐ Apply sunscreen when outside.

- ○ Drowning
  - ■ Tell parents to:
    - ☐ Reinforce to adolescents how to swim.
    - ☐ Encourage adolescents not to swim alone.

- ○ Motor-vehicle injuries
  - ■ Instruct parents to:
    - ☐ Encourage attendance at driver education courses. Emphasize the need for adherence to seat belt use.
    - ☐ Insist on helmet use with bicycles, motorcycles, skateboards, rollerblades, and snowboards.
    - ☐ Discourage use of cell phones, talking or texting, while driving and enforce laws regarding use.
    - ☐ Reinforce the dangers of combining substance abuse with driving.
    - ☐ Role-model desired behavior.

- ○ Substance abuse
  - ■ Tell parents to:
    - ☐ Monitor for signs of substance abuse in adolescents who are at risk.
    - ☐ Reinforce to adolescents to say "no" to illegal drugs and alcohol.
    - ☐ Present a no-tolerance attitude.

- ○ Sexually transmitted diseases (STDs)
  - ■ Provide information and resources for treatment.

- ○ Pregnancy prevention
  - ■ Provide information.

Ⓐ APPLICATION EXERCISES

1. Place the following steps of sexual maturation in adolescent males in the correct order of occurrence by numbering 1 to 6.

   _____ Voice changes

   _____ Pubic hair appears

   _____ Testes and scrotum increase in size

   _____ Downy hair appears on upper lip

   _____ Growth of axillary hair

   _____ Rapid growth of genitalia occurs

2. A mother is concerned because her son was always the first one up in the home until this past year. He now sleeps late into the morning and she asks if this is common. What guidance can the nurse offer this parent?

3. Adolescents are in Erickson's psychosocial development stage of _____.

4. Which of the following are common causes of motor-vehicle injuries among adolescents? (Select all that apply.)

   _____ Using a cell phone while driving

   _____ Not wearing helmets while skateboarding

   _____ Drinking alcohol while driving

   _____ Using seat belts

   _____ Attending driver-education classes

APPLICATION EXERCISES ANSWER KEY

1. Place the following steps of sexual maturation in adolescent males in the correct order of occurrence by numbering 1 to 6.

    __6__ Voice changes

    __2__ Pubic hair appears

    __1__ Testes and scrotum increase in size

    __5__ Downy hair appears on upper lip

    __4__ Growth of axillary hair

    __3__ Rapid growth of genitalia occurs

 NCLEX® Connection: Health Promotion and Maintenance, Data Collection Techniques

2. A mother is concerned because her son was always the first one up in the home until this past year. He now sleeps late into the morning and she asks if this is common. What guidance can the nurse offer this parent?

    Sleep habits change with puberty due to increased metabolic needs and the rapid changes in growth that occur during the adolescent years. Typical changes in sleep habits include staying up late, sleeping until late morning, and needing more hours of sleep than during the school-age period.

NCLEX® Connection: Health Promotion and Maintenance, Aging Process

3. Adolescents are in Erickson's psychosocial development stage of **identity versus role confusion.**

NCLEX® Connection: Health Promotion and Maintenance, Developmental Stages and Transitions

4. Which of the following are common causes of motor-vehicle injuries among adolescents? (Select all that apply.)

    __X__ **Using a cell phone while driving**

    __X__ **Not wearing helmets while skateboarding**

    __X__ **Drinking alcohol while driving**

    _____ Using seat belts

    _____ Attending driver-education classes

    Motor-vehicle related injuries often occur when adolescents use a cell phone or drink alcohol while driving, and do not wear a helmet when on a skateboard. The use of seat belts and attending driver education classes can prevent motor-vehicle injuries.

 NCLEX® Connection: Safety and Infection Control, Accident/Error/Injury Prevention

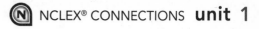

UNIT 1: FOUNDATIONS OF NURSING CARE OF CHILDREN

Section: Special Considerations of Nursing Care of Children

- Safe Administration of Medication

- Pain Management

- Hospitalization, Illness, and Play

- Death and Dying

NCLEX® CONNECTIONS

When reviewing the chapters in this section, keep in mind the relevant sections of the NCLEX® outline, in particular:

CLIENT NEEDS: BASIC CARE AND COMFORT

Relevant topics/tasks include:
- Nonpharmacological Comfort Interventions
  - Identify client need for palliative/comfort care.
  - Assist in planning comfort interventions for client who have impaired comfort.

CLIENT NEEDS: PHARMACOLOGICAL THERAPIES

Relevant topics/tasks include:
- Adverse Effects/Contraindications/Side Effects/Interactions
  - Identify a contraindication to the administration of prescribed over-the-counter medication to the client.
- Dosage Calculation
  - Use clinical decision making when calculating doses.
- Medication Administration
  - Follow the rights of medication administration.

UNIT 1	FOUNDATIONS OF NURSING CARE OF CHILDREN
Section:	Special Considerations of Nursing Care of Children
Chapter 8	Safe Administration of Medication

Overview

- Organ system immaturity affects drug sensitivity in infants and children.

- Variations

    o Newborns and young infants may be more sensitive to medications than adults due to organ system immaturity.

    o In comparison to adults, medications administered by IM injection are absorbed more slowly in newborns, but faster in infants.

    o Topical medications administered to young children may be absorbed at a greater rate than in older children and adults.

    o Infants are highly sensitive to medications that affect the CNS and are metabolized by the liver.

    o Newborns and infants have limited renal excretion abilities. Therefore, they must have reduced dosages of medications that are eliminated by the renal system.

    o Starting at 1 year of age, children's pharmacokinetic responses to medication will start to be similar to those of adults, with the exception of a faster metabolism until age 12.

- Pediatric dosages are based on body weight or body surface area (BSA).

- Nurses should be particularly alert when administering medications to children due to the high risk for medication error.

    o Adult medication forms and concentrations may require dilution, calculation, preparation, and administration of very small doses. Certain medications should be double-checked by another nurse. Nurses should be aware of those medications and follow facility policies on administration.

- Six Rights of Safe Medication Administration

  o Right client – Verify the client's identification each time a medication is administered.

    ▪ The Joint Commission requires that two client identifiers be used when administering medications. Acceptable identifiers include the client's name, an assigned identification number, a telephone number, a birth date, or another person-specific identifier. Nurses cannot rely on infants and young children to identify themselves. Young children may answer to any name that is called. A parent or guardian can be asked to identify an infant or young child.

  o Right medication – Correctly interpret the medication prescription (verify completeness and clarity). Read the label three times: when container is selected, when removing dose from container, and when container is replaced. Leave unit-dose medication in its package until administration.

  o Right dose – Calculate the correct medication dose. Check medication reference to ensure the dose is within usual range. Have a second nurse check if unsure or if facility policy requires it. Use a cutting device to break a scored tablet.

  o Right time – Administer the medication on time to maintain consistent therapeutic blood levels. It is generally acceptable to give the medication 0.5 hr before or after the scheduled time. However, refer to the medication reference or facility policy for exceptions. PRN medications should not be given sooner than the interval specified by the provider.

  o Right route – Select the correct preparation for the prescribed route (otic versus ophthalmic, topical ointment, or drops). Understand how to safely and correctly administer the medication. Administer injections only from preparations designed for parenteral use. If the route is not designated, or if a specified route is not recommended, contact the provider for clarification.

  o Right documentation – Immediately record pertinent information, including the client's response to the medication.

Factors Influencing Medication Administration

- Organ system immaturity is the greatest factor that affects medication response in children.

- Psychosocial variables affecting medication responses in children

  o Health-illness beliefs of the child and family

  o Previous experiences with medications

  o Knowledge base

  o Cultural beliefs

  o Developmental stage

  o Social support/financial status

Data Collection

- Medication and food allergies

- Medication dose appropriate for child's weight

- Child's ability to cooperate with medication administration

- Tissue and skin integrity when administering intramuscular and topical medications

- IV patency when administering IV medications

Nursing Interventions

- Check dosage calculation with another nurse

  o Question dosages that seem too large

- Administration of Oral Medications

  o Consider the oral route as the preferred route for children and milliliters (mL) as the preferred measurement (5 mL = 1 tsp, 30 mL = 1 oz).

  o Use plastic, needleless syringes for measurement and administration of small doses of medications.

  o Use only appropriate devices for administration, such as an oral syringe for oral medications.

  o Use only a small amount of liquid or soft food when mixing medications to ensure the total dose is given.

  o Do not crush enteric-coated or time-released tablets. Divide tablets only if scored.

  o Strategies for administering oral medications to infants

    ▪ Do not mix a medication with formula because infants may not take all of the formula, which will result in them not receiving the full dose of medication. This may also alter the taste of the formula, which may cause infants to refuse to drink it in the future.

    ▪ Hold infants in a semi-upright or semi-Fowler's position to prevent aspiration.

    ▪ Use a medicine cup once infants are able to drink from a cup.

    ▪ Place the medication into nipples from which infants can suck.

  o Administering oral medications via a feeding tube or a gastrostomy tube

    ▪ Check tube placement before administering any medication.

    ▪ Use liquid forms of medications.

    ▪ Check the compatibility of medications before mixing.

- Do not mix medications with enteral feedings.
- Flush the tubing with warm water before and after each medication. Amount of flush solution depends on the length and gauge of tubing. Determine this amount, which is usually 1.5 times the tubing volume, before administering medication.

- Rectal Medication Administration

  o This route is used as a substitute for oral administration (for children with nausea/vomiting or difficult oral administration).

  o Acetaminophen (Tylenol), sedatives, morphine, and some antiemetics are available in suppository form.

  o Cut the suppository lengthwise for partial dosing due to the irregular shaping of the suppository.

  o Insert suppository with the apex (pointed end) entering first, then gently push beyond rectal sphincter and hold the buttocks together until the urge to expel has passed (5 to 10 min).

- Other Medication Administration Routes

  o Optic, otic, and nasal administration

    - Procedures for these routes are similar to adult administration.

    - Pull the auricle down and back when instilling otic solutions for children up to 3 years of age. Pull the auricle up and back for older children.

    - Strategies to gain the child's cooperation

      □ Allow parents to be present. Parents may also hold their children.

      □ Warm otic solutions to room temperature before instilling.

      □ Hyperextend the child's neck for nasal medication administration to prevent the medication from sliding down into the child's throat.

- Subcutaneous (SQ) and Intradermal Medication Administration

  o These administration techniques are very similar for children and adults.

  o Strategies to decrease pain

    - Apply a eutectic mixture of local anesthetics (EMLA) in the form of a cream or disk 60 min prior to injection.

    - Use an appropriately sized needle.

    - Change the needle if used to puncture the rubber top of a vial.

    - Ensure that the amount of medication injected is appropriate for the child's muscle size (approximately 0.5 mL in infants and 2.0 mL in children).

SUBCUTANEOUS	INTRADERMAL

• Insert the needle at a 90° angle, or a 45° angle for a child with minimal subcutaneous tissue.
• Sites
  ○ Upper arm (lateral aspect, center third)
  ○ Abdomen (avoid umbilicus)
  ○ Anterior thigh (center third)
• Common uses
  ○ Insulin administration
  ○ Allergy desensitization
  ○ Hormone replacement
  ○ Immunizations
	• Insert the needle at a 15° angle, injecting the medication to form a bleb (a small bubble) just beneath the surface of the skin.
	• The intradermal site is the inside surface of the forearm, not the medial surface.
	• Common uses
	  ○ Local anesthetic
	  ○ Tuberculosis (TB) skin testing
	  ○ Allergy testing

- Intramuscular (IM) Medication Administration

  o Strategies to decrease pain

    ▪ Apply a eutectic mixture of local anesthetics (EMLA) in the form of a cream or disk a minimum of 60 min, preferably 2 to 2.5 hr, prior to injection.

    ▪ Change the needle if used to puncture the rubber top of a vial.

    ▪ Use the smallest gauge possible.

  o Considerations when selecting a site

    ▪ Medication amount, viscosity, and type

    ▪ Muscle mass, condition, access of site, and potential for contamination

    ▪ Treatment course frequency and number of injections

    ▪ Ability to obtain proper positioning of the child

  o General considerations for IM medication administration

    ▪ The vastus lateralis site is usually the recommended site for infants and children less than 2 years of age (it can accommodate fluid up to 0.5 mL in infants and 2 mL in children).

    ▪ After age 2, the ventral gluteal site can be used (it can accommodate fluid up to 0.5 mL in infants and 2 mL in children).

    ▪ The deltoid site has a smaller muscle mass and can only accommodate up to 0.5 mL of fluid in infants and 1 mL in children.

 View Media Supplement: Pediatric IM Injections (Video)

SITE	NEEDLE SIZES	POSITIONS	COMMENTS
Vastus Lateralis	• 22 to 25 gauge • 0.625 to 1 inch	• Supine • Side lying • Sitting	• Recommended site for infants and children less than 2 years of age • May be used for toddlers and older children
Ventrogluteal	• 22 to 25 gauge • 0.625 to 1 inch	• Supine • Side lying • Prone	• Can be used for children ages 2 and older • Less painful than vastus lateralis • Free of any nerves or blood vessels
Deltoid	• 22 to 25 gauge • 0.625 to 1 inch	• Supine • Side lying • Sitting	• Not as painful as vastus lateralis • Less local side effects than with vastus lateralis • Should not be used in infants/children with underdeveloped muscles • If muscle size is appropriate, it may be used for immunization of toddlers and children

- Intravenous (IV) Medication Administration
  - Peripheral venous access devices
    - Use for continuous and intermittent IV medication administration.
    - Children who require short-term therapy may be discharged with a peripheral line that is maintained by a home health care nurse.
  - Central venous access devices (VADs)
    - Long-term central VADs may be tunneled or implanted infusion ports.
    - If a child is to go home with a VAD, discharge instructions should include how to prepare and inject medication, flush the line, and perform dressing changes.
    - Short-term, or nontunneled, catheters are inserted into large veins and are used in acute care, emergency situations and intensive care units.
    - Peripherally inserted central catheters (PICCs) are used for short- to moderate-length therapy. PICCs are the least costly and have the fewest incidences of complications.

Ⓐ APPLICATION EXERCISES

1. List three interventions, including rationales, that a nurse can use to decrease the risk of medication errors when administering medications to children.

2. When instilling an otic solution into a toddler's ear, what technique should the nurse use?

3. Which of the following are appropriate interventions when administering medications via a nasogastric or gastrostomy tube? (Select all that apply.)

_____ Mix medication with a small amount of enteral feeding.

_____ Use liquid forms of medications.

_____ Question if the volume of medication seems too large.

_____ Verify tube placement before administering medication.

_____ Flush tube with cold water after administering medication.

4. When administering an IM injection to a toddler, which of the following interventions should the nurse take? (Select all that apply.)

_____ Insert the needle at a 15-degree angle.

_____ Use the smallest needle gauge possible.

_____ Change to a new needle after withdrawing medication from a rubber topped vial.

_____ Select the inside aspect of the forearm for the injection.

_____ Apply EMLA cream to the injection site.

(A) **APPLICATION EXERCISES ANSWER KEY**

1. List three interventions, including rationales, that a nurse can use to decrease the risk of medication errors when administering medications to children.

INTERVENTION	RATIONALE
Have a second nurse verify dosage calculation.	Dosage calculations may be more complex because pediatric medication formulations may require dilution, calculation, and preparation of very small doses.
Obtain accurate weight of child.	Dosages are based on weight or body surface area.
Mix medications with small amounts of liquid or soft foods.	If the medication is mixed in large amounts of liquid or foods, the child may refuse to finish the dose.

 NCLEX® Connection: Safety and Infection Control, Accident/Injury Prevention

2. When instilling an otic solution into a toddler's ear, what technique should the nurse use?

Pull the auricle down and back for children up to 3 years of age. Pull the auricle up and back for older children and adults. This helps open the ear canal and facilitate administration of the medication.

(N) NCLEX® Connection: Pharmacological Therapies, Medication Administration

3. Which of the following are appropriate interventions when administering medications via a nasogastric or gastrostomy tube? (Select all that apply.)

  _____ Mix medication with a small amount of enteral feeding.
  ___X___ **Use liquid forms of medications.**
  ___X___ **Question if the volume of medication seems too large.**
  ___X___ **Verify tube placement before administering medication.**
  _____ Flush tube with cold water after administering medication.

When administering medication, it should be in liquid form to prevent clogging of the tube. If the volume seems too large, question the provider regarding the dosage to prevent a medication error. Verify tube placement before giving medication to ensure the medication will be administered into the appropriate location. Do not mix medication with enteral feeding to prevent clogging of the tube. Flush the tube with warm water after the medication is administered so the water is close to body temperature.

(N) NCLEX® Connection: Pharmacological Therapies, Medication Administration

4. When administering an IM injection to a toddler, which of the following interventions should the nurse take? (Select all that apply.)

        _____   Insert the needle at a 15-degree angle.

        X   **Use the smallest needle gauge possible.**

        X   **Change to a new needle after withdrawing medication from a rubber topped vial.**

        _____   Select the inside aspect of the forearm for the injection.

        X   **Apply EMLA cream to the injection site.**

The nurse should change the needle after withdrawing medication from a rubber-topped vial to prevent injury from any fibers from the vial top that may cling to the needle. The nurse should use the smallest gauge possible to minimize pain. The nurse should apply EMLA cream to the injection site 60 min prior to the injection. Either a 90- or 45-degree angle is used when inserting the needle for an IM injection. The inner aspect of the forearm is an appropriate site for an intradermal injection.

(N) NCLEX® Connection: Pharmacological Therapies, Medication Administration

UNIT 1	FOUNDATIONS OF NURSING CARE OF CHILDREN
Section:	Special Considerations of Nursing Care of Children
Chapter 9	Pain Management

 Overview

- Identification of pain in children is complex and challenging.

- Children have a right to appropriate pain management. The nurse's role is to advocate for children and families and educate about proper pain management.

- Pain is whatever the child says it is, and it exists whenever the child says it does. The child's report of pain is the most reliable diagnostic measurement of pain. Behavioral and physiological measures are also used to evaluate pain.

- The type of pain children experience includes procedure-related pain, operative and trauma-associated pain, and/or acute and chronic pain from illness or injury.

- Perform pain assessments and record frequently. Consider pain the fifth vital sign.

- Evaluate the effectiveness of treatment in a timely manner (15 min after IV pain medication administration, 30 min after IM pain medication, 30 to 60 min after oral medication administration and nonpharmacologic therapies).

    ○ Children from 3 to 7 years of age may comprehend how to use a pain rating scale, and self-report using pain scales may be useful with children over 7 years of age. However, each child's ability should be determined. Verification with parents will validate data.

- Proper pain management includes the use of pharmacological and nonpharmacological pain management therapies, such as guided imagery.

- Monitor children receiving opioid medications closely for respiratory depression.

(M) View Media Supplement: Pain Evaluation in Children (Video)

Influential Factors

- Age can influence how pain is perceived and how it can be communicated.

- Fatigue, anxiety, and fear can increase sensitivity to pain.

- Genetic sensitivity can increase or decrease the amount of pain tolerated.

- Cognitive impairment may impact a child's ability to report pain or report it accurately.

- Prior experiences can increase or decrease sensitivity depending on whether or not adequate relief was obtained, especially in older children and adolescents.

- Family and friends may decrease sensitivity to pain by staying with the child.

- Culture may influence how children express pain or the meaning given to it.

Data Collection

- Subjective data may be obtained using a symptom analysis. Nurses should adapt questions to the appropriate developmental level of the child.

SYMPTOMS	QUESTIONS TO ASK
• Location is described using anatomical terminology and landmarks.	• "Where is your pain?" • "Does it hurt anywhere else?" • "Can you point to where it hurts?"
• Quality refers to how the pain feels. • Feelings of pain include: sharp, dull, aching, burning, stabbing, pounding, throbbing, shooting, gnawing, tender, heavy, tight, tiring, exhausting, sickening, terrifying, torturing, nagging, annoying, intense, and/or unbearable.	• "What does the pain feel like?" • "Is the pain throbbing, burning, or stabbing?"

• Intensity, strength, and severity are measures of the pain. Pain assessment tools (description scale, number rating scale) can be used to:
  ○ Measure pain.
  ○ Monitor pain.
  ○ Evaluate effectiveness of interventions.
	• "Can you rate your pain on a scale of 0 to 10?"
	• "How much pain do you have now?"
	• "What is the worst/best the pain has been?"

• The timing of pain includes the onset, duration, and frequency. ○ This may be difficult for a younger child to understand. An older child or adolescent may have a better understanding of time.	• "When did the pain start?" • "How long does the pain last?" • "How often does the pain occur?" • "Is the pain constant or intermittent?"
• Setting has to do with where the child is or what he is doing when the pain occurs.	• "Where are you when you feel pain?" • "What are you doing when you feel pain?"
• Associated symptoms may include fatigue, depression, nausea, and anxiety, and they should be noted.	• "Do you feel tired or sad when you are in pain?"
• Aggravating/relieving factors are things that make the pain feel better or worse.	• "What makes the pain better?" • "What makes the pain worse?"

- Objective Data

  o Behaviors complement self-report and assist in pain assessment of children who are unable to verbalize their feelings.

    ■ Facial expressions (grimace, wrinkled forehead) and body movements (restlessness, pacing, guarding)

    ■ Moaning and crying

    ■ Decreased attention span

  o Physiologic measures of blood pressure, pulse, and respiratory rate will be temporarily increased by acute pain. Eventually, increased vital signs will return to normal despite the persistence of pain. Therefore, physiologic indicators may not be an accurate measure of pain over time.

  o Common pain scales

PAIN ASSESSMENT TOOL	FORM OF EVALUATION	AGE OF CHILD

CRIES Neonatal Postoperative Scale	• Pain rated on a scale of 0 to 10
	• Behavior indicators
	  o Crying
	  o Changes in vital signs
	  o Changes in expression
	  o Altered sleeping patterns
		32 weeks of gestation to 20 weeks post-term

Faces, Legs, Activity, Cry, and Consolability (FLACC) Postoperative Pain Tool	• Behavior indicators
	  o Facial expressions
	  o Position of legs
	  o Activity
	  o Crying
	  o Ability to be consoled
		2 months to 7 years

FACES Pain Rating Scale	• Rating scale uses drawings of happy and sad faces to depict levels of pain.	3 years and older
Visual Analog Scale (VAS)	• Pain is rated on a scale of 0 to 10. • Child points to the number that best describes the pain he is experiencing.	7 years and older (may be effective with children as young as 4.5 years)

Noncommunicating Children's Pain Checklist	• Pain is rated on a scale of 0 to 18.
	• Behavior indicators
	  o Vocalization
	  o Socialization
	  o Facial expressions
	  o Activity level
	  o Movement of extremities
	  o Physiologic changes
		3 to 18 years of age (for children with or without cognitive impairments)

Nursing Interventions

- Interventions should be determined in conjunction with children and their families. Severity of the pain will also guide the choice of treatment.

- Pharmacological measures

  o Give medications routinely versus PRN (as needed) to manage pain that is expected to last for an extended period of time.

  o Use caution when administering medications to newborns less than 2 to 3 months of age because of immature liver function.

  o Combine adjuvant medications (steroids, antidepressants, sedatives, antianxiety medications, muscle relaxants, anticonvulsants) with other analgesics.

  o Use nonopioid and opioid medications.

    ■ Acetaminophen (Tylenol) and NSAIDs are acceptable for mild to moderate pain.

    ■ Opioids are acceptable for moderate to severe pain. Medications used include morphine sulfate, oxycodone (OxyContin), and fentanyl (Duragesic).

    ■ Combining a nonopioid and an opioid medication treats pain peripherally and centrally. This offers greater analgesia with less adverse effects (respiratory depression, constipation, nausea).

- Appropriate Routes

ROUTE	NURSING IMPLICATIONS
Oral	• The oral medication route is preferred due to its convenience, cost, and ability to maintain steady blood levels. • Oral medications take 1 to 2 hr to reach peak analgesic effects. Therefore, these medications are not suited for children experiencing pain that requires rapid relief or pain that is fluctuating in nature.

Topical/transdermal	• One type of topical/transdermal medication is a eutectic mixture of local anesthetics (EMLA), which contains equal quantities of lidocaine and prilocaine in the form of a cream or disk.
	  ○ Use EMLA for any procedure in which the skin will be punctured (IV insertion, biopsy) 60 min prior to a superficial puncture and 2 hr prior to a deep puncture.
	  ○ Place an occlusive dressing over the cream after application.
	  ○ Prior to the procedure, remove the dressing or disk and clean the skin. An indication of an adequate response is reddened or blanched skin.
	  ○ Demonstrate to children that the skin is not sensitive by tapping or scratching lightly.
	  ○ Instruct parents to apply EMLA at home prior to coming to a health care facility for the procedure.
	• Use 4% lidocaine cream (LMX4) 30 min prior to a procedure.
	• Fentanyl
	  ○ Use for children older than 12 years of age.
	  ○ Use to provide continuous pain control. It has an onset of 12 to 24 hr and a duration of 72 hr.
	  ○ Use an immediate-release opioid for breakthrough pain.
	  ○ Notify charge nurse of respiratory depression for administration of naloxone (Narcan).

Continuous intravenous (IV)	• Monitor children who are receiving continuous intravenous (IV) medication administration which provides stable blood levels. • Notify the charge nurse of respiratory depression for administration of naloxone (Narcan).
Patient-controlled analgesia (PCA)	• Monitor children who are receiving parenteral PCA to control pain from injury and chronic conditions. • Medications used include morphine, fentanyl, and hydromorphone (Dilaudid) via PCA. • Allow children to control PCA if appropriate.

- Nonpharmacological Measures
  - Positioning
  - Reinforcing breathing and relaxation techniques
  - Splinting
  - Maintaining a calm environment (low noise, reduced lighting)
  - Providing ice to swollen or injured area
  - Offering warm blankets
  - Assisting with guided imagery
  - Offering distractions (video games, cartoons, videos)
  - Providing comfort with physical contact (holding, rocking)
  - Administering sucrose pacifiers for infants during procedures

Ⓐ APPLICATION EXERCISES

1. The Visual Analog Scale (VAS) is an appropriate pain assessment tool for which of the following?

   A. 6-week-old infant

   B. 2-year-old toddler

   C. 3-year-old preschool-aged child

   D. 8-year-old school-aged child

2. When should a nurse plan to use a topical or transdermal pain medication?

3. A nurse is caring for a 14-year-old client following cardiac surgery who has a patient-controlled analgesia (PCA) pump for pain management. Which of the following comments by the client's parent indicates the need for clarification regarding the use of the pump?

   A. "My son is in control of the pump."

   B. "I'll push the button if I think my son is in too much pain."

   C. "The medication in this pump needs to be monitored by the nurses."

   D. "My son won't have to call the nurse when he needs medication."

4. Offering a sucrose pacifier to an infant during a circumcision is considered

   A. adjuvant pain control.

   B. a nonpharmacological approach.

   C. an oral pain medication.

   D. mind-body management approach.

5. A nurse is assigned to care for an adolescent who had surgery to repair a fractured femur. The adolescent calls the nurse into his room and states, "My leg hurts really bad and I need my pain medicine!" Which of the following is subjective data related to pain that the nurse should obtain prior to medicating the client? (Select all that apply.)

   _____ The anatomical location

   _____ A detailed description of the type

   _____ The pulse rate and characteristic

   _____ The intensity using a rating scale

   _____ The client's facial expressions

APPLICATION EXERCISES ANSWER KEY

1. The Visual Analog Scale (VAS) is an appropriate pain assessment tool for which of the following?

   A. 6-week-old infant

   B. 2-year-old toddler

   C. 3-year-old preschool-aged child

   D. 8-year-old school-aged child

   The VAS scale is appropriate for an 8-year-old because it is typically used for children age 7 and older. The CRIES Neonatal Postoperative Scale is used for newborns and young infants. The FLACC scale is used for infants and children up to age 7. The FACES scale is appropriate for age 3 and older.

 NCLEX® Connection: Basic Care and Comfort, Nonpharmacological Comfort Interventions

2. When should a nurse plan to use a topical or transdermal pain medication?

   Apply topical or transdermal pain medication prior to a biopsy, the insertion of an IV catheter, an injection, or any puncture of the skin. Use topical or transdermal pain medication for continuous pain control or break-through pain.

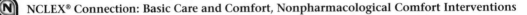 NCLEX® Connection: Pharmacological Therapies, Pharmacological Pain Management

3. A nurse is caring for a 14-year-old client following cardiac surgery who has a patient-controlled analgesia (PCA) pump for pain management. Which of the following comments by the client's parent indicates the need for clarification regarding the use of the pump?

   A. "My son is in control of the pump."

   B. "I'll push the button if I think my son is in too much pain."

   C. "The medication in this pump needs to be monitored by the nurses."

   D. "My son won't have to call the nurse when he needs medication."

   The child should control the PCA and a 14-year-old should be able to do so. Remind the parents that they are not to control the pump. The medication is monitored by the nurse and the client should not need to call the nurse since he will control his dosage of pain medication.

   NCLEX® Connection: Pharmacological Therapies, Pharmacological Pain Management

4. Offering a sucrose pacifier to an infant during a circumcision is considered

    A. adjuvant pain control.

    B. a nonpharmacological approach.

    C. an oral pain medication.

    D. mind-body management approach.

    Non-pharmacological pain management includes offering sucrose pacifiers to infants during procedures. Adjuvant pain control involves the use of combination drug therapies. Sucrose is not considered an oral pain medication. The mind-body management approach is a specific class of complementary and alternative medicine.

(N) NCLEX® Connection: Basic Care and Comfort, Nonpharmacological Comfort Interventions

5. A nurse is assigned to care for an adolescent who had surgery to repair a fractured femur. The adolescent calls the nurse into his room and states, "My leg hurts really bad and I need my pain medicine!" Which of the following is subjective data related to pain that the nurse should obtain prior to medicating the client? (Select all that apply.)

    __X__ **The anatomical location**

    __X__ **A detailed description of the type**

    _____ The pulse rate and characteristic

    __X__ **The intensity using a rating scale**

    _____ The client's facial expressions

    Subjective data is what the client describes as his experience with pain. The nurse should ask the client to describe the anatomical location of the pain, the type or quality of the pain (throbbing, burning), and to rate the pain using an appropriate rating scale. Objective data is what the nurse can collect, which includes the pulse rate and characteristic, and the patient's facial expressions.

(N) NCLEX® Connection: Health Promotion and Maintenance, Data Collection Techniques

---

UNIT 1	FOUNDATIONS OF NURSING CARE OF CHILDREN
Section:	Special Considerations of Nursing Care of Children
Chapter 10	Hospitalization, Illness, and Play

Overview

- A nurse is likely to encounter children who are ill and/or hospitalized. When caring for these children, it is important to know what play activities are considered appropriate.

HOSPITALIZATION AND ILLNESS

Overview

- Families and children may experience major stress related to hospitalization. The nurse should be alert to signs of stress and intervene as appropriate.

- Consider families as clients when children are ill, and use family-centered care when providing care for the hospitalized child.

- Separation anxiety during hospitalization manifests in three behavioral responses:

  ○ Protest (screaming)

  ○ Despair (developmental regression)

  ○ Detachment (lack of interaction with unfamiliar people)

- Each child's understanding of illnesses and hospitalization is dependent on the child's stage of development and cognitive ability.

Impact Based on Development

AGE	LEVEL OF UNDERSTANDING	IMPACT OF HOSPITALIZATION
Infants	• Inability to describe symptoms and follow directions • Lack of understanding of the need for therapeutic procedures	• Experience stranger anxiety between 6 to 18 months of age • Display physical behaviors as expressions of discomfort due to inability to verbalize • May experience sleep deprivation due to strange noises, monitoring devices, and procedures

AGE	LEVEL OF UNDERSTANDING	IMPACT OF HOSPITALIZATION
Toddlers	• Limited ability to describe symptoms • Poorly developed sense of body image and boundaries • Limited understanding of the need for therapeutic procedures • Limited ability to follow directions	• Experience separation anxiety • May exhibit an intense reaction to any type of procedure due to the intrusion of boundaries
Preschoolers	• Limited understanding of the cause of illness but knows what illness feels like • Limited ability to describe symptoms • Fears related to magical thinking • Ability to understand cause and effect inhibited by concrete thinking	• May experience separation anxiety • May harbor fears of bodily harm • May believe illness and hospitalization are a punishment
School-age children	• Beginning awareness of body functioning • Ability to describe pain symptoms • Increasing ability to understand cause and effect	• Fear loss of control • Seek information as a way to maintain a sense of control • May sense when not being told the truth • May experience stress related to separation from peers and regular routine
Adolescents	• Increasing ability to understand cause and effect • Perceptions of illness severity are based on the degree of body image changes	• Develop body-image disturbance • Attempt to maintain composure but are embarrassed about losing control • Experience feelings of isolation from peers • Worry about outcome and impact on school/activities • May not adhere to treatments/medication regimen due to peer influence

Family Responses

- Fear and guilt regarding not bringing children in for care earlier

- Frustration due to the perceived inability to care for their children.

- Altered family roles

- Worry regarding finances if work is missed

- Worry regarding care of other children within the household

- Fear related to lack of knowledge regarding illness or treatments

Data Collection

- Child's and family's understanding of the illness or the reason for hospitalization

- Stressors unique to children and their families (needs of other children in the family, socioeconomic situation, health of other extended family members)

- Past experiences with hospitalization and illness

- Developmental level and needs of children/families

- Parenting role and the family's perception of role changes

- Support available to the children/families

Nursing Interventions

- Tell children and families what to expect during hospitalization.

- Encourage parents or family members to stay with the child during the hospital experience to reduce the stress.

- Attempt to maintain routine as much as possible.

AGE-RELATED INTERVENTIONS	
AGE	INTERVENTIONS
Infants	<ul><li>Place infants whose parents are not in attendance close to nursing stations so that their needs may be quickly met.</li><li>Provide consistency in assigning caregivers.</li></ul>
Toddlers	<ul><li>Encourage parents to provide routine care for the child, such as changing diapers and feeding the child.</li><li>Encourage the child's autonomy by giving the child appropriate choices.</li><li>Provide consistency in assigning caregivers.</li></ul>

AGE-RELATED INTERVENTIONS	
AGE	**INTERVENTIONS**
Preschoolers	• Explain all procedures using simple, clear language. Avoid medical jargon and terms that can be misinterpreted by children. • Encourage the child's independence by letting the child provide self-care. • Encourage children to express feelings. • Validate the child's fears and concerns. • Provide toys that allow for emotional expression, such as a pounding board to release feelings of protest. • Provide consistency in assigning caregivers. • Give choices when possible, such as "Do you want your medicine in a cup or a spoon?" • Allow younger children to handle equipment if it is safe.
School-age Children	• Provide factual information. • Encourage children to express feelings. • Try to maintain a normal routine for long hospitalizations, including time for school work. • Encourage contact with peer group.
Adolescents	• Provide factual information. • Include adolescents in the planning of care to relieve feelings of powerlessness and lack of control. • Encourage contact with peer group.

View Media Supplement: Interventions for Hospitalization (Video)

PLAY

 Overview

- Play allows children to express feelings and fears.

- Play facilitates mastery of developmental stages and assists in the development of problem-solving abilities.

- Play allows children to learn socially acceptable behaviors.

- Play is a means of protection from everyday stressors.

- Make play activities specific to each child's stage of development.

- Use play to teach children.

Content of Play

- Social affective – Taking pleasure in relationships

- Sense-pleasure – Objects in the environment catching the child's attention

- Skill – Demonstrating new abilities

- Unoccupied behavior – Focusing attention on something of interest

- Dramatic – Pretending and fantasizing

- Games – Imitative, formal, or competitive

Social Character of Play

- Onlooker – Children observing others

- Solitary – Children playing alone

- Parallel – Children playing independently but among other children, which is characteristic of toddlers

- Associative – Children playing together without organization, which is characteristic of preschoolers

- Cooperative play – Organized playing in groups, which is characteristic of school-age children

Functions of Play

- Play helps in the development of the following types of skills:

  o Intellectual

  o Sensorimotor

  o Social

    - Self-awareness

    - Creativity

    - Therapeutic and moral values

Play Activities Related to Age

- Infants

  o Birth to 3 months – Visual and auditory stimuli

  o 3 to 6 months – Noise-making objects and soft toys

  o 6 to 9 months – Teething toys and social interaction

  o 9 to 12 months – Large blocks, toys that pop apart, and push-and-pull toys

- Toddlers
  - Cloth books
  - Large crayons and paper
  - Push-and-pull toys
  - Tricycles
  - Balls
  - Puzzles with large pieces
  - Educational television
  - Videos for children
- Preschoolers
  - Associative, imitative, and imaginative play
  - Drawing, painting, riding a tricycle, swimming, jumping, and running
  - Educational television and videos
- School-age children
  - Games that can be played alone or with another person
  - Team sports
  - Musical instruments
  - Arts and crafts
  - Collections
- Adolescents
  - Team sports
  - School activities
  - Reading and listening to music
  - Peer interactions

Therapeutic Play

- Makes use of dolls and/or stuffed animals
- Encourages the acting out of feelings of fear, anger, hostility, and sadness
- Enables children to learn coping strategies in a safe environment
- Assists in gaining cooperation for medical treatment

Data Collection

- Developmental level of the child

- Motor skills

- Level of activity tolerance

- Child's preferences

Nursing Interventions

- Select activities that enhance development.

- Observe the child's play for clues to the child's fears or anxieties.

- Encourage parents to bring one favorite toy from home.

- Use dolls and/or stuffed animals to demonstrate a procedure before it is done.

- Provide play opportunities that meet the child's level of activity tolerance.

- Allow children to go to the play room if able.

- Encourage the adolescent's peers to visit.

Ⓐ APPLICATION EXERCISES

1. A 4-year-old child is admitted to the hospital following surgical repair of a fractured arm after falling from a swing. The child is receiving IV fluids, pain medications, and antibiotics while his arm is in a fiberglass cast which is elevated on a pillow. Which of the following interventions should the nurse implement to assist the parent and child in managing the stress of hospitalization? (Select all that apply.)

   _____ Offer pillows, blankets, and a day-bed for parents to sleep on.

   _____ Encourage parents to have children from the child's play group visit.

   _____ Explain medications in simple terms the child can understand.

   _____ Ask the child to plan bathing and hygiene routine.

   _____ Plan for the same nurses to care for the child during hospitalization.

2. Which of the following actions should the nurse plan to take when contributing to the plan of care for a 14-year-old child hospitalized for an extended time while receiving antibiotics by intermittent IV bolus?

   A. Wear IV access hospital gowns as much as possible.

   B. Discuss having a tutor assist with school activities.

   C. Write out a schedule for the day's events.

   D. Restrict family visiting hours.

3. What is the purpose of play for children?

4. Which of the following activities is considered therapeutic play? (Select all that apply.)

   _____ Reading a book to the child that is about children being hospitalized.

   _____ Using a doll with anatomical parts to explain the disease process.

   _____ Giving the child a stuffed animal that has a cast on it, in the same location as the child's cast.

   _____ Walking the child in the hall.

   _____ Allowing the child to sit at the nurses' station and draw pictures.

5. Match the following play activities with the appropriate age group.

   _____ A. Mobile with brightly colored fish   1. Adolescents

   _____ B. Stringing and painting bead necklaces.   2. 3 to 6 months

   _____ C. Toy stove with pots and pans   3. Preschool

   _____ D. Shooting basketballs   4. Toddler

   _____ E. Riding big-wheel tricycle   5. School-age

(A) APPLICATION EXERCISES ANSWER KEY

1. A 4-year-old child is admitted to the hospital following surgical repair of a fractured arm after falling from a swing. The child is receiving IV fluids, pain medications, and antibiotics while his arm is in a fiberglass cast which is elevated on a pillow. Which of the following interventions should the nurse implement to assist the parent and child in managing the stress of hospitalization? (Select all that apply.)

   __X__ **Offer pillows, blankets, and a day-bed for parents to sleep on.**

   _____ Encourage parents to have children from the child's play group visit.

   __X__ **Explain medications in simple terms the child can understand.**

   _____ Ask the child to plan bathing and hygiene routine.

   __X__ **Plan for the same nurses to care for the child during hospitalization.**

   Maintaining home-like routines and encouraging parents to remain at night can reduce stress for both the child and parents. For the preschool-age child, explaining procedures in simple terms and providing for consistency in caregivers are helpful in allaying stress. Having contact with peers and planning for care routines are appropriate for the school-age child and adolescent, not the preschool-age child.

    NCLEX® Connection: Health Promotion and Maintenance, Aging Process

2. Which of the following actions should the nurse plan to take when contributing to the plan of care for a 14-year-old child hospitalized for an extended time while receiving antibiotics by intermittent IV bolus?

   A. Wear IV access hospital gowns as much as possible.

   B. Discuss having a tutor assist with school activities.

   C. Write out a schedule for the day's events.

   D. Restrict family visiting hours.

   The adolescent worries about the impact of missing school/activities so integrating a tutor into the hospital routine, when possible, is appropriate. Body image is a concern of the adolescent and wearing hospital gowns does not recognize the child's need for self-expression and to maintain control. Involve adolescents in planning the schedule of activities. Encourage the family to visit as much as possible to reduce stress in both the parent and adolescent.

   NCLEX® Connection: Health Promotion and Maintenance, Developmental Stages and Transitions

3. What is the purpose of play for children?

Play allows children to express feelings and fears; facilitates meeting developmental needs; allows for socialization and learning socially appropriate behaviors; is a learning tool; and can relieve stress.

(N) NCLEX® Connection: Health Promotion and Maintenance, Developmental Stages and Transitions

4. Which of the following activities is considered therapeutic play? (Select all that apply.)

__X__ **Reading a book to the child that is about children being hospitalized.**

__X__ **Using a doll with anatomical parts to explain the disease process.**

__X__ **Giving the child a stuffed animal that has a cast on it, in the same location as the child's cast.**

_____ Walking the child in the hall.

__X__ **Allowing the child to sit at the nurses' station and draw pictures.**

Therapeutic play includes reading about hospitalization with a child. This encourages the child to recognize appropriate coping strategies in a safe environment. Using dolls or stuffed animals to demonstrate procedures and explain what is happening to the child is also therapeutic play. Allowing the child in the nurses' station gains his cooperation and reduces feelings of fear and sadness. Walking the child in the hall has physiological benefits, but is not considered play.

(N) NCLEX® Connection: Health Promotion and Maintenance, Health Promotion/Disease Prevention

5. Match the following play activities with the appropriate age group.

__2__	A. Mobile with brightly colored fish	1. Adolescents
__5__	B. Stringing and painting bead necklaces.	2. 3 to 6 months
__3__	C. Toy stove with pots and pans	3. Preschool
__1__	D. Shooting basketballs	4. Toddler
__4__	E. Riding big-wheel tricycle	5. School-age

(N) NCLEX® Connection: Health Promotion and Maintenance, Aging Process

UNIT 1   FOUNDATIONS OF NURSING CARE OF CHILDREN

Section: Special Considerations of Nursing Care of Children

Chapter 11   Death and Dying

Overview

- The death of a child may be traumatic and devastating for a family.

- Parental grief may last a lifetime, place stress on marital relations, and impact a parent's ability to assist siblings in dealing with their grief.

- Children, regardless of age, will experience grief and loss, which is expressed sporadically through behavior and play and is present for a long period of time. Grief in children is expressed and dealt with in an individual manner. Children who have sustained the loss of siblings may experience physical symptoms (sleep disturbances, depression) or may display behaviors like trying to be perfect or acting out for attention.

- Dysfunctional grief is a type of complicated grief that persists for more than a year after the loss. This type of grief presents with the following characteristics: intense and prolonged feelings of loneliness, emptiness, and yearnings; distractive thoughts; an inability to sleep; lowered self-esteem; and loss of interest in daily activities.

- Family-centered care is required to meet the needs of each individual family member who is experiencing grief.

- Palliative care (end-of-life care)

  o Palliative care is a multidisciplinary approach that focuses on the process of dying rather than prolonging life in cases in which cures are no longer possible.

  o Pain control, symptom management, and support of the child and family must be given top priority in the terminal stages of illness.

  o Palliative care uses education, support, and honest communication to foster a therapeutic environment.

- End-of-life decisions require honest information regarding prognosis, disease progression, treatment options, and the impact of the treatments. These decisions are made during a highly stressful time. It is important that all health care personnel are aware of the child and family's decisions.

- Nurses may experience personal grief when caring for children with whom they have developed rapport and intimacy. A debriefing of the entire staff by professional grief/mental health counselors may be indicated.

Factors Influencing Loss, Grief, and Coping Ability

- Interpersonal relationships and social support networks

- Type and significance of loss

- Culture and ethnicity

- Spiritual and religious beliefs and practices

- Prior experience with loss

- Socioeconomic status

- Current stage of development

AGE	RELEVANT FACTORS
Infants/Toddlers (birth to 3 years)	- Have little to no concept of death - Have egocentric thinking that prevents them from understanding death (toddlers) - Mirror parental emotions (sadness, anger, depression, anxiety) - React in response to the changes brought about by being in the hospital (change of routine, painful procedures, immobilization, less independence, separation from family) - May regress to an earlier stage of behavior
Preschool children (3 to 6 years)	- Have egocentric thinking - Have magical thinking that allows them to believe that their thoughts can cause an event such as death (As a result, they may feel guilty and shameful.) - Interpret separation from parents as punishment for bad behavior - View dying as temporary because they have no concept of time and because they still believe the dead person has attributes of the living (sleeping, eating, breathing)
School-age children (6 to 12 years)	- Start to respond to logical or factual explanations - Begin to have an adult concept of death (inevitable, irreversible, universal), which generally applies to school-age children who are older (9 to 12 years) - Experience fear of the disease process, the death process, the unknown, and loss of control ○ Fear is often displayed through uncooperative behavior - May be curious about funeral services and what happens to the body after death

AGE	RELEVANT FACTORS
Adolescents (12 to 20 years)	• May have an adult-like concept of death • May have difficulty accepting death because they are discovering who they are, establishing an identity, and dealing with issues of puberty • Rely more on their peers rather than the influence of their parents, which may cause the reality of a serious illness to make the adolescent feel isolated. • May be unable to relate to peers and communicate with their parents • May become more stressed by changes in physical appearance from the medications or illness than the prospect of death • May experience guilt and shame

- Factors that may increase the family's potential for dysfunctional grieving following the death of a child include:

    o Lack of a support system

    o Presence of poor coping skills

    o Association of violence or suicide with the death of the child

    o Sudden and unexpected death of the child

    o Lack of hope or presence of pre-existing mental health issues

Data Collection

- Knowledge regarding diagnosis, prognosis, and care

- Perceptions and desires regarding diagnosis, prognosis, and care

- Nutritional status, as well as growth and development patterns

- Activity and energy level of child and siblings

- Parents' wishes regarding the child's end-of-life care

- Presence of a do-not-resuscitate (DNR) order

- Family coping and available support

- The stage of grief children and families are experiencing

- Symptoms of normal grief, which may include:

    o Feelings of sadness, denial, anxiety, and/or yearning

    o Feelings of guilt and/or anger toward the deceased

    o Somatic reports of chest pain, palpitations, headaches, nausea, changes in sleep patterns, or fatigue

    o Experience of hearing the deceased person's voice

Nursing Interventions

- Care for terminally ill children.

CARE	FOCUS
Hospital care	• Children cannot be managed at home (families do not want or are not able to provide necessary care, children require intensive nursing care).
Home care	• Home care agency nurses perform data collection and provide treatments, medications, supplies, and equipment under the direction of the health care provider.
Hospice care	• Management of the psychological, spiritual, physical, and social needs of children and families is conducted by hospice teams. • The hospice team provides support to family members who provide most of the care • Pain and symptom control is the priority. • Support to families will continue post death.

- Allow an opportunity for anticipatory grieving, which impacts the way a family will cope with the death of a child.

- Offer strategies specific to developmental level.

AGE GROUP	DEVELOPMENTAL APPROACH
Infants and toddlers	• Encourage parents to stay with their children. • Attempt to maintain a normal environment.
Preschoolers	• Encourage parents to stay with their children. • Communicate with children in honest, simple terms. • Be aware of medical jargon that may frighten children.
School-age children	• Encourage parents to stay with their children. • Use language that is clear regarding the disease, medications, procedures, and expectations. • Encourage self-care to promote independence and self-esteem. • Allow participation in plans for funeral services.
Adolescents	• Be honest and respectful when communicating. • Encourage self-care to promote independence and self-esteem. • Allow participation in plans for funeral services. • Encourage parents or other family members to stay with adolescents.

- Palliative Care

  - Consider the child, siblings, and parents as the units of care.

  - Provide an environment that is as close to being like home as possible.

  - Consult with children and families for desired measures.

  - Respect the family's cultural and religious preferences and rituals.

  - Provide and clarify information and explanations.

  - Encourage physical contact; address feelings; and show concern, empathy, and support.

  - Provide comfort measures (warmth, quiet, noise control, dry linens).

  - Provide adequate nutrition and hydration.

  - Control pain.

    - Give medications on a regular schedule.

    - Treat breakthrough pain.

    - Increase doses as necessary to control pain.

    - Encourage use of relaxation, imagery, and distraction to help manage pain.

- Care for grieving families during the dying process

  - Provide information to children and families about the disease, medications, procedures, and expected events.

  - Encourage and support parents to participate in caring for their children.

  - Encourage parents to remain near their children as much as possible.

  - Encourage the child's independence and control as developmentally and physically appropriate.

  - Allow for visitation of family and friends as desired.

  - Emphasize open, honest communication among children, families, and the health care team.

  - Provide support to children and families with decision-making.

  - Provide opportunities for children and families to ask questions.

  - Assist children with completion of unfinished tasks.

  - Assist parents to cope with their feelings and help them to understand their children's behaviors.

  - Use books, movies, art, music, and play therapy to stimulate discussions and provide an outlet for emotions.

  - Provide and encourage professional support and guidance from a trusted member of the health care team.

○ Remain neutral and accepting.

○ Give reassurance that the child is not in pain and that all efforts are being made to maintain comfort and support of the child's life.

○ Recognize and support the individual differences of grieving. Advise families that each member may react differently on any given day.

○ Give families privacy, unlimited time, and opportunities for any cultural or religious rituals. Respect the family's decisions regarding care of the child.

○ Encourage discussion of special memories and people, reading of favorite books, providing favorite toys/objects, physical contact, sibling visits, and continued verbal communication, even if the child seems unconscious.

○ After death, validate the loss.

 ■ The nurse should express his own feelings of loss and sadness to someone who can offer support.

 ■ Issues and decisions to be addressed at the time of death include the following:

  □ Organ and/or tissue donation if applicable

  □ Autopsy

  □ Viewing of the body

  □ Sibling attendance at the funeral

APPLICATION EXERCISES

1. Which of the following nursing interventions is appropriate when working with a school-age child who has a terminal illness?

   A. Offer factual explanations about the disease, medications, and procedures.

   B. Set a schedule for the child to complete personal care.

   C. Tell the child that everything will be okay.

   D. Reinforce that being in the hospital is not a punishment for behavior.

2. What are some causes of dysfunctional grieving in a family following the death of a child?

3. A nurse is talking with parents about how children experience grief and loss. Which of the following behaviors occur in children? (Select all that apply.)

   _____ Each child deals with grief and loss in his own way.

   _____ Sleep may be difficult.

   _____ Seeking attention is typical.

   _____ Activities become a focus of their daily routine.

   _____ Grief is usually a short-lived experience.

4. What data should the nurse collect when admitting a child who is terminally ill?

(A) APPLICATION EXERCISES ANSWER KEY

1. Which of the following nursing interventions is appropriate when working with a school-age child who has a terminal illness?

   A. Offer factual explanations about the disease, medications, and procedures.

   B. Set a schedule for the child to complete personal care.

   C. Tell the child that everything will be okay.

   D. Reinforce that being in the hospital is not a punishment for behavior.

   School-age children should be given clear, factual information. It is not necessary for a child with a terminal illness to perform self-care on a schedule; the child should be allowed to rest when necessary. Telling the child that everything will be okay is giving false reassurance and will not promote a trusting relationship with the child or family. A preschool-age child typically believes that actions can cause bad things to happen.

   (N) NCLEX® Connection: Psychosocial Integrity, Grief and Loss

2. What are some causes of dysfunctional grieving in a family following the death of a child?

   Causes of dysfunctional grieving can include inadequate support systems, poor coping skills, the child having died by violence or suicide, sudden and unexpected death, loss of hope, and long-term health issues.

   (N) NCLEX® Connection: Psychosocial Integrity, Grief and Loss

3. A nurse is talking with parents about how children experience grief and loss. Which of the following behaviors occur in children? (Select all that apply.)

   __X__ Each child deals with grief and loss in his own way.

   __X__ Sleep may be difficult.

   __X__ Seeking attention is typical.

   _____ Activities become a focus of their daily routine.

   _____ Grief is usually a short-lived experience.

   Children experience grief and deal with it in an individual manner. Grief may be present for a long period of time. Children may have sleep disturbances, act out for attention, and become depressed and less involved in daily activities.

   (N) NCLEX® Connection: Psychosocial Integrity, Grief and Loss

4. What data should the nurse collect when admitting a child who is terminally ill?

Data to be collected include the current level of knowledge of the parent/child and their perceptions and desires regarding the diagnosis, prognosis and expected care; nutrition status; growth and development pattern; activity and energy level; parents' preferences regarding end-of-life care; the presence of a do-not-resuscitate (DNR) order; family coping and support available; stage of grief of the parent and child, and symptoms being experienced.

(N) NCLEX® Connection: Psychosocial Integrity, Grief and Loss

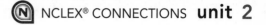

UNIT 2: NURSING CARE OF CHILDREN WITH SYSTEM DISORDERS

Section: Neurosensory Disorders

- Acute Neurological Disorders

- Seizures

- Visual and Hearing Impairments

NCLEX® CONNECTIONS

When reviewing the chapters in this section, keep in mind the relevant sections of the NCLEX® outline, in particular:

CLIENT NEEDS: PHARMACOLOGICAL THERAPIES

Relevant topics/tasks include:
- Adverse Effects/ Contraindications/Side Effects/Interactions
  - Reinforce client teaching on possible effects of medications.
- Expected Actions/ Outcomes
  - Reinforce education to client regarding medications.
- Medication Administration
  - Administer a medication by ear, eye, nose, rectum, vagina or skin route.

CLIENT NEEDS: REDUCTION OF RISK POTENTIAL

Relevant topics/tasks include:
- Diagnostic Tests
  - Reinforce client teaching about diagnostic test.
- Potential for Alterations in Body Systems
  - Perform neurological checks.
- Potential for Complications of Diagnostic Tests/ Treatments/Procedures
  - Reinforce teaching to prevent complications due to client diagnostic tests/treatments/ procedures.

CLIENT NEEDS: PHYSIOLOGICAL ADAPTATION

Relevant topics/tasks include:
- Alterations in Body Systems
  - Provide care to client who has experienced a seizure.
- Basic Pathophysiology
  - Identify signs and symptoms related to acute or chronic illness.
- Unexpected Response to Therapies
  - Respond to a client life-threatening situation.

UNIT 2	NURSING CARE OF CHILDREN WITH SYSTEM DISORDERS
Section:	Neurosensory Disorders

Chapter 12   Acute Neurological Disorders

Overview

- Meningitis is an inflammation of the meninges, which are the membranes that protect the brain and spinal cord.

- Reye syndrome is a life-threatening disease that leads to multisystem failure.

- Meningitis and Reye syndrome have similar symptoms and are both often preceded by viral infections. Therefore, testing may be necessary to differentiate between the two.

- Head injuries can be classified as open (skull integrity is compromised – penetrating trauma) or closed (skull integrity is maintained – blunt trauma). Head injuries are also classified as mild, moderate, or severe, depending upon Glasgow Coma Scale (GCS) ratings and length of loss of consciousness.

MENINGITIS

Overview

- Viral or aseptic meningitis usually requires only supportive care for recovery.

- Bacterial, or septic, meningitis is a contagious infection. The prognosis depends on how quickly care is initiated.

Data Collection

- Risk Factors

  o Viral Meningitis

    ▪ Viral illnesses (mumps, measles, herpes)

  o Bacterial Meningitis

    ▪ Upper respiratory infections (otitis media, tonsillitis) caused by bacterial agents (Neisseria meningitides [meningococcal], Streptococcus pneumonia [pneumococcal], Haemophilus influenzae, Escherichia coli)

    ▪ Immunosuppression

- ■ Injuries that provide direct access to cerebrospinal fluid (skull fracture, penetrating head wound)
        - ■ Overcrowded living conditions
- • Subjective Data
    - ○ Children may report photophobia or headache
    - ○ Parents may report that children are irritable, have vomited, and are drowsy.
- • Objective Data
    - ○ Physical Assessment Findings
        - ■ Newborns
            - □ No illness is present at birth, but it progresses within a few days.
            - □ Clinical signs may be vague and difficult to diagnose.
                - ‣ Poor muscle tone, weak cry, and poor feeding
                - ‣ Fever or hypothermia
            - □ Nuchal rigidity is not usually present.
            - □ Bulging fontanels are a late sign.
        - ■ 2 months to 2 years
            - □ Seizures with a high-pitched cry
            - □ Fever and irritability
            - □ Bulging fontanels
            - □ Possible nuchal rigidity
            - □ Poor feeding
            - □ Vomiting
            - □ Brudzinski's sign and Kernig's sign do not assist with the diagnosis.
        - ■ 2 years through adolescence
            - □ Seizures (often initial sign)
            - □ Nuchal rigidity
            - □ Positive Brudzinski's sign (flexion of extremities occurring with deliberate flexion of the child's neck)
            - □ Positive Kernig's sign (resistance to extension of the child's leg from a flexed position)
            - □ Fever and chills
            - □ Headache
            - □ Vomiting
            - □ Photophobia

- □ Irritability and restlessness that may progress to drowsiness, delirium, stupor, and coma

- □ Petechia or purpuric type rash (seen with meningococcal infection)

- □ Involvement of joints (seen with meningococcal and Haemophilus influenza)

- □ Chronic draining ear (seen with pneumococcal infection)

- o Laboratory Tests

  - ▪ Perform a blood culture and sensitivity test to identify an appropriate broad-spectrum antibiotic.

  - ▪ Complete blood counts should be taken.

  - ▪ Cerebrospinal fluid (CSF) should be collected.

    - □ Results indicative of meningitis

      - ▸ CSF that appears cloudy (bacterial) or clear (viral)

      - ▸ Elevated WBC

      - ▸ Elevated protein levels

      - ▸ Decreased glucose (bacterial)

      - ▸ Elevated CSF pressure

- o Diagnostic Procedures

  - ▪ Cerebrospinal fluid (CSF) analysis

    - □ This is the best diagnostic test for meningitis.

    - □ The collection of CSF with a lumbar puncture (performed by a health care provider)

    - □ Nursing Actions

      - ▸ Have children empty the bladder if appropriate.

      - ▸ Place children in the fetal position and assist in maintaining the position. Older children may be placed in the sitting position.

      - ▸ Administer sedatives as prescribed.

      - ▸ Apply a eutectic mixture of local anesthetics (EMLA), which contains equal quantities of lidocaine and prilocaine, over the area between L3 and L5 60 min prior to the procedure.

      - ▸ Appropriately label the three test tubes of CSF and deliver them to the laboratory.

      - ▸ Monitor the site for hematoma and/or infection.

    - □ Client Education

      - ▸ Children should be encouraged to remain in bed for 4 to 8 hr in a flat position to prevent leakage and a resulting spinal headache. This may not be possible for infants, toddlers, or preschoolers.

- CT or MRI scans
  - These may be performed to identify increased intracranial pressure (ICP) and/or an abscess.
  - Nursing Actions
    - Assist with positioning.
    - Administer sedatives as prescribed.

Collaborative Care

- Nursing Care

  - The presence of petechia or a purpuric-type rash requires immediate medical attention.

  - Isolate children as soon as meningitis is suspected.

  - Maintain isolation precautions (droplet precautions) per facility protocol. This requires a private room or a room with cohorts, the wearing of a surgical mask within 3 feet of children, appropriate hand hygiene, and the use of designated equipment, such as blood pressure cuff and thermometer. Continue for 24 hr after the first antibiotic has been administered.

  - Apply cardiac monitor and monitor status.

  - Monitor for signs and symptoms of increased intracranial pressure (severe headache, deteriorating level of consciousness, restlessness, irritability, agitation).

  - Continue frequent monitoring of vital signs, urine output, fluid status, pain level, neurologic status, and head circumference (for infants).

  - Monitor I&O hourly for children receiving IV fluids.

  - Maintain NPO status if children have a decreased level of consciousness. As the child's condition improves, advance to clear liquids and then to a diet that the child can tolerate.

  - Decrease environmental stimuli.
    - Provide a quiet environment.
    - Minimize the child's exposure to bright light (natural and electric).

  - Provide comfort.
    - Keep the child's room cool.
    - Position children without a pillow and slightly elevate the head of the bed. Children may prefer a side-lying position to take pressure off the neck.
    - Maintain safety (keep the bed in a low position, implement seizure precautions).
    - Keep the family informed of the child's condition.

- Medications

    o Antibiotics – usually a cephalosporin

        ▪ Administer for bacterial infections via an IV route. Length of therapy is determined by the child's condition and CSF results (normal blood glucose levels, negative culture). Therapy may last as long as 10 days.

        ▪ Nursing Considerations

            □ Check for allergies.

            □ Monitor children receiving IV infusions.

        ▪ Client Education

            □ Provide support for children and families.

            □ Educate the family about the need to complete the entire course of medication.

    o Corticosteroids – Dexamethasone (Decadron)

        ▪ Administer to prevent neurologic complications for children with bacterial meningitis.

        ▪ Nursing Considerations

            □ Check for effectiveness of medication.

        ▪ Client Education

            □ Provide support for children and their families.

            □ Educate on the administration of the medication and side effects that may occur.

    o Anticonvulsants – Phenytoin (Dilantin) or fosphenytoin (Cerebyx)

        ▪ Prophylaxis for seizures

        ▪ Nursing Considerations

            □ Watch for effectiveness of the medication.

            □ Monitor therapeutic medication levels.

        ▪ Client Education

            □ Instruct children and their families about the need to administer the medication on schedule.

    o Analgesics

        ▪ Nonopioids should be used to avoid masking changes in the level of consciousness.

        ▪ Nursing Considerations

            □ Monitor respiratory status.

            □ Monitor level of consciousness.

        ▪ Client Education

            □ Provide support for children and their families.

- Care After Discharge

  - Client Education

    - Recommend early and complete treatment for upper respiratory infections.

    - Encourage parents to maintain appropriate immunizations for children. Children should receive the Haemophilus influenza Type B vaccine (Hib); the pneumococcal conjugate vaccine (PCV) at 2, 4, and 6 months of age and then again between 12 and 15 months of age; and the meningococcal vaccine (MCV4) between 11 and 12 years of age.

- Client Outcomes

  - The child will experience minimal neurologic deficits.

REYE SYNDROME

Overview

- Reye syndrome primarily affects the liver and brain, causing:

  - Liver dysfunction

    - Bleeding and poor blood clotting

  - Cerebral edema (with increased intracranial pressure).

    - Lethargy progressing to coma

    - Potential for cerebral herniation

  - Hypoglycemia

  - Shock

- Reye syndrome has been mistaken for a variety of other disorders, including encephalitis, meningitis, poisoning, sudden infant death syndrome (SIDS), diabetes mellitus, and psychiatric illness.

- The prognosis for Reye syndrome is best with early recognition and aggressive treatment.

Data Collection

- Risk Factors

  - The cause of Reye syndrome is unknown. However, research has revealed an association between using aspirin (salicylate) products for treating viral infections and the development of Reye syndrome.

  - Peak incidence occurs in January, February, and March. The symptoms most often appear at the end of a viral illness (viral upper respiratory infection, varicella) but may occur earlier in the illness.

- Subjective Data

  - History of recent viral illness or recent use of aspirin

- Objective Data
  - Physical Assessment Findings
    - Reye syndrome presents in five clinical stages. Each stage contains intensified signs and symptoms of the previous stage.

STAGE	MANIFESTATIONS
I	<ul><li>Lethargy</li><li>Vomiting</li><li>Anorexia</li><li>Early liver dysfunction</li><li>Brisk pupillary reaction</li><li>Ability to follow commands</li></ul>
II	<ul><li>Confusion/disorientation/delirium</li><li>Combativeness</li><li>Hyperventilation</li><li>Hyperactive reflexes</li><li>Sluggish pupillary response</li><li>Response to painful stimuli</li></ul>
III	<ul><li>Coma</li><li>Seizures</li><li>Decorticate (extension) posturing</li></ul>
IV	<ul><li>Deeper coma</li><li>Decerebrate (flexion) posturing</li><li>Fixed, large pupils, and loss of corneal reflexes</li><li>Brainstem dysfunction</li><li>Minimal liver dysfunction</li></ul>
V	<ul><li>Hypotonia</li><li>Seizures</li><li>Respiratory arrest</li><li>Absence of liver dysfunction</li></ul>

  - Laboratory Tests
    - Liver enzymes (alanine aminotransferase [ALT], aspartate aminotransferase [AST]) – Elevated
    - Serum ammonia level – Elevated
    - Serum electrolytes – Altered electrolytes due to cerebral edema and liver changes
    - Serum blood glucose – Hypoglycemia
    - CBC may indicate low Hgb, Hct, and platelets.
    - Coagulation times may be extended.

- o Diagnostic Procedures
  - ▪ Nursing Actions
    - □ Liver biopsy – A piece of liver tissue is taken using a large-bore needle and sent to the pathology department.
      - ‣ Maintain NPO status prior to the procedure.
      - ‣ Monitor for hemorrhage postprocedure.
      - ‣ Monitor vital signs frequently postprocedure.
    - □ Client Education
      - ‣ Encourage the parents to limit the child's postprocedure activities to decrease the risk of hemorrhage.
  - ▪ Cerebrospinal fluid (CSF) analysis
    - □ A lumbar puncture should be performed to collect CSF and rule out meningitis as a cause of symptoms (performed by a provider, usually a physician).

Collaborative Care

- • Nursing Care
  - o Maintain hydration.
    - ▪ Monitor IV fluids as prescribed.
    - ▪ Maintain accurate I&O.
    - ▪ Insert indwelling urinary catheter as ordered.
  - o Position children to avoid extreme flexion, extension, or rotation.
    - ▪ Maintain the head in a midline neutral position.
    - ▪ Keep the head of the bed elevated 30°.
  - o Monitor appropriateness of coagulation.
    - ▪ Note unexplained or prolonged bleeding.
    - ▪ Apply pressure after procedures.
    - ▪ Prepare to administer vitamin K.
  - o Monitor pain status and response to painful stimuli. Administer pain medications when appropriate.
  - o Insert a nasogastric tube as ordered.
  - o Take seizure precautions.
  - o Keep the family informed of the child's status.
  - o Provide private time for families to be with their children if death is imminent.
  - o Contact support for families.

- Medications

  - Osmotic diuretic – Mannitol (Osmitrol)

    - To decrease cerebral swelling

    - Nursing Considerations

      - Monitor children for increased intracranial pressure.

  - Insulin

    - Administer to increase glucose metabolism.

    - Nursing Considerations

      - Monitor blood glucose levels prior to insulin administration and periodically.

    - Client Education

      - Provide support for children.

- Interdisciplinary Care

  - Occupational and physical therapy to be involved with children who have neurologic deficits post-Reye syndrome.

  - Dietician to be involved if indicated.

- Care After Discharge

  - Client Education

    - Remind parents to avoid giving salicylates for pain or fever in children.

    - Recommend to parents to read labels of over-the-counter medications to check for the presence of salicylates.

- Client Outcomes

  - The child will experience minimal neurologic deficits.

HEAD INJURY

Overview

- Open head injuries pose a high risk for infection.

- Skull fractures are often accompanied by brain injury. Damage to brain tissue may be the result of decreased oxygen supply, direct impact from the skull fracture, or an instrument that caused the trauma. The glucose levels in the brain are negatively affected, resulting in an alteration in neurologic synaptic ability.

- Head injuries may or may not be associated with hemorrhage (epidural, subdural, and intracerebral). Cerebrospinal fluid leakage is also possible. Any collection of fluid or foreign object that occupies space within the confines of the skull poses a risk for cerebral edema, cerebral hypoxia, and brain herniation.

- Cervical spine injury should always be suspected when head injury occurs and must be ruled out prior to removing any devices used to stabilize the cervical spine.

Data Collection

- Risk Factors
  - ○ Lack of supervision
  - ○ Poor/absent safety practices
  - ○ Improper use of safety devices (helmets, seat belts)
- Subjective Data
  - ○ History of events leading up to the injury, including any reports of dizziness, headache, diplopia, and/or vomiting
  - ○ Amnesia (loss of memory) before or after injury
  - ○ Alcohol or drug ingestion
- Objective Data
  - ○ Physical Assessment Findings
    - ■ Loss of consciousness – The length of time the client is unconscious is significant
    - ■ Signs of increased intracranial pressure and brainstem involvement
      - □ Severe headache
      - □ Deteriorating level of consciousness, restlessness, irritability, and agitation
      - □ Dilated and fixed, constricted and fixed, slow to react, or nonreactive pupils
      - □ Alteration in breathing pattern, such as deep, fast, and intermittent gasping respirations
      - □ Abnormal posturing
        - ▸ Decorticate (dysfunction of the cerebral cortex) – Demonstrates the arms, wrists, and fingers flexed and bent inward onto the chest and the legs extended and adducted
        - ▸ Decerebrate (dysfunction at the midbrain) – Demonstrates a backward arching of the head and arms with legs rigidly extended and toes pointing downward

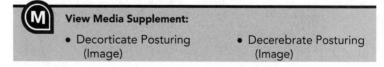

View Media Supplement:
- Decorticate Posturing (Image)
- Decerebrate Posturing (Image)

        - ▸ Flaccidity – Demonstrates no muscle tone
      - □ It is considered a medical emergency when a child is comatose and has asymmetric pupils or one pupil that is dilated and nonreactive.
      - □ Cushing's reflex is a late sign characterized by severe hypertension with widening pulse pressure (systolic – diastolic) and bradycardia.

- Cerebrospinal fluid (CSF) leakage from the nose and ears.
  - A sample of fluid that makes a yellow stain (halo sign) surrounded by blood on a paper towel and tests positive for glucose indicates CSF leakage.
- Seizure activity
- Other signs
  - Difficulty waking up
  - Odd behavior
  - Visual disturbances, such as double or blurred vision
  - Uncoordinated movements and difficulty walking
  - Bulging fontanels and inconsolable crying (in infants)
- Glasgow Comma Scale (GCS)
  - GCS scores of 8 or less are associated with severe head injury and coma.
  - GCS scores between 9 and 12 indicate moderate head injury.
  - GCS scores of 13 or greater reflect minor head trauma.

- Laboratory Tests
  - Arterial blood gases (ABGs)
  - Alcohol level and drug screen
  - CBC with differential
- Diagnostic Procedures
  - Cervical spine films
    - Rule out cervical spine injury.
  - CT and/or MRI scans of head and/or neck
    - Perform with and without contrast if indicated.
  - Measurement of ICP
    - The expected reference range is 10 to 15 mm Hg.
    - Client Education
      - Provide support to the children and their families.

Collaborative Care

- Nursing Care
  - Ensure the child's spine is stabilized until spinal cord injury is ruled out.
  - Monitor the child's vital signs, level of consciousness, pupils, ICP, motor activity, sensory perception, and verbal responses at frequent intervals. Use the Glasgow Coma Scale as indicated.
  - Maintain a patent airway. Monitor children receiving mechanical ventilation.

- ○ Administer oxygen as indicated to maintain an O_2 saturation level greater than 95%.

- ○ Hyperventilate children to keep the $PaCO_2$ between 30 and 35 mm Hg (this reduces cerebral blood flow).

- ○ Maintain c-spine stability if indicated.

- ○ Implement actions that will decrease ICP.

    - ■ Keep the head of the bed elevated to 30°, which will also promote venous drainage.

    - ■ Avoid extreme flexion, extension, or rotation of the head and maintain in midline neutral position.

    - ■ Keep the child's body in alignment, avoiding hip flexion/extension.

    - ■ Minimize endotracheal or oral suctioning.

    - ■ Instruct the child to avoid coughing and blowing her nose, because these activities increase ICP.

- ○ Restrain extremities as indicated to prevent pulling on tubes.

- ○ Implement measures to prevent complications of immobility (turn every 2 hr, maintain foot alignment and splints). Use specialty beds if indicated.

- ○ Insert and maintain an indwelling urinary catheter.

- ○ Administer stool softener to prevent straining (Valsalva maneuver).

- ○ Report to the provider the presence of CSF from nose or ears.

- ○ Provide a calm, restful environment (limit visitors, minimize noise).

- ○ Use energy conservation measures. Alternate activities with rest periods.

- ○ Implement seizure precautions.

- ○ Monitor fluid and electrolyte values and osmolarity to detect changes in sodium regulation, the onset of diabetes insipidus, or severe hypovolemia.

- ○ Provide adequate fluids to maintain cerebral perfusion. When a large amount of IV fluids is ordered, monitor the child carefully for excess fluid volume, which may increase ICP.

- ○ Maintain the child's safety (side rails up, padded side rails, call light within reach).

- ○ Provide nutritional support (enteral nutrition).

- ○ Maintain ongoing communication with children.

- ○ Instruct families on effective ways to communicate with the child (touching, talking, assisting with care as appropriate).

- • Medications

    - ○ Corticosteroids – Dexamethasone (Decadron) and methylprednisolone (Solu-Medrol)

        - ■ Decrease cerebral edema

- Nursing Considerations
  - Monitor for signs of infection.
- Mannitol (Osmitrol)
  - Osmotic diuretic used to treat cerebral edema
  - Nursing Considerations
    - Monitor children receiving IV infusion to treat acute cerebral edema.
    - Insert an indwelling urinary catheter to monitor fluid status and renal function.
- Phenytoin (Dilantin) or fosphenytoin (Cerebyx)
  - Used to prevent or treat seizures that may occur
  - Nursing Considerations
    - Monitor therapeutic medication levels.
    - Check for medication interactions.
- Analgesics – Morphine sulfate and fentanyl citrate (Sublimaze)
  - Control pain and restlessness.
  - Nursing Considerations
    - Monitor children receiving opioids if the child is receiving ventilation.

- Interdisciplinary Care

  - Care for the child who has a head injury should include professionals from other disciplines as indicated. These may include physical, occupational, recreational and/or speech therapists.

  - Social services should be involved to provide links to social service agencies and schools.

  - Rehabilitation services may be needed if indicated.

- Surgical Interventions

  - Craniotomy

    - A craniotomy is removal of nonviable brain tissue that allows for expansion and/or removal of epidural or subdural hematomas. It involves drilling a burr hole or creating a bone flap to permit access to the affected area.

    - Nursing Actions

      - Initially, care will focus on the prevention of complications, maximizing cerebral function, and supporting other physiologic systems to include mechanical ventilation and parenteral nutrition.

      - Postoperative treatment will depend upon the neurologic status of the child after surgery.

- Care After Discharge

  o Client Education

    ▪ Instruct children to wear helmets when skateboarding, riding a bike or motorcycle, skiing, playing football, and participating in any other sport that may lead to head injury. Helmets that are appropriate for the sport should be worn.

    ▪ Remind children and adolescents to wear seat belts when driving or riding in a car.

    ▪ Encourage children and adolescents to avoid dangerous activities (riding a bicycle at night without a light, driving faster than the speed limit or while under the influence of alcohol or drugs).

- Client Outcomes

  o The child will experience minimal neurologic deficits.

  o The child will be able to perform ADLs independently or with assistive devices.

  o The child will be able to ambulate independently or with assistive devices.

Complications

- Increased ICP

  o Could lead to brain damage

  o Nursing Actions

    ▪ Monitor for signs of increased intracranial pressure.

      □ Infants – Bulging or tense fontanels, increased head circumference, high-pitched cry, distended scalp veins, irritability, bradycardia, and respiratory changes

      □ Children – Increased irritability, headache, nausea, vomiting, diplopia, seizures, bradycardia, and respiratory changes

    ▪ Provide interventions to reduce ICP (positioning, avoidance of coughing, straining, and bright lights, environmental stimuli).

APPLICATION EXERCISES

1. A nurse is caring for a child with photophobia. Which of the following should the nurse do to reduce sensitivity?

   A. Avoid using the television.

   B. Lower the volume of the child's portable CD player.

   C. Lower the room temperature.

   D. Keep the door to the closet open at night.

2. Match the following physical findings with the correct term.

_____	Nasal drainage making a yellow stain on white pillowcase	A. Kernig's sign
_____	Arms, wrists, and fingers flexed and bent inward onto chest, chest and legs extended and adducted	B. Brudzinski's sign
_____	Extremities flex when neck deliberately flexed	C. Decerebrate posture
_____	Backward arch of head and arms, legs rigid and extended, toes pointed downward	D. Halo sign
_____	Child resists when extending leg from flexed position	E. Decorticate posture

3. A nurse is caring for a 12-year-old child who is to have a lumbar puncture. Place the following steps in the correct order related to the procedure.

   _____ Monitor the puncture site for hematoma formation.

   _____ Have the child empty his bladder.

   _____ Administer prescribed oral sedative.

   _____ Place prescribed local anesthetic over puncture site.

   _____ Have the child remain flat for 4 to 6 hr.

   _____ Place the child in a sitting position.

4. A nurse in a clinic is caring for a child with suspected Reye syndrome. Which of the following questions should be asked of the parents when collecting data that will assist in confirming the diagnosis? (Select all that apply.)

   _____ Have you given your child ibuprofen?

   _____ Has your child had chickenpox recently?

   _____ Did your child receive aspirin in the last few days?

   _____ Does your child have a history of any recent upper respiratory infections?

   _____ Does your child drink adequate fluids?

5. The _____ is a rating system used to monitor a client who has sustained a head injury for signs of increasing intracranial pressure.

6. A nurse is caring for a toddler who has meningitis. Which of the following is the skin change that may be seen in bacterial meningitis?

  A. Discrete rose-pink macules or papules first appearing on the trunk, and then spreading outward.

  B. Red pinhead-sized lesions mostly in the skin folds which then scab over and slough in 5-7 days.

  C. Reddish-purple, non-raised, bruise-like areas that appear under the skin; may be pinpoint at first and then spread rapidly.

  D. Begins as a macule, becomes a papule, and finally a vesicle which is highly pruritic and then crusts over.

APPLICATION EXERCISES ANSWER KEY

1. A nurse is caring for a child with photophobia. Which of the following should the nurse do to reduce sensitivity?

   A. Avoid using the television.

   B. Lower the volume of the child's portable CD player.

   C. Lower the room temperature.

   D. Keep the door to the closet open at night.

   Photophobia is an abnormal sensitivity to light. Keeping the television off, closing window curtains, and using minimal lighting will decrease light exposure. Regulating the volume of sounds, lowering the room temperature, and keeping the closet door open at night will not affect light sensitivity.

    NCLEX® Connection: Reduction of Risk Potential, Potential for Alterations in Body Systems

2. Match the following physical findings with the correct term.

D	Nasal drainage making a yellow stain on white pillowcase	A. Kernig's sign
E	Arms, wrists, and fingers flexed and bent inward onto chest, chest and legs extended and adducted	B. Brudzinski's sign
A	Extremities flex when neck deliberately flexed	C. Decerebrate posture
C	Backward arch of head and arms, legs rigid and extended, toes pointed downward	D. Halo sign
B	Child resists when extending leg from flexed position	E. Decorticate posture

    NCLEX® Connection: Health Promotion and Maintenance, Data Collection Techniques

3. A nurse is caring for a 12-year-old child who is to have a lumbar puncture. Place the following steps in the correct order related to the procedure.

    6 Monitor the puncture site for hematoma formation.

    2 Have the child empty his bladder.

    3 Administer prescribed oral sedative.

    1 Place prescribed local anesthetic over puncture site.

    5 Have the child remain flat for 4 to 6 hr.

    4 Place the child in a sitting position.

    The local anesthetic is applied 60 min prior to the procedure. Have the child empty his bladder before giving a sedative to reduce the risk of injury. Give the oral sedative 30 min prior to the procedure to allow time for its effects. Place the child in a sitting position during the procedure and have him remain flat for 4 to 6 hr after the lumbar puncture. Monitor the puncture site for hematoma and infection.

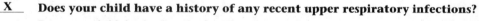 NCLEX® Connection: Reduction of Risk Potential, Diagnostic Tests

4. A nurse in a clinic is caring for a child with suspected Reye syndrome. Which of the following questions should be asked of the parents when collecting data that will assist in confirming the diagnosis? (Select all that apply.)

    _____ Have you given your child ibuprofen?

    X **Has your child had chickenpox recently?**

    X **Did your child receive aspirin in the last few days?**

    X **Does your child have a history of any recent upper respiratory infections?**

    _____ Does your child drink adequate fluids?

    The cause of Reye syndrome is unknown but there is an association with having taken aspirin for treatment of a viral infection. The symptoms most often appear at the end of a viral illness (upper respiratory infection, varicella) and peak incidence is during the months of January through March. There is no known association with ingesting ibuprofen and inadequate fluid intake.

NCLEX® Connection: Reduction of Risk Potential, Potential for Alterations in Body Systems

5. The **Glasgow Coma Scale** is a rating system used to monitor a client who has sustained a head injury for signs of increasing intracranial pressure.

   NCLEX® Connection: Reduction of Risk Potential, Diagnostic Tests

6. A nurse is caring for a toddler who has meningitis. Which of the following is the skin change that may be seen in bacterial meningitis?

   A. Discrete rose-pink macules or papules first appearing on the trunk, and then spreading outward.

   B. Red pinhead-sized lesions mostly in the skin folds which then scab over and slough in 5-7 days.

   C. Reddish-purple, non-raised, bruise-like areas that appear under the skin; may be pinpoint at first and then spread rapidly.

   D. Begins as a macule, becomes a papule, and finally a vesicle which is highly pruritic and then crusts over.

   Purpura and/or petechia are seen with meningococcal meningitis. This skin change is characterized as a reddish-purple, non-raised, bruise-like area that appears under the skin. It may begin as pinpoint areas which then spread rapidly. Roseola rash is characterized by rose-pink macules which spread. The rash of scarlet fever appears as pinhead-sized lesions mostly in skin folds which then slough. Chickenpox rash begins as macules, then papules and finally progresses to vesicles.

   NCLEX® Connection: Reduction of Risk Potential, Potential for Alterations in Body Systems

UNIT 2	NURSING CARE OF CHILDREN WITH SYSTEM DISORDERS
Section:	Neurosensory Disorders

Chapter 13   Seizures

Overview

- Seizures are abrupt, abnormal, excessive, and uncontrolled electrical discharges of neurons within the brain that may cause alterations in level of consciousness and/or changes in motor and sensory abilities and/or behavior. Seizures can be abrupt in nature or slow and insidious in onset.

- Epilepsy is the term used to define the medical disorder characterized by chronic, recurring abnormal brain electrical activity.

- The three major categories of seizures include generalized, partial (focal/local), and unclassified (idiopathic).

Data Collection

- Risk Factors

  - Genetic predisposition

  - Rapid increase or decrease in body temperature (acute febrile state), particularly among infants and children under the age of 2

  - Head trauma, cerebral edema, brain tumor

  - Abrupt cessation of antiepileptic medications (AEDs)

  - Infection, metabolic disorders, hypoxia, fluid and electrolyte imbalances

  - Exposure to toxins, such as lead and insecticides

  - Triggering factors

    - Increased physical activity

    - Excessive stress

    - Overwhelming fatigue

    - Acute alcohol ingestion

    - Exposure to flashing lights

    - Specific substances such as alcohol, caffeine, cocaine, aerosols, and glue products

- Subjective and Objective Data

  - Generalized seizures – Loss of consciousness occurs with involvement of both cerebral hemispheres

  - Tonic-clonic seizure – A 15- to 20-second episode of loss of consciousness, followed by a 1- to 2-min episode of rhythmic jerking of the extremities, and then a recovery period of several hr

    - It may begin with an aura (alteration in vision, smell, or emotional feeling).

    - Tonic phase – A 15- to 20-second episode of stiffening of muscles, loss of consciousness, cessation of breathing, dilated pupils and development of cyanosis.

    - Clonic phase – A 1- to 2-min episode of rhythmic jerking of the extremities, irregular respirations, biting of the cheek or tongue and bladder and bowel incontinence may occur.

    - Postictal phase – May last for several hr. Unconsciousness may last for 30 min at which time client awakens slowly and is usually confused and disoriented. Reports of headache, fatigue and muscle aches are not uncommon. Client may have no memory of what happened just before the seizure.

    - Absence seizure

      - The seizure consists of a loss of consciousness lasting a few seconds accompanied by blank staring (appears to be daydreaming) and associated automatisms (behaviors that clients are unaware of, such as lip-smacking or picking at clothes).

      - Baseline neurological function is resumed after seizures, with no apparent sequela.

      - Clients are often unaware seizure is occurring

  - Partial (focal/local)

    - Complex partial seizure

      - Complex partial seizures have associated automatisms (behaviors that children are unaware of, such as lip-smacking or picking at clothes).

      - The seizure can cause a loss of consciousness that lasts for several minutes.

      - Amnesia may occur immediately prior to and after the seizure.

    - Simple partial seizure

      - Consciousness is maintained throughout the event.

      - Seizure activity may consist of unusual sensations, a sense of déjà vu, autonomic abnormalities (changes in heart rate and abnormal flushing, unilateral abnormal extremity movements, pain, offensive smell).

  - Unclassified (idiopathic)

    - These seizures do not fit into other categories; they account for half of all seizure activity and occur for no known reason.

- ○ Laboratory Tests
  - ■ Laboratory tests should include alcohol and illicit drug levels and screens for the presence of excessive toxins, if suspected. In addition, cerebrospinal fluid may be obtained for analysis.
- ○ Diagnostic Procedures
  - ■ Electroencephalogram (EEG)
    - □ An EEG records electrical activity and may identify the origin of seizure activity.
    - □ Nursing Actions
      - ‣ Administer sedatives as prescribed.
      - ‣ Assist with positioning.
    - □ Client Education
      - ‣ Instruct children to avoid caffeine for 6 to 9 hr prior to the procedure.
      - ‣ Instruct children to wash hair before (no oils or sprays) and after (to remove electrode gel) the procedure.
      - ‣ Inform children that they may be asked to take deep breaths and/or be exposed to flashes of light during the procedure.
      - ‣ If prescribed, instruct parents to withhold sleep prior to test.
        - ▷ Inform children that they may be allowed to sleep during the test. Sleep may be withheld prior to test and may be induced during the test.
      - ‣ Inform children that the test will not be painful.
  - ■ MRI, CT, PET scans, and skull x-rays may all be used to identify or rule out potential causes of seizures.

Collaborative Care

- • Nursing Care
  - ○ During a seizure
    - ■ Protect children from injury (move furniture away, hold head in lap if on the floor).
    - ■ Position children to provide a patent airway.
    - ■ Be prepared to suction oral secretions.
    - ■ Turn children to the side (decreases risk of aspiration).
    - ■ Loosen restrictive clothing.
    - ■ Do not attempt to restrain children.
    - ■ Do not attempt to open the jaw or insert an airway during seizure activity (this may damage teeth, lips, or tongue). Do not use padded tongue blades.

- o Post seizure

  - Maintain children in a side-lying position to prevent aspiration and to facilitate drainage of oral secretions.

  - Check vital signs.

  - Check for injuries.

  - Perform neurologic checks.

  - Allow children to rest if necessary.

  - Reorient and calm children (they may be agitated or confused).

  - Institute seizure precautions, including placing the bed in the lowest position and padding the side rails to prevent future injury.

  - Encourage children to describe the period before, during, and after the seizure activity.

  - Determine if children experienced an aura, which may indicate the origin of seizure in the brain.

  - Try to determine the possible trigger, such as fatigue or stress.

  - Document onset and duration of seizure and client findings/observations prior to, during, and following the seizure (level of consciousness, apnea, cyanosis, motor activity, incontinence).

- Medications

  - o Antiepileptic drugs (AEDs) – Diazepam (Valium), phenytoin (Dilantin), carbamazepine (Tegretol), valproic acid (Depakene), gabapentin (Neurontin) and fosphenytoin sodium (Cerebyx)

    - Seizure control

    - Nursing Considerations

      - □ Monitor therapeutic serum medication levels.

    - Client Education

      - □ Advise children to take medications at the same time every day to enhance effectiveness.

      - □ Instruct clients to avoid taking any non-prescribed medications and to be aware of medication and food interactions that are specific to each medication.

- Interdisciplinary Care

  - o Social service agencies should be asked to assist with school support.

- Surgical Interventions

  o Vagal nerve stimulator

    ▪ This procedure is performed under general anesthesia.

    ▪ The device is implanted into the left chest wall. It is connected to an electrode that is placed at the left vagus nerve. The device is then programmed to administer intermittent vagal nerve stimulation at a rate specific to the child's needs.

    ▪ In addition to routine stimulation, children may initiate vagal nerve stimulation by holding a magnet over the implantable device at the onset of seizure activity. This will either abort the seizure or lessen its severity.

    ▪ Care after Discharge

      □ Educate children/family about the importance of periodic laboratory testing to monitor AED levels.

      □ Encourage medication adherence.

      □ Encourage children to wear a medical alert bracelet or necklace at all times.

- Client Outcomes

  o The child will experience a decreased incidence of seizures.

  o The child will be compliant with the medication regimen.

Complications

- Status Epilepticus

  o This is prolonged seizure activity occurring over a 30-min time frame. The complications associated with this condition are related to decreased oxygen levels, inability of the brain to return to normal functioning, and continued assault on neuronal tissue.

  o Nursing Actions

    ▪ Call for assistance.

    ▪ Maintain an airway, provide oxygen, and monitor pulse oximetry.

    ▪ Assist with emergency care as appropriate.

  o Client Education

    ▪ Provide support for the family.

Ⓐ **APPLICATION EXERCISES**

1. A teacher is talking to the school nurse about a student in her classroom. The teacher states, "He stares at the top of his desk, taps his pencil loudly and rhythmically, but when I call on him he usually responds. When I talk to him about his behavior, he doesn't remember doing this. I'm wondering if he's seeking attention." The nurse suspects the child is experiencing

   A. a tonic-clonic seizure.

   B. an absence seizure.

   C. a complex partial seizure.

   D. a simple partial seizure.

2. Which of the following is the priority intervention a nurse should take when caring for a child who just experienced a generalized seizure?

   A. Keep the child in a side-lying position.

   B. Take the child's vital signs.

   C. Reorient the child by calling his name.

   D. Check the child for injuries.

3. A mother brings her 12-year-old son who has a seizure disorder to the clinic because of increasing seizure activity. She states, "I don't understand what is going on. Every time he plays with his model-building kits, he has a seizure." What data should the nurse collect?

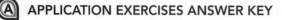

APPLICATION EXERCISES ANSWER KEY

1. A teacher is talking to the school nurse about a student in her classroom. The teacher states, "He stares at the top of his desk, taps his pencil loudly and rhythmically, but when I call on him he usually responds. When I talk to him about his behavior, he doesn't remember doing this. I'm wondering if he's seeking attention." The nurse suspects the child is experiencing

   A. a tonic-clonic seizure.

   B. an absence seizure.

   C. a complex partial seizure.

   D. a simple partial seizure.

   An absence seizure is characterized by a loss of consciousness for a few seconds with blank staring and an associated automatic behavior, such as pencil-tapping. The client is unaware of the seizure activity. A tonic-clonic seizure has tonic, clonic, and post-ictal phases and is characterized by a 15- to 20-second episode of loss of consciousness, followed by a 1- to 2-min episode of rhythmic jerking of the extremities, and then a recovery period of several hours. A complex partial seizure lasts for several minutes and may result in loss of consciousness. A simple partial seizure does not involve a loss of consciousness.

   NCLEX® Connection: Reduction of Risk Potential, Potential for Alterations in Body Systems

2. Which of the following is the priority intervention a nurse should take when caring for a child who just experienced a generalized seizure?

   A. Keep the child in a side-lying position.

   B. Take the child's vital signs.

   C. Reorient the child by calling his name.

   D. Check the child for injuries.

   The greatest risk to the child is injury from aspiration. The priority intervention during the postictal phase is to keep the child in a side-lying position so secretions can drain from the mouth. The other interventions are important, but are not the priority at this time.

   NCLEX® Connection: Physiological Adaptation, Medical Emergencies

3. A mother brings her 12-year-old son who has a seizure disorder to the clinic because of increasing seizure activity. She states, "I don't understand what is going on. Every time he plays with his model-building kits, he has a seizure." What data should the nurse collect?

   The nurse should ask about triggers that might provoke a seizure, in this case the use of glue products or aerosol paint spray in building models or other specific substances. Possible triggers include significant stress, excessive physical activity, feeling overly fatigued, exposure to flashing lights, or the possibility of alcohol ingestion.

   NCLEX® Connection: Health Promotion and Maintenance, Data Collection Techniques

Overview

- Sensory impairments in children most commonly affect the eyes and ears. Adequate vision and hearing is necessary for normal growth and development. Therefore, it is important to identify any impairment early in life.

VISUAL IMPAIRMENTS

Overview

- Common types of visual impairment in children include strabismus (misalignment of eyes), refractive errors (nearsightedness, farsightedness, astigmatism), and amblyopia (decreased acuity in one eye).

- Children may also experience cataracts and glaucoma.

Data Collection

- Risk Factors

  o Visual impairment may result from prenatal or postnatal infections, retinopathy of prematurity, trauma, or chronic illnesses (such as sickle cell anemia or juvenile rheumatoid arthritis).

- Subjective and Objective Data

  o Visual screening using age-appropriate tools (E Snellen chart used for children who cannot read, alphabet Snellen chart used for children who can read)

  o Visual acuity of 20/70 to 20/200 is considered partially sighted.

  o Visual acuity of 20/200 or less and/or a visual field of 20° or less in the better eye is considered legal blindness, which has legal implications for the child's care.

VISUAL IMPAIRMENT	SIGNS AND SYMPTOMS
Myopia (nearsightedness)	• Sees close objects clearly, but not objects in the distance • Headaches and dizziness • Eye rubbing • Difficulty reading • Clumsiness (frequently walking into objects) • Poor school performance
Hyperopia (farsightedness)	• Sees distant objects clearly, but not objects that are close • Normal vision until about age 7 • Children are usually able to accommodate.
Astigmatism	• Uneven vision in which only parts of letters on a page may be seen • Headache and vertigo • The appearance of normal vision because tilting the head enables all letters to be seen
Strabismus	• Misaligned eyes • Frowning or squinting • Difficulty seeing print clearly • One eye closed to enable better vision • Head tilted to one side • Headache, dizziness, diplopia, photophobia, and crossed eyes
Amblyopia (lazy eye)	• Reduced visual acuity in one eye

Collaborative Care

- Nursing Care

    o Maintain normal to bright lighting for children when reading, writing, or participating in any activity that requires close vision.

    o Identify safety hazards.

    o Inform children and families about corrective measures.

      ▪ Myopia may be corrected with biconcave lenses that help focus light rays on the retina.

      ▪ Hyperopia may be corrected using convex lenses that help focus light rays on the retina.

      ▪ Astigmatism may be corrected with a special lens to correct refractive errors.

      ▪ Strabismus may be corrected with eye exercises or patching of the strong eye.

- Surgical Interventions

    o Surgical repair of strabismus

      ▪ Increases visual stimulation to the weaker eye

- Care After Discharge

  - Client Education

    - Encourage the family to work with the child's school to meet educational needs.

- Client Outcomes

  - The child will maintain visual acuity.

  - The child will be free of injury.

HEARING IMPAIRMENTS

Overview

- Hearing impairments affect the ability to clearly process linguistic sounds and impact speech.

Data Collection

- Risk Factors

  - Hearing defects may be caused by a variety of conditions, including anatomic malformation, maternal ingestion of toxic substances during pregnancy, perinatal asphyxia, perinatal infection, chronic ear infection, and/or ototoxic medications.

  - Hearing defects are associated with chronic conditions such as Down syndrome and/or cerebral palsy.

    - Conductive losses involve interference of sound transmission, which may result from otitis media, external ear infection, foreign bodies or excessive earwax.

    - Sensorineural losses involve interference of the transmission along the nerve pathways, which may result from congenital defects or secondary to acquired conditions (infection, ototoxic medication, exposure to constant noise – as in an NICU).

    - Central auditory imperception involves all other hearing losses (aphasia, agnosia [inability to interpret sounds]).

- Subjective and Objective Data

  - Infants

    - Lack of startle reflex

    - Failure to respond to noise

    - Absence of vocalization

    - Delayed verbal development

- o Older children

  - Speaking in monotone

  - Need for repeated conversation

  - Speaking loudly for situation

Collaborative Care

- Nursing Care

  - o Use an interpreter when working with children who are hearing impaired. Always remember to talk to children, not the interpreter.

  - o Observe gait/balance for instability.

  - o Adjust environment for physiologic symptoms.

  - o Identify safety hazards.

  - o Encourage use of a hearing aid for conductive loss.

- Care After Discharge

  - o Client Education

    - Help families identify community resources for children who are hearing impaired.

    - Encourage parents to learn strategies to communicate with their children.

    - Encourage parents to work with the child's school to assist with meeting educational needs.

    - Teach children and families to avoid further damage and hearing loss.

    - Encourage children to avoid exposure to hazardous noise.

    - Encourage children to wear ear protection if loud environmental noise cannot be avoided.

- Client Outcomes

  - o The child will learn strategies to communicate effectively.

  - o The child will remain free of injury.

Complications

- Delayed growth and development

  - o Visual and hearing impairments may prevent children from appropriate speech and motor development. Identifying the impairment early may minimize this.

  - o Nursing Actions

    - Encourage self-care and optimal independence.

  - o Client Education

    - Assist families to obtain and access appropriate assistive devices.

Ⓐ APPLICATION EXERCISES

1. A school health nurse is performing a vision screening clinic for kindergarten children. Explain why the nurse should use the E Snellen chart to assess vision in kindergarten children.

2. A nurse observes a group of children in the play area of a pediatric clinic waiting room and focuses on one particular child. Which of the following findings indicates to the nurse that this child might have myopia?

    A. Squinting when looking across the room

    B. Closes one eye to read.

    C. Turns head to one side when playing with toys

    D. Holds book at an extended distance when turning pages

3. Which of the following data noted in a health history might alert the nurse that an infant is at risk for impaired hearing? (Select all that apply.)

    _____ Nuchal cord present at birth.

    _____ Maternal herpes lesions present at 7 months gestation

    _____ Infant placed on soy formula due to lactose intolerance

    _____ Positive Babinski reflex noted at 2 month well-baby check

    _____ Large for gestational age at birth

4. A foreign object in the ear canal or impacted cerumen could be a possible cause of _____.

5. A newborn who received large doses of ototoxic medications is at risk for _____.

(A) **APPLICATION EXERCISES ANSWER KEY**

1. A school health nurse is performing a vision screening clinic for kindergarten children. Explain why the nurse should use the E Snellen chart to assess vision in kindergarten children.

   A kindergarten student may not be able to distinguish the letters of the alphabet yet. They should be able to distinguish directions by pointing after brief instructions from the nurse.

(N) NCLEX® Connection: Health Promotion and Maintenance, Data Collection Techniques

2. A nurse observes a group of children in the play area of a pediatric clinic waiting room and focuses on one particular child. Which of the following findings indicates to the nurse that this child might have myopia?

   A. Squinting when looking across the room
   B. Closes one eye to read.
   C. Turns head to one side when playing with toys
   D. Holds book at an extended distance when turning pages

   Myopia or nearsightedness involves difficulty seeing objects in the distance. A child might squint in an attempt to focus when looking across the room. A child who has strabismus may close one eye to read better or turn his head to the side to improve vision. A child who has hyperopia may hold a book at a distance to improve vision.

(N) NCLEX® Connection: Reduction of Risk Potential, System Specific Assessment

3. Which of the following data noted in a health history might alert the nurse that an infant is at risk for impaired hearing? (Select all that apply.)

   __X__ **Nuchal cord present at birth.**
   __X__ **Maternal herpes lesions present at 7 months gestation**
   _____ Infant placed on soy formula due to lactose intolerance
   _____ Positive Babinski reflex noted at 2 month well-baby check
   _____ Large for gestational age at birth

   Hypoxia at birth due to nuchal cord and perinatal herpes infection are risk factors for hearing loss. Lactose intolerance and an LGA infant are not risk factors associated with hearing loss. A positive Babinski in an infant is a normal reflex response.

(N) NCLEX® Connection: Physiological Adaptations, Basic Pathophysiology

4. A foreign object in the ear canal or impacted cerumen could be a possible cause of **conductive hearing loss.**

   Conductive hearing loss involves the interference in sound transmission due to blockage of the ear canal. This would occur with a foreign object, excessive earwax, otitis media, or an external ear infection.

(N) NCLEX® Connection: Physiological Adaptations, Basic Pathophysiology

5. A newborn who received large doses of ototoxic medications is at risk for **sensorineural hearing loss.**

> Sensorineural hearing loss involves interference in sound wave transmission along the nerve pathways. Causes may be primary due to a congenital defect or secondary due to exposure to ototoxic medications, infection, an acquired condition, or exposure to high-decibel noises that occur to the neonate in the NICU.

 NCLEX® Connection: Pharmacological Therapies, Adverse Effects/Contraindications/Side Effects/Interactions

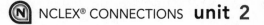

UNIT 2: NURSING CARE OF CHILDREN WITH SYSTEM DISORDERS

Section: Respiratory Disorders

- Oxygen and Inhalation Therapy

- Acute and Infectious Respiratory Illnesses

- Asthma

- Cystic Fibrosis

NCLEX® CONNECTIONS

When reviewing the chapters in this section, keep in mind the relevant sections of the NCLEX® outline, in particular:

CLIENT NEEDS: SAFETY AND INFECTION CONTROL

Relevant topics/tasks include:
- Standard Precautions/ Transmission-Based Precautions/Surgical Asepsis
  - Reinforce appropriate infection control procedures with client and staff members.

CLIENT NEEDS: REDUCTION OF RISK POTENTIAL

Relevant topics/tasks include:
- Diagnostic Tests
  - Perform diagnostic testing.
- Laboratory Values
  - Identify laboratory values for ABGs, BUN, cholesterol, glucose, hematocrit, hemoglobin, glycosylated hemoglobin, platelets, potassium, sodium, WBC, creatinine, PT, PTT, and APTT.
- Potential for Complications of DiagnosticTests/ Treatments/Procedures
  - Evaluate client respiratory status by measuring oxygen (O_2) saturation.

CLIENT NEEDS: PHYSIOLOGICAL ADAPTATION

Relevant topics/tasks include:
- Alterations in Body Systems
  - Identify signs and symptoms of an infection.
- Basic Pathophysiology
  - Consider general principles of client disease process when providing care.
- Medical Emergencies
  - Reinforce teaching of emergency intervention explanations to client.

UNIT 2	NURSING CARE OF CHILDREN WITH SYSTEM DISORDERS
Section:	Respiratory Disorders
Chapter 15	**Oxygen and Inhalation Therapy**

Overview

- Oxygen is used to maintain adequate cellular oxygenation. It is used in the treatment of many acute and chronic respiratory problems (hypoxemia, cystic fibrosis, asthma). Supplemental oxygen may be delivered using a variety of methods, depending on individual circumstances.

- Pulse oximetry is used to monitor the effectiveness of inhalation therapies.

- Common treatment methods for children with respiratory issues (acute or chronic)

    o Nebulized aerosol therapy

    o Metered-dose inhaler (MDI) or dry powder inhaler (DPI)

    o Chest physiotherapy (CPT)

    o Oxygen therapy

    o Suctioning

    o Artificial airways

Pulse Oximetry

- This is a noninvasive measurement of the oxygen saturation of the blood.

- A pulse oximeter is a device that is operated by a battery or electricity and has a sensor probe that is attached securely to the child's fingertip, toe, bridge of nose, earlobe, or forehead with a clip or band.

- A pulse oximeter measures arterial oxygen saturation (SaO_2) via a wave of infrared light that measures light absorption by oxygenated and deoxygenated hemoglobin in arterial blood. SaO_2 and SpO_2 are used interchangeably.

- Indications

    o Pulse oximetry is used for a variety of situations in which quick assessments of a child's respiratory status are needed.

- ○ Client Presentation
  - ▪ Children who present with the following signs and symptoms will benefit from pulse oximetry:
    - ☐ Increased work of breathing
    - ☐ Wheezing
    - ☐ Coughing
    - ☐ Cyanosis

- • Interpretation of Findings
  - ○ The expected reference range for SaO_2 is 95% to 100%. Acceptable levels may range from 91% to 100%. Some illnesses may allow for an SaO_2 of 85% to 89%.
  - ○ Results less than 91% require nursing intervention to assist the child to regain normal SaO_2 levels. An SaO_2 of less than 86% is a life-threatening emergency. The lower the SaO_2 level, the less accurate the value.

- • Preprocedure
  - ○ Nursing Actions
    - ▪ Perform hand hygiene and provide privacy.
    - ▪ Find an appropriate probe site. The probe site must be dry and have adequate circulation.
    - ▪ Be sure the child is in a comfortable position and that the arm is supported if a finger is used as a probe site.

- • Intraprocedure
  - ○ Nursing Actions
    - ▪ Apply the sensor probe to the site.
    - ▪ Press the power switch on the oximeter.
    - ▪ Note the pulse reading and compare it with the child's radial pulse. Any discrepancy warrants further data collection.
    - ▪ Allow time for the readout to stabilize, then record the value as the oxygen saturation.
    - ▪ Remove the probe, turn off the oximeter, and store it appropriately.
    - ▪ If continuous monitoring is required, make sure the alarms are set for a low and a high limit, the alarms are functioning, and the sound is audible. Check the condition of the skin when changing the placement of the probe every 3 to 4 hr. Change the placement of the probe more frequently for children with poor perfusion or sensitive skin.

- Postprocedure
  - Nursing Actions
    - Document the findings and report abnormal findings to the provider.
    - If a child's SaO_2 is less than 90% (indicating hypoxemia):
      - Confirm that the sensor probe is properly placed.
      - Confirm that the oxygen delivery system is functioning and that the child is receiving prescribed oxygen levels.
      - Place the child in a semi-Fowler's or Fowler's position to maximize ventilation.
      - Encourage deep breathing.
      - Report significant findings to the provider.
      - Remain with the child and provide emotional support to decrease anxiety.

Nebulized Aerosol Therapy

- The process of nebulization breaks up medications (bronchodilators, mucolytic agents) into minute particles that are then dispersed throughout the respiratory tract. These droplets are much finer than those created by inhalers.
  - Medication may be given through a hand-held nebulizer that is held by the child. The hand-held nebulizer is a small machine that changes a medication solution into a mist.
- Indications
  - Diagnoses
    - Respiratory conditions that necessitate bronchodilators or corticosteroids
- Client Outcomes
  - The child will maintain a patent airway.
  - The child will maintain an oxygen saturation of 95% to 100%
- Nursing Actions
  - Preparation of the Client
    - Inform the child and family that the treatment may take 10 to 15 min.
    - Determine if the child is able to hold the mouthpiece or if a mask should be used.
    - Perform a preprocedure evaluation, including vital signs.
    - Pour the medication into the small container, and attach the device to an air or oxygen source.
  - Ongoing Care
    - Encourage the child to take slow, deep breaths through an open mouth.
    - Monitor the child during the treatment.

- - Obtain vital signs, oxygen saturation, and lung sounds at the completion of treatment.
  - Inform the family that a portable device may be rented for home use.
- Complications
  - Tachycardia
    - Nursing Actions
      - Check the client's vital signs.
      - Stop the medication.
    - Client Education
      - Inform the parents that the child may experience jitteriness or an increased heart rate during the treatment.

Metered-Dose Inhaler (MDI) or Dry Powder Inhaler (DPI)

- These are hand-held devices that allow children to self-administer medications on an intermittent basis.
- Indications
  - Diagnoses
    - Respiratory conditions that necessitate bronchodilators or corticosteroids
- Client Outcomes
  - The child will maintain a patent airway.
  - The child will maintain an oxygen saturation of 95% to 100%
- Nursing Actions
  - Provide instructions to the child and parents for use of an MDI.

 View Media Supplement: Metered-Dose Inhaler (Animation)

- - Remove the cap from the inhaler.
  - Shake the inhaler five to six times.
  - Hold the inhaler with the mouthpiece at the bottom.
  - Hold the inhaler with the thumb near the mouthpiece and the index and middle fingers at the top.
  - Hold the inhaler approximately 2 to 4 cm (1 to 2 in) away from the front of the mouth.
  - Take a deep breath and then exhale.

- Tilt the head back slightly, and press the inhaler. While pressing the inhaler, begin a slow, deep breath that lasts for 3 to 5 seconds to facilitate delivery to the air passages.

- Hold the breath for 10 seconds to allow the medication to deposit in the airways.

- Take the inhaler out of the mouth and slowly exhale through pursed lips.

- Resume normal breathing.

  o Instruct the child to use a spacer to keep the medication in the device longer, thereby increasing the amount of medication delivered to the lungs and decreasing the amount of the medication in the oropharynx.

  - If a spacer is used, instruct the child to:

    □ Remove the covers from the mouthpieces of the inhaler and of the spacer

    □ Insert the MDI into the end of the spacer.

    □ Shake the inhaler five to six times.

    □ Exhale completely and then close the mouth around the spacer mouthpiece

    □ Continue as with an MDI.

  o Provide instructions to the child and parents for the use of a DPI.

  - Do not shake the device.

  - Take the cover off the mouthpiece.

  - Follow the directions of the manufacturer, such as turning the wheel of the inhaler, for preparing the medication.

  - Exhale completely.

  - Place the mouthpiece between the lips, and take a deep breath through the mouth.

  - Hold breath for 5 to 10 seconds.

  - Take the inhaler out of the mouth, and slowly exhale through pursed lips.

  - Resume normal breathing.

  o If more than one puff is prescribed, instruct the child to wait the length of time directed before administering the second puff.

  o Instruct the child to remove the canister and rinse the inhaler, cap, and spacer once a day with warm running water. Instruct the child to dry the inhaler before using it again.

- Complications

  o Fungal infections

  - Fungal infections of the oral cavity may occur with corticosteroid use.

  - Nursing Actions

    □ Administer cool liquids.

- Client Education
  - Instruct the child and parents to clean the MDI and spacer after each use and to have the child rinse his mouth and gargle with warm water after administration.

Chest Physiotherapy (CPT)

- Chest physiotherapy is the use of a set of techniques that include percussion, vibration, and postural drainage. Gravity and positioning loosen respiratory secretions and move them into the central airways where they can be removed by coughing or suctioning to promote removal of excessive secretions from specific areas of the lungs.

- Indications
  - Client Presentation
    - Thick secretions with an inability to clear the airway
    - Contraindication – Decreased cardiac reserves, pulmonary embolism, or increased intracranial pressure

- Client Outcomes
  - The child will maintain a patent airway.
  - The child will maintain an oxygen saturation of 95% to 100%.

- Preprocedure
  - Nursing Actions
    - Schedule treatments 1 hr before meals or 2 hr after meals and at bedtime to decrease the likelihood of vomiting or aspirating.
    - Administer a bronchodilator medication or nebulizer treatment 30 min to 1 hr prior to postural drainage if prescribed.
    - Offer the child an emesis basin and facial tissues

- Intraprocedure
  - Nursing Actions
    - Perform hand hygiene, provide privacy, and explain the procedure to the child and parents.
    - Ensure proper positioning of the child to promote drainage of specific areas of the lungs.
      - Apical sections of the upper lobes – Fowler's position
      - Posterior sections of the upper lobes – Side-lying position
      - Right lobe – On the left side with a pillow under the chest wall
      - Left lobe – Trendelenburg position

- Apply manual percussion by using cupped hand or a special device to clap rhythmically on the chest wall to break up secretions.

- Place hands on the affected area, tense hand and arm muscles, and move the heel of the hands to create vibrations as the child exhales to help remove secretions. Have the client cough after each set of vibrations.

- Have the child remain in each postural drainage position for 10 to 15 min to allow time for percussion, vibration, and postural drainage.

- Discontinue the procedure if the child reports faintness or dizziness.

- Postprocedure

  - Nursing Actions

    - Perform lung auscultation, and check the amount, color, and character of the expectorated secretions.

    - Document interventions, and repeat the procedure as prescribed (typically 2 to 3 times per day).

- Complications

  - Hypoxia

    - Decrease in SaO_2

    - Nursing Actions

      - Monitor respiratory status during the procedure.

      - Discontinue the procedure if the child experiences dyspnea.

Oxygen Therapy

- Oxygen therapy increases the oxygen concentration of the air that is being breathed.

  - Humidification of oxygen will moisten the airways, which promotes loosening and mobilization of pulmonary secretions and prevents drying and injury of respiratory structures.

- Indications

  - Diagnoses

    - Hypoxemia

      - Hypoxemia develops when there is an inadequate level of oxygen in the blood. Hypovolemia, hypoventilation, and interruption of arterial flow can lead to hypoxemia.

EARLY SIGNS	LATE SIGNS
• Tachypnea • Tachycardia • Restlessness • Pallor of the skin and mucous membranes • Elevated blood pressure • Symptoms of respiratory distress (use of accessory muscles, nasal flaring, tracheal tugging, adventitious lung sounds)	• Confusion and stupor • Cyanosis of skin and mucous membranes • Bradypnea • Bradycardia • Hypotension • Cardiac dysrhythmias

- Client Outcomes

  - The child will maintain a patent airway.

  - The child will maintain an SaO_2 of 95% to 100%.

- Nursing Actions

  - Preparation of the Client

    - Warm oxygen to prevent hypothermia.

    - Use a calm, nonthreatening approach.

    - Explain all procedures to the child and parents.

    - Place the child in a semi-Fowler's or Fowler's position to facilitate breathing and to promote chest expansion.

    - Ensure that all equipment is working properly.

  - Ongoing Care

    - Provide oxygen therapy at the lowest liter flow that will correct hypoxemia.

    - Monitor lung sounds and respiratory rate, rhythm, and effort to determine the child's need for supplemental oxygen.

      - Signs and symptoms of hypoxemia are shortness of breath, anxiety, tachypnea, tachycardia, restlessness, pallor or cyanosis of skin and/or mucous membranes, adventitious breath sounds, and confusion.

      - Signs and symptoms of hypercarbia (elevated levels of CO_2) are restlessness, hypertension, and headache.

    - Do not allow oxygen to blow directly onto the faces of infants.

    - Change linens and clothing frequently.

    - Monitor temperature for hypothermia.

    - Avoid placing toys that could induce sparks in the tent.

    - Monitor oxygenation status with pulse oximetry and arterial blood gases (ABGs).

    - Apply the oxygen delivery device prescribed.

- Promote good oral hygiene, and provide as needed.
- Promote turning, coughing, deep breathing, and use of incentive spirometry and suctioning.
- Promote rest, and decrease environmental stimuli.
- Provide emotional support to the child who appears anxious.
- Monitor nutritional status, and provide supplements as prescribed.
- Monitor the child's skin integrity. Provide moisture and pressure-relief devices as indicated.
- Monitor and document the child's response to oxygen therapy.
- Maintain oxygen flow as prescribed.
- Discontinue oxygen gradually.

DELIVERY SYSTEM	NURSING IMPLICATIONS
Oxygen hood – Small plastic hood that fits over the infant's head	• Use a minimum flow rate of 4 to 5 L/min to prevent carbon dioxide buildup. • Ensure that the child's neck, chin, or shoulders do not rub against the hood. • Secure a pulse oximeter to the child for continuous SaO_2 monitoring.

Oxygen tent – Large plastic tent that fits over the crib or bed and can provide oxygen and humidity if prescribed	• Use for children older than 2 to 3 months.
	• Set the tent on a high flow rate to flood the tent with oxygen. Then, adjust flow meter to the desired amount prior to placing children into the tent. Repeat if the tent has been opened for an extended period of time.
	• Attempt to maintain an oxygen level greater than 30% to 50% FiO_2.
	   o Keep the tent around the perimeter of the bed.
	   o Plan care to minimize how often the tent is opened.
	• Monitor the temperature inside the tent to ensure that it is appropriate.
	• Use plastic or vinyl toys, avoiding soft toys and toys that are mechanical or electrical.
	• Keep children warm and dry.

DELIVERY SYSTEM	NURSING IMPLICATIONS
Nasal cannula – Disposable plastic tube with two prongs for insertion into the nostrils that delivers an oxygen concentration of 24% to 40% FiO$_2$ at a flow rate of 1 to 6 L/min	• Safe, easy to apply, and well tolerated. • Use so children are able to eat, talk, and ambulate while receiving oxygen. • Use for infants and older children who are cooperative. • Check the patency of the nares. • Ensure that the prongs fit in the nares properly. • Monitor for skin breakdown and dry mucous membranes. • Supply children with a water-soluble gel if the nares are dry. • Provide humidification for flow rates greater than 4 L/min. • Monitor the children frequently for dislodged nasal cannula prongs.
Pediatric face mask – Pediatric-size mask that covers the child's nose and mouth	• Face masks are not tolerated well by children. • Explain the procedure to gain cooperation from older children.

- Complications
    - Combustion
        - Oxygen is combustible.
        - Nursing Actions
            - Place "No Smoking" or "Oxygen in Use" signs to alert others of the fire hazard.
            - Know where the closest fire extinguisher is located.
            - Have children wear a cotton gown, because synthetics or wools may create sparks of static electricity.
            - Ensure that all electric devices (razors and heating pads) are in working condition.
            - Ensure that all electric machinery (monitors, suction machines) are well grounded.
            - Avoid toys that may induce a spark.
            - Do not use volatile, flammable materials (alcohol, acetone) near children who are receiving oxygen.
        - Client Education
            - Educate children and others about the fire hazards of smoking with oxygen use.

- ○ Oxygen toxicity
  - ▪ Oxygen toxicity may result from high concentrations of oxygen (typically 50%), long duration of oxygen therapy (typically greater than 24 to 48 hr), and the child's degree of lung disease.
    - ▢ Signs and symptoms include a nonproductive cough, substernal pain, nasal stuffiness, nausea and vomiting, fatigue, headache, sore throat, and hypoventilation.
  - ▪ Nursing Actions
    - ▢ Use the lowest level of oxygen necessary to maintain an adequate SaO_2.
    - ▢ Monitor ABGs, and notify the provider if SaO_2 levels rise outside of the expected reference range.
    - ▢ Use an oxygen mask with continuous positive airway pressure (CPAP), bilevel positive airway pressure (BiPAP), or positive end-expiratory pressure (PEEP) while a child is on a mechanical ventilator to decrease the amount of oxygen needed.
    - ▢ Decrease the amount of oxygen gradually.

Suctioning

- • Suctioning can be accomplished orally, nasally, or endotracheally.
- • Indications
  - ○ Diagnosis
    - ▪ Hypoxemia
  - ○ Client Presentation
    - ▪ Early signs of hypoxemia (restlessness, tachypnea, tachycardia, decreased SaO_2 levels, adventitious breath sounds, visualization of secretions, cyanosis, absence of spontaneous cough)
- • Client Outcomes
  - ○ The child will maintain a patent airway.
  - ○ The child will maintain an SaO_2 of 95% to 100%.
- • Endotracheal suctioning (ETS)
  - ○ Preprocedure
    - ▪ Nursing Actions
      - ▢ Perform hand hygiene, provide privacy, and explain the procedure to the child.
      - ▢ Don the required personal protective equipment.
      - ▢ Assist the child to a high-Fowler's or Fowler's position for suctioning if possible.

- □ Perform ETS through a tracheostomy or an endotracheal tube. Obtain a suction catheter with an outer diameter of no more than 1 cm (0.5 in) of the internal diameter of the endotracheal tube.

- □ Ask for assistance if necessary.

- □ Hyperoxygenate the child using a bag-valve-mask (BVM) resuscitator or specialized ventilator function with an FiO_2 of 100%.

- □ Obtain baseline breath sounds and vital signs, including oxygen saturation (SaO_2) by pulse oximeter. Oxygen saturation may be monitored continually during the procedure.

- ○ Intraprocedure

  - ■ Nursing Actions

    - □ Open the sterile suction package using surgical aseptic technique.

    - □ Place the sterile drape or towel on the child's chest.

    - □ Set up the container, touching only the outside.

    - □ Pour approximately 100 mL of sterile water or 0.9% sodium chloride (NaCl) into the container.

    - □ Don sterile gloves.

      - ▸ Use the clean/nondominant hand to hold the connecting tube; this glove protects the nurse.

      - ▸ Use the sterile/dominant hand to hold the sterile catheter; this glove protects the child.

    - □ Connect the suction catheter to the wall unit's tubing.

    - □ Set the suction pressure to no higher than 110 mm Hg for children, and 95 mm Hg for infants. Use the lowest amount of pressure possible.

    - □ Test the suction setup by aspirating sterile water/0.9% NaCl solution from the cup. If the unit is operating properly, continue with the procedure.

    - □ Insert the catheter into the lumen of the airway. First remove the bag or ventilator from tracheostomy or endotracheal tube if necessary). Advance the catheter until resistance is met. The catheter should reach the level of the carina (location of bifurcation into the mainstem bronchi).

    - □ Pull the catheter back 0.5 cm (0.2 in) prior to applying suction to prevent mucosal damage.

    - □ Apply suction intermittently by covering and releasing the suction port with the thumb for 5 seconds at a time.

    - □ Apply suction only while withdrawing the catheter and rotating it with the thumb and forefinger.

    - □ Limit each suction attempt to no longer than 5 seconds to avoid hypoxemia and the vagal response. Limit suctioning to two to three attempts.

- □ Reattach the BVM or ventilator and supply the child with 100% inspired oxygen.

- □ Clear the catheter and tubing.

- □ Allow time, usually 30 to 60 seconds, for the child to recover between sessions.

- □ Repeat as necessary.

- □ Once suctioning is complete, clear the suction tubing by aspirating sterile water/0.9% NaCl solution.

  - o Postprocedure

    - ■ Nursing Actions

      - □ Document the child's response.

- Complications

  - o Hypoxia

    - ■ A decrease in SaO_2 or cyanosis

    - ■ Nursing Actions

      - □ Stop the procedure.

      - □ Limit each suction attempt to no longer than 10 to 15 seconds.

      - □ Limit suctioning to two to three attempts.

      - □ Allow the child 30 to 60 seconds for recovery between suction passes.

      - □ Hyperoxygenate children before and after each suctioning pass.

Artificial Airways

- A tracheotomy is a sterile surgical incision into the trachea through the skin and muscles for the purpose of establishing an airway.

- A tracheotomy can be performed as an emergency procedure or as a scheduled surgical procedure.

- A tracheostomy is the stoma/opening that results from a tracheotomy to provide and secure a patent airway. A tracheostomy can be permanent or temporary.

- Artificial airways can be placed orotracheally, nasotracheally, or through a tracheostomy to assist with respiration.

  - o Pediatric tracheostomy tubes made of plastic have a more acute angle than adult tubes. Pediatric tracheostomy tubes soften with body temperature to shape to the contour of the child's trachea. No inner cannula is necessary, because this material resists the accumulation of dried secretions.

  - o Pediatric tubes made of metal have an inner cannula. These tubes have a decreased risk of causing an allergic reaction.

- Indications

  - Client Presentation

    - Indications for artificial airways include artificial ventilation and obstruction of the upper airway.

- Client Outcomes

  - The child will maintain a patent airway.

  - The child will maintain an oxygen saturation of 95% to 100%.

- Nursing Actions

  - Preparation of the Client

    - Use an uncuffed endotracheal tube for children younger than 8 years of age.

    - Explain the procedure.

    - Place child in semi-Fowler's or Fowler's position.

    - Keep the following at the child's bedside: two extra tracheostomy tubes (one that is the child's size and one that is a size smaller, in case of accidental decannulation), the obturator for the existing tube, an oxygen source, suction catheters and a suction source, and a manual resuscitation bag.

    - Provide the child with methods to communicate with staff (paper and pen, dry-erase board).

  - Ongoing Care

    - Monitor

      - Oxygenation, ventilation (respiratory rate, effort, SaO_2), and vital signs hourly

      - Thickness, quantity, odor, and color of mucous secretions

      - The stoma and the skin surrounding the stoma for signs of inflammation or infection (redness, swelling, or drainage)

    - Provide adequate humidification and hydration to thin secretions and decrease the risk of mucus plugging.

    - Do not suction routinely, because this may cause mucosal damage, bleeding, and bronchospasm.

    - Monitor the need for suctioning. Suction on a PRN basis when findings indicate the need to do so (audible/noisy secretions, crackles, restlessness, tachypnea, tachycardia, and mucus in the airway).

    - Maintain surgical aseptic technique when suctioning to prevent infection.

    - Provide emotional support to the child and parents.

    - Give frequent oral care, usually every 2 hr.

    - For cuffed tubes, keep the pressure below 20 mm Hg to reduce the risk of tracheal necrosis due to prolonged compression of tracheal capillaries.

- Provide tracheostomy care every 8 hr.
  - If necessary, suction the tracheostomy tube using sterile suctioning supplies.
  - Remove old dressings and excess secretions.
  - Apply the oxygen source loosely if the child's oxygen saturation level decreases during the procedure.
  - Use cotton-tipped applicators and gauze pads to clean the exposed outer cannula surfaces. Begin with half-strength (mixed with sterile 0.9% sodium chloride) or full-strength hydrogen peroxide followed by 0.9% sodium chloride. Clean in a circular motion from stoma site outward.
  - Use surgical aseptic technique to remove and clean the inner cannula (use half-strength or full strength hydrogen peroxide to clean the cannula and sterile 0.9% sodium chloride to rinse it). Reinsert a multi-use inner cannula or replace the inner cannula with a new one if it is disposable.
  - Clean the stoma site and then the tracheostomy plate with half-strength or full strength hydrogen peroxide followed by sterile 0.9% NaCl.
  - Place split dressings that are 4 inches by 4 inches around the tracheostomy.
  - Change tracheostomy ties if they are soiled. Secure new ties in place before removing soiled ones to prevent accidental decannulation.
  - If a knot is needed, tie a square knot that is visible on the side of the neck. Check that one or two fingers fit between the tie tape and the neck.
  - Document the type and amount of secretions, the general condition of the stoma and surrounding skin, the child's response to the procedure, and any instructions or learning.
- Change multi-use tracheostomy tubes every 6 to 8 weeks or per protocol.
- Reposition the child every 2 hr to prevent atelectasis and pneumonia.
  - Client Education
    - Provide discharge instructions regarding the following:
      - Tracheostomy care
      - Signs and symptoms that the family should immediately report to the health care provider (signs of infection or copious secretions)
      - Ways to achieve good nutrition

- Complications
  - Accidental decannulation
    - Accidental decannulation in the first 72 hr after surgery is an emergency because the tracheostomy tract has not matured and replacement may be difficult.
    - Nursing Actions
      - Always have an additional staff member present when moving the tube or during any situation in which decannulation may occur.

- Client Education
  - □ Instruct families when caring for the tube at home, have a second tube on hand to use as a replacement in the event of dislodgement.
  - □ Have scissors available to cut the old strings in an emergency.
- ○ Occlusion
  - Occlusion is a situation in which the tube is clogged with secretions and prevents adequate air exchange.
  - Nursing Actions
    - □ Maintain a patent airway with suctioning.
  - Client Education
    - □ Instruct the parents about the need to suction to prevent occlusion.

(A) APPLICATION EXERCISES

1. Match each child based on age and disorder with the most efficient oxygen delivery system.

   _____ A. Infant with congenital heart defect   1. Nasal cannula

   _____ B. Active toddler with pneumonia   2. Face mask

   _____ C. School-age child with asthma exacerbation   3. Oxygen hood

   _____ D. Adolescent with fractured femur   4. Oxygen tent

2. Place the following steps in the correct order for administration of a medication via a metered-dose inhaler (MDI) or dry powder inhaler (DPI) to a 10-year-old child.

   _____ Ask the child to hold breath for 10 seconds.

   _____ Place the MDI in the correct position.

   _____ Ask the child to take a deep breath and exhale.

   _____ Remove the cap and shake the MDI five to six times.

   _____ Ask the child to slowly exhale after the MDI is removed.

   _____ Ask the child to depress the MDI when taking a slow, deep breath.

3. What is the purpose of using a spacer with a metered-dose inhaler (MDI)?

4. In which of the following situations should the nurse use nebulizer aerosol therapy?

   A. Administering antibiotics to a child who has a lung abscess.

   B. Administering antireflux medications to a child who has GERD.

   C. Administering a flu immunization to a child who has a cold sore.

   D. Administering a bronchodilator to a child who has asthma.

5. When performing chest physiotherapy to facilitate drainage in the left lobe, the nurse should place the child in which of the following positions?

   A. Side-lying

   B. Trendelenburg

   C. Fowler's position

   D. Left side with pillow under chest wall

6. A nurse is caring for an 8-year-old child who is receiving oxygen therapy following surgery. When collecting data, the nurse identifies early onset hypoxemia. Which of the following nursing actions is appropriate in caring for the child? (Select all that apply.)

   _____ Titrate the rate of oxygen flow to maintain SaO_2 at or above 95%.

   _____ Place the child in the supine position.

   _____ Have the child use the incentive spirometer every hour while awake.

   _____ Encourage the child to cough and deep breathe while splinting the incision.

   _____ Check blood pressure once a shift.

7. A nurse recognizes the need to suction a child with a tracheostomy when assessment findings include which of the following? (Select all that apply.)

_____ Bradycardia

_____ Crackles upon auscultation

_____ Audible noisy secretions

_____ Restlessness

_____ Capillary refill of 3 seconds

(A) APPLICATION EXERCISES ANSWER KEY

1. Match each child based on age and disorder with the most efficient oxygen delivery system.

    3   A. Infant with congenital heart defect   1. Nasal cannula

    4   B. Active toddler with pneumonia   2. Face mask

    2   C. School-age child with asthma exacerbation   3. Oxygen hood

    1   D. Adolescent with fractured femur   4. Oxygen tent

    The most effective way to deliver oxygen to an infant is by a plastic oxygen hood. Place the toddler in a mist/oxygen tent allowing him to play and move around without restriction. The school-age child may be able to tolerate a face mask and should be encouraged to do so until the exacerbation is resolved. The adolescent should be able to comply with directions given to maintain oxygen administration via nasal cannula.

 NCLEX® Connection: Reduction of Risk Potential, Therapeutic Procedures

2. Place the following steps in the correct order for administration of a medication via a metered-dose inhaler (MDI) or dry powder inhaler (DPI) to a 10-year-old child.

    5   Ask the child to hold breath for 10 seconds.

    2   Place the MDI in the correct position.

    3   Ask the child to take a deep breath and exhale.

    1   Remove the cap and shake the MDI five to six times.

    6   Ask the child to slowly exhale after the MDI is removed.

    4   Ask the child to depress the MDI when taking a slow, deep breath.

(N) NCLEX® Connection: Pharmacological Therapies, Medication Administration

3. What is the purpose of using a spacer with a metered-dose inhaler (MDI)?

    The use of a spacer increases the amount of medication delivered to the lungs and decreases the amount of medication in the oropharynx.

(N) NCLEX® Connection: Pharmacological Therapies, Medication Administration

4. In which of the following situations should the nurse use nebulizer aerosol therapy?

    A. Administering antibiotics to a child who has a lung abscess.

    B. Administering antireflux medications to a child who has GERD.

    C. Administering a flu immunization to a child who has a cold sore.

    D. Administering a bronchodilator to a child who has asthma.

    Nebulizer aerosol therapy should be utilized in respiratory conditions being treated by the administration of bronchodilators and corticosteroids. Antibiotics and antireflux medications are not administered in this route. The flu vaccine is given by nasal spray.

(N) NCLEX® Connection: Pharmacological Therapies, Medication Administration

5. When performing chest physiotherapy to facilitate drainage in the left lobe, the nurse should place the child in which of the following positions?

    A. Side-lying

    B. Trendelenburg

    C. Fowler's position

    D. Left side with pillow under chest wall

    Place the child in Trendelenburg position to promote drainage of the left lobe. Place the child in the side-lying position to drain the posterior sections of the upper lobes, place the child in Fowler's position for apical sections of the upper lobes, and place the child on the left side with a pillow under the chest wall to drain the right lobe.

 NCLEX® Connection: Reduction of Risk Potential, Therapeutic Procedures

6. A nurse is caring for an 8-year-old child who is receiving oxygen therapy following surgery. When collecting data, the nurse identifies early onset hypoxemia. Which of the following nursing actions is appropriate in caring for the child? (Select all that apply.)

X	**Titrate the rate of oxygen flow to maintain SaO$_2$ at or above 95%.**
___	Place the child in the supine position.
X	**Have the child use the incentive spirometer every hour while awake.**
X	**Encourage the child to cough and deep breathe while splinting the incision.**
___	Check blood pressure once a shift.

    The goal is to reverse the signs of hypoxemia and to maintain a SaO$_2$ of 95% or higher at the lowest oxygen flow rate that is needed. Using incentive spirometry and having the child cough and deep breathe opens airways and improves oxygenation status. The child should be placed in semi-Fowler's or Fowler's position to ease breathing and promote chest expansion. Blood pressure should be monitored at least every 1 to 2 hr or more often as needed, since one of the early signs of hypoxemia is elevated blood pressure.

 NCLEX® Connection: Physiological Adaptations, Alterations in Body Systems

7. A nurse recognizes the need to suction a child with a tracheostomy when assessment findings include which of the following? (Select all that apply.)

___	Bradycardia
X	**Crackles upon auscultation**
X	**Audible noisy secretions**
X	**Restlessness**
___	Capillary refill of 3 seconds

    Assessment findings that indicate the need to suction a tracheostomy include crackles upon auscultation, audible/noisy secretions, restlessness, tachycardia, tachypnea, and mucus in the airway. A capillary refill of 3 seconds is within the expected range of findings.

 NCLEX® Connection: Reduction of Risk Potential, Potential for Alterations in Body Systems

Overview

○   Acute and infectious respiratory illnesses that are prevalent in children include tonsillitis, nasopharyngitis, pharyngitis, croup syndromes, bacterial tracheitis, bronchitis, bronchiolitis, allergic rhinitis, and pneumonia.

TONSILLITIS AND TONSILLECTOMY

Overview

- Tonsils are masses of lymph-type tissue found in the pharyngeal area. They filter pathogenic organisms (viral and bacterial), which helps to protect the respiratory and gastrointestinal tracts. In addition, they contribute to antibody formation.

- Palatine tonsils are located on both sides of the oropharynx. These are the tonsils removed during a tonsillectomy.

- Other tonsils are the pharyngeal tonsils, also known as the adenoids. These are removed during an adenoidectomy.

- Tonsils are highly vascular, which helps them to perform their function of protecting against infection because foreign materials, such as viral or bacterial organisms, enter the body through the mouth.

- In some instances, enlarged tonsils can block the nose and throat. This can interfere with normal breathing, nasal and sinus drainage, sleeping, swallowing, and speaking.

- Enlarged tonsils can also disrupt the normal functioning of the eustachian tube, which can impede hearing.

- Acute tonsillitis occurs when the tonsils become inflamed and reddened. Small patches of yellowish pus also may become visible. Acute tonsillitis may become chronic.

Data Collection

- Risk Factors

    ○   Exposure to a viral or bacterial agent

    ○   Immature immune systems (found in younger children)

- Subjective Data
  - Reports of sore throat with difficulty swallowing
  - History of otitis media and hearing difficulties
- Objective Data
  - Physical Assessment Findings
    - Mouth odor
    - Mouth breathing
    - Snoring
    - Nasal qualities in the voice
    - Fever
    - Tonsil inflammation with redness and edema
  - Laboratory Tests
    - Throat culture for group A β-hemolytic streptococci (GABHS)
    - Preoperative CBC to assess for anemia and infection

Collaborative Care

- Nursing Care
  - Tonsillitis
    - Provide symptomatic treatment for viral tonsillitis (rest, cool fluids, warm salt-water gargles).
    - Administer antibiotic therapy for bacterial tonsillitis.
- Medications
  - Antipyretics – Acetaminophen (Tylenol)
    - Antipyretics decrease fever.
    - Nursing Considerations
      - Be aware of allergies.
    - Client Education
      - Advise about appropriate dosing for acetaminophen.
  - Antibiotics – Amoxicillin (Amoxil)
    - Nursing Considerations
      - Be aware of allergies.
    - Client Education
      - Tell parents to administer antibiotics for the full course of treatment.

○ Analgesics – Acetaminophen (Tylenol) and codeine

■ Nursing Considerations

□ Provide pain control on a regular schedule.

□ Monitor for side effects.

■ Client Education

□ Instruct parents to monitor for side effects.

□ Instruct children and families about proper dosing to prevent overdose.

□ Advise parents to keep children away from others for 24 hr after starting the antibiotic.

□ Advise parents to wash the child's eating utensils and dishes with boiling water and antimicrobial dish soap for 24 hr after starting the antibiotic.

- Therapeutic Procedures

○ Tonsillectomy

■ Nursing Actions

□ Preoperatively

▸ Encourage the use of warm salt-water gargles and throat lozenges.

▸ Encourage fluid intake and monitor hydration status of the child (until required NPO status).

□ Postoperatively

NURSING CONSIDERATION	NURSING ACTIONS
Positioning	• Position children on their side to facilitate drainage. • Elevate the head of the child's bed when he is fully awake.
Data Collection	• Observe children for signs of bleeding, which include frequent swallowing, clearing the throat, restlessness, bright red emesis, tachycardia, and/or pallor. • Monitor the child's airway and vital signs. • Monitor children for any difficulty breathing related to oral secretions, edema, and/or bleeding.
Comfort measures	• Provide an ice collar and analgesics. • Keep the child's throat moist. • Administer pain medication on a regular schedule.
Diet	• Encourage clear liquids and fluids after a return of the gag reflex, avoiding red-colored liquids and milk-based foods initially. • Advance the child's diet with soft, bland foods.
Instruction	• Discourage coughing, throat clearing, and nose blowing in order to protect the surgical site. • Refrain from placing pointed objects in the back of the mouth. • Alert parents that there may be clots or blood-tinged mucus in vomitus.

- Client Education
  - □ Instruct families to notify the provider if signs of bleeding occur.
  - □ Encourage children to rest.

- Care After Discharge
  - ○ Client Education
    - Instruct the parents to contact the provider if children experience difficulty breathing, bright red bleeding, lack of oral intake, an increase in pain, and/or any signs of infection.
    - Tell the parents to ensure that children do not put anything sharp (ice-cream stick, straw, any pointed object) into the mouth.
    - Advise the parents to administer pain medications for discomfort.
    - Encourage fluid intake and diet advancement to a soft diet with no spicy foods or hard, sharp foods like corn chips.
    - Instruct children and their families to limit strenuous activity and physical play with no swimming for 2 weeks.
    - Instruct children and their families that full recovery usually occurs within 10 days to 2 weeks.

- Client Outcomes

  - ○ The child will recover from surgery without complications, such as hemorrhage.

Complications

- Hemorrhage
  - ○ Nursing Actions
    - Use a good light source and possibly a tongue depressor to directly observe the child's throat.
    - Observe children for signs of bleeding (tachycardia, repeated swallowing and clearing of throat, hemoptysis). Hypotension is a late sign of shock.
    - Contact the provider immediately if there is any indication of bleeding.
  - ○ Client Education
    - Instruct families to report signs of bleeding (frequent swallowing, clearing the throat, restlessness, bright red emesis, tachycardia, pallor).

- Chronic infection

  o Chronically infected tonsils may pose a potential threat to other parts of the body. Some children who have tonsillitis frequently may develop other diseases, such as rheumatic fever and kidney infection.

  o Client Education

    ▪ Instruct families to seek medical attention when children present with symptoms of tonsillitis.

COMMON RESPIRATORY ILLNESSES

Overview

- Disorders can affect both the upper (nasopharynx, pharynx, larynx, and upper part of the trachea) and lower (lower trachea, mainstem bronchi, segmental bronchi, subsegmental bronchioles, terminal bronchioles, and alveoli) respiratory tracts.

- Infections of the respiratory tract may affect more than one area.

- Infectious agents include Group A β-hemolytic streptococci (GABHS), respiratory syncytial virus (RSV), *Haemophilus influenzae*, *Streptococcus pneumoniae*, and *Mycoplasma pneumoniae*. Autumn & Early winter

Data Collection

- Risk Factors

  o Age

    ▪ Infants between 3 and 6 months of age are at an increased risk due to the decrease of maternal antibodies acquired at birth and the lack of antibody protection.

    ▪ Viral infections are more common in toddlers and preschoolers. The incidence of these infections decreases by age 5.

    ▪ GABHS and *Mycoplasma pneumoniae* infection rates increase after age 5.

    ▪ Certain viral agents can cause serious illness during infancy, but will only cause a mild illness in older children.

  o Anatomy

    ▪ A short, narrow airway can become easily obstructed with mucus or edema.

    ▪ A short respiratory tract allows infections to travel quickly to the lower airways.

    ▪ Infants and young children have small surface areas for gas exchange.

    ▪ Infectious agents have easy access to the middle ear through the short and open eustachian tubes of infants and young children.

- o Decreased resistance due to:
  - Compromised immune system
  - Anemia
  - Nutritional deficiencies
  - Allergies
  - Chronic medical conditions (asthma, cystic fibrosis, congenital heart disease)
  - Exposure to second-hand smoke
- o Seasonal variables
  - Children with asthma have a greater incidence of respiratory infections during cold weather.
  - RSV and other common respiratory infections are more common during the winter and spring.
  - Infections caused by Mycoplasma pneumoniae are more frequent during autumn and early winter.
- Subjective Data
  - o Nursing history that includes recent infections, medications taken, immunization status, and family coping
  - o Reports of sore throat, decreased activity level, chest pain, fatigue, difficulty breathing, shortness of breath, and decreased appetite
- Objective Data
  - o Physical Assessment Findings

RESPIRATORY ILLNESS	SIGNS/SYMPTOMS
• Nasopharyngitis (common cold) o Self-limiting virus that persists for 7 to 10 days	• Nasal inflammation, rhinorrhea, cough, dry throat, sneezing, and nasal qualities heard in voice • Fever, decreased appetite, and irritability
• Pharyngitis (strep throat) o Caused by GABHS	• Inflamed throat with exudate, pain with swallowing • Headache, fever, and abdominal pain • Cervical lymphadenopathy • Truncal, axillary, and perineal rash
• Bacterial tracheitis o Infection of the lining of the trachea	• Thick, purulent drainage from the trachea that can obstruct the airway and cause respiratory distress

RESPIRATORY ILLNESS	SIGNS/SYMPTOMS

• Bronchitis (tracheobronchitis)
  o Associated with an upper respiratory infection (URI) and inflammation of large airways
  o Self-limiting and requires symptomatic relief
	• Persistent cough as a result of inflammation

• Bronchiolitis
  o Mostly caused by the respiratory syncytial virus (RSV)
  o Primarily affects the bronchi and bronchioles
  o Occurs at the bronchiolar level
	• Rhinorrhea – Pharyngitis, intermittent fever, cough, and wheezing
	• Coughing that progresses toward wheezing, increased respiratory rate, nasal flaring, retractions, and cyanosis

• Allergic rhinitis o Caused by seasonal reaction to allergens most often in the autumn or spring	• Watery rhinorrhea; nasal congestion; itchiness of the nose, eyes, and pharynx; itchy, watery eyes; nasal quality of the voice; dry, scratchy throat; snoring; poor sleep leading to poor performance in school; and fatigue
• Pneumonia (RSV, *Streptococcus pneumoniae*, *Haemophilus influenzae*, *Mycoplasma pneumoniae*)	• High fever • Cough that may be unproductive or productive of white sputum • Retractions and nasal flaring • Rapid, shallow respirations • Chest pain • Adventitious breath sounds (rhonchi, crackles) • Pale color that progresses to cyanosis • Irritability, anxiety, agitation, and fatigue • Abdominal pain, diarrhea, lack of appetite, and vomiting • Sudden onset, usually following a viral infection (bacterial pneumonia)

RESPIRATORY ILLNESS	SIGNS/SYMPTOMS
Croup Syndromes	

• Bacterial epiglottitis (acute supraglottitis)
  ○ Medical emergency
  ○ Caused by *Haemophilus influenzae*
	• Sitting with chin pointing out, mouth opened, and tongue protruding
	• Drooling
	• Anxiety with respiratory distress
	• Absence of spontaneous coughing
	• Dysphonia (hoarseness or difficulty speaking)
	• Dysphagia (difficulty swallowing)
	• Inspiratory stridor (noisy inspirations)
	• Sore throat, high fever, and restlessness

• Acute laryngitis ○ Self-limiting viral infection	• Hoarseness as the only symptom
• Acute laryngotracheobronchitis ○ Causative agents include RSV, influenza A and B, and *Mycoplasma pneumoniae*	• Low-grade fever, restlessness, hoarseness, barky cough, inspiratory stridor, and retractions
• Acute spasmodic laryngitis ○ Self-limiting illness that may result from allergens	• Barky cough, restlessness, difficulty breathing, hoarseness, and nighttime episodes of laryngeal obstruction

 View Media Supplement: Laryngotracheobronchitis (Croup) (Animation)

- ○ Laboratory Tests
  - ▪ Throat culture for GABHS
  - ▪ Blood samples
    - □ Elevated serum antistreptolysin-O (ASO) titer
    - □ Elevated C-reactive protein (CRP) or erythrocyte sedimentation rate (ESR) in response to an inflammatory reaction
  - ▪ CBC to assess for anemia and infection
  - ▪ Sputum culture and sensitivity to detect infection
- ○ Diagnostic Procedures
  - ▪ Collection of direct aspiration of nasal secretions
    - □ Collect secretions for immunofluorescence analysis to detect RSV. One to 3 mL of NS is instilled into one of the child's nostrils. The fluid is then aspirated for evaluation.

▫ Nursing Actions

▸ Place children in a supine position.

▸ Use a sterile syringe without a needle.

▫ Client Education

▸ Caregivers should be educated about the potential need for isolation, dependent on the results of laboratory tests.

■ Chest x-ray

▫ Identifies infiltration in pneumonia

▫ Nursing Actions

▸ Ensure children are positioned correctly to avoid the need for a repeat x-ray.

▫ Client Education

▸ Inform adolescents of childbearing age of the need for confirmation of nonpregnant status.

Collaborative Care

- Nursing Care

  ○ Closely monitor progression of illness and ensuing respiratory distress. Observe for increased heart and respiratory rate, retractions, nasal flaring, and restlessness.

  ○ Make emergency equipment for intubation readily accessible.

  ○ Do not attempt to use a tongue depressor or take a throat culture if epiglottitis is suspected.

  ○ Use oxygen and high humidity for infants and young children with hoods or tents.

  ○ Use postural drainage and/or chest physiotherapy (CPT) to help mobilize and remove fluid from the lungs.

  ○ Maintain adequate hydration by offering preferred fluids at frequent intervals.

  ○ Monitor rate of IV fluids.

  ○ Allow for the child to be held in an upright position.

- Medications

  ○ Epinephrine

    ■ Nebulized (racemic) epinephrine may be prescribed to decrease subglottic edema.

    ■ Nursing Considerations

      ▫ Observe children for 3 hr after administration of medication.

    ■ Client Education

      ▫ Inform children that they may feel an acceleration in heart rate during the administration of this medication.

- ○ Corticosteroids – Dexamethasone (Decadron) and budesonide (Rhinocort)
  - ▪ Administer to decrease inflammation.
  - ▪ Nursing Considerations
    - □ Administer orally via nebulizer or IV route.
  - ▪ Client Education
    - □ Assist children to rinse the mouth after nebulizer treatment.
- ○ Antipyretics – Acetaminophen (Tylenol)
  - ▪ Administer to decrease fever.
  - ▪ Nursing Considerations
    - □ Be aware of allergies.
  - ▪ Client Education
    - □ Educate children and their families about the proper dose of medication.
- ○ Mild analgesics
  - ▪ Administer to decrease pain.
  - ▪ Nursing Considerations
    - □ Monitor for safety while using analgesics.
  - ▪ Client Education
    - □ Advise the parents of proper dosing and safety considerations.
- ○ Antibiotics
  - ▪ Administer to treat bacterial infection.
  - ▪ Nursing Considerations
    - □ Be aware of allergies.
  - ▪ Client Education
    - □ Advise parents that the child should finish the full course of antibiotics.
- • Care After Discharge
  - ○ Recommend parents use a cool-air vaporizer to provide humidity.
  - ○ Suggest children rest during febrile illness.
  - ○ Instruct parents to assist children to maintain adequate fluid intake. Give infants commercially prepared oral rehydration solutions, and older children sports drinks.
  - ○ Instruct parents to limit use of nose drops or sprays to 3 days to prevent rebound congestion.
  - ○ Instruct parents to apply an ice bag or heating pad to the neck to decrease pain from enlarged cervical nodes.

○ Tell parents to administer medications using accurate dosages and appropriate time intervals.

○ Reinforce strategies to decrease the spread of infection. Strategies include performing good hand hygiene; covering the nose and mouth with tissues when sneezing and coughing; properly disposing of tissues; not sharing cups, eating utensils, and towels; and keeping infected children from contact with children who are well.

○ Instruct parents to seek further medical attention for children if symptoms worsen or respiratory distress occurs.

- Client Outcomes

○ The child and family will adhere to the medication regimen.

○ The child will be free of infection.

Complications

- Airway Obstruction

○ May result from progression of respiratory infectious process or foreign body aspiration

○ Nursing Actions

■ Ensure proper body alignment. Position the child (prone, semiprone, side lying) to promote lung expansion, promote gas exchange, and prevent aspiration.

■ Perform suctioning of airways if indicated, limiting each attempt to 5 seconds.

■ Do not examine the child's throat with a tongue blade or take a throat culture if epiglottitis is suspected.

■ Administer medications as prescribed to include epinephrine and corticosteroids.

■ Carry out CPT.

■ Assist children to deep breathe with the use of a splint, and expectorate sputum.

■ Ensure availability of emergency equipment.

○ Client Education

■ Instruct parents to keep small objects away from children.

■ Instruct parents to identify respiratory distress (increased heart and respiratory rate, nasal flaring, chest retractions, increased restlessness) and to seek medical attention.

Ⓐ APPLICATION EXERCISES

1. A nurse is assessing a child who may have bacterial epiglottitis. Which of the following manifestations is likely to be present? (Select all that apply.)

    _✓_ Hoarseness when speaking

    _✓_ Difficulty swallowing

    _____ Low-grade fever

    _✓_ Drooling

    _✓_ Stridor

2. A nurse is reinforcing teaching to the parents of a 6-month-old infant who is brought to the pediatric clinic frequently with upper respiratory illnesses. Which of the following should the nurse include in a discussion of risk factors for respiratory disorders? (Select all that apply.)

    _✓_ Exposure to smoke in the home

    _✓_ Eustachian tubes are short and open

    _✓_ Winter and spring months are the usual period for RSV

    _____ Maternal antibodies are peaking, overwhelming the infant's immune system

    _____ Inadequate insulation in the home

3. Match the following respiratory illness with their cause.

    X B (D) Rhinitis   A. Respiratory syncytial virus (RSV)

    _E_ Bacterial epiglottitis   B. Influenza A or B

    _A_ Bronchiolitis   C. Group B streptococcus

    _C_ Pharyngitis   D. Allergens

    X D (B) Laryngotracheobronchitis   E. Haemophilus influenza

4. Describe the discharge instructions a nurse should review with the parents of a child following a tonsillectomy.

5. Place the following steps for collecting nasal secretions for analysis in the correct order.

    _____ Instill 1 to 3 mL of 0.9% sodium chloride into one of the nares using a sterile needleless syringe.

    _____ Place the child in a supine position.

    _____ Transfer secretions to sterile specimen container for transport to the laboratory.

    _____ Aspirate the secretions using a clean bulb syringe.

(A) **APPLICATION EXERCISES ANSWER KEY**

1. A nurse is assessing a child who may have bacterial epiglottitis. Which of the following manifestations is likely to be present? (Select all that apply.)

     X   **Hoarseness when speaking**

     X   **Difficulty swallowing**

          Low-grade fever

     X   **Drooling**

     X   **Stridor**

   A child who is ill with epiglottitis typically exhibits dysphonia (hoarseness or difficulty speaking), dysphagia (difficulty swallowing), drooling, and anxiety with respiratory distress. Inspiratory stridor (noisy inspirations) is also common. The child usually has a high fever and a cough is not present.

   (N) NCLEX® Connection: Health Promotion and Maintenance, Data Collection Techniques

2. A nurse is reinforcing teaching to the parents of a 6-month-old infant who is brought to the pediatric clinic frequently with upper respiratory illnesses. Which of the following should the nurse include in a discussion of risk factors for respiratory disorders? (Select all that apply.)

     X   **Exposure to smoke in the home**

     X   **Eustachian tubes are short and open**

     X   **Winter and spring months are the usual period for RSV**

          Maternal antibodies are peaking, overwhelming the infant's immune system

          Inadequate insulation in the home

   Risk factors for common respiratory illnesses include exposure to second-hand smoke, short, open eustachian tubes and short respiratory tract of infants and young children, the winter and spring seasonal aspects of illnesses such as RSV, nutritional deficiencies, allergies, and altered immune response. At 6 months of age, the infant's maternal antibodies are decreased, which places him at a higher risk. Inadequate insulation in the home is not a risk factor.

   (N) NCLEX® Connection: Physiological Adaptations, Alterations in Body Systems

3. Match the following respiratory illness with their cause.

D	Rhinitis	A. Respiratory syncytial virus (RSV)
E	Bacterial epiglottitis	B. Influenza A or B
A	Bronchiolitis	C. Group B streptococcus
C	Pharyngitis	D. Allergens
B	Laryngotracheobronchitis	E. Haemophilus influenza

   (N) NCLEX® Connection: Physiological Adaptations, Basic Pathophysiology

       PN NURSING CARE OF CHILDREN

4. Describe the discharge instructions a nurse should review with the parents of a child following a tonsillectomy.

   Contact the provider if the child experiences difficulty breathing, bright red bleeding, a lack of oral intake, and increased pain or signs of infection.

   Avoid placing any sharp objects in the mouth, such as straws, oral thermometer, or an ice cream stick.

   Give pain medications for discomfort.

   Limit strenuous physical activities and play, including swimming, for 2 weeks.

   Expect recovery to take 10 to 14 days.

   Ⓝ NCLEX® Connection: Reduction of Risk Potential, Therapeutic Procedures

5. Place the following steps for collecting nasal secretions for analysis in the correct order.

   __2__ Instill 1 to 3 mL of 0.9% sodium chloride into one of the nares using a sterile needleless syringe.

   __1__ Place the child in a supine position.

   __4__ Transfer secretions to sterile specimen container for transport to the laboratory.

   __3__ Aspirate the secretions using a clean bulb syringe.

   Nasal secretions are collected by placing the child in a supine position, and using a sterile needleless syringe, instilling 1 to 3 mL of normal saline into one of the nares. The secretions are then aspirated using a clean bulb syringe and placed in a sterile specimen container for transport to the laboratory.

   Ⓝ NCLEX® Connection: Reduction of Risk Potential, Laboratory Values

UNIT 2	NURSING CARE OF CHILDREN WITH SYSTEM DISORDERS
Section:	Respiratory Disorders

Chapter 17   Asthma

Overview

- Asthma is a chronic inflammatory disorder of the airways that results in intermittent and reversible airflow obstruction of the bronchioles.

- The obstruction occurs either by inflammation or airway hyper-responsiveness.

- The cause of asthma is unknown.

- Manifestations of asthma

    o Mucosal edema

    o Bronchoconstriction

    o Excessive secretion production

    (M) View Media Supplement: Asthma (Video)

- Asthma diagnoses are based on symptoms and classified into one of the following four categories.

    o Mild intermittent – Symptoms occur less than twice a week.

    o Mild persistent – Symptoms occur more than twice a week, but not daily.

    o Moderate persistent – Daily symptoms occur in conjunction with exacerbations twice a week.

    o Severe persistent – Symptoms occur continually, along with frequent exacerbations that limit the child's physical activity and quality of life.

Data Collection

- Risk Factors

    o Young children are more susceptible to infections.

    o The presence of secondhand smoke increases the risk for asthma.

- Subjective Data
  - Anxiety
  - Stress
  - Chest tightness
  - History regarding current and previous asthma exacerbations
    - Onset and duration
    - Precipitating factors (stress, exercise, exposure to irritant)
    - Changes in medication regimen
    - Medications that relieve symptoms
    - Other medications taken
    - Self-care methods used to relieve symptoms
- Objective Data
  - Physical Assessment Findings
    - Dyspnea
    - Coughing
    - Wheezing
    - Diminished lung sounds
    - Mucus production
    - Use of accessory muscles
    - Poor oxygen saturation (low SaO_2)
    - Tachycardia and premature ventricular contractions (PVCs)
  - Laboratory Tests
    - ABGs
      - Hypoxemia (decreased PaO_2 of less than 80 mm Hg)
      - Hypocarbia (decreased $PaCO_2$ of less than 35 mm Hg early in attack)
      - Hypercarbia (increased $PaCO_2$ of greater than 45 mm Hg later in attack)
    - Sputum cultures
      - Bacteria may be present, indicating infection.

o Diagnostic Procedures

- Pulmonary function tests (PFTs) are the most accurate tests for diagnosing asthma and its severity.

  □ Forced vital capacity (FVC) is the volume of air exhaled from full inhalation to full exhalation.

  □ Forced expiratory volume (FEV_1) is the volume of air able to be blown out as quickly as possible during the first second of a forceful exhalation after inhaling fully.

  □ Peak expiratory flow rate (PEFR), measured using a peak expiratory flow meter (PEFM), is the maximum airflow exhaled forcefully in 1 second.

  □ A decrease in FEV_1 or PEFR by 15% to 20% below the expected value is common in children with asthma. An increase in these values by 12% following the administration of bronchodilators is diagnostic for asthma.

- A chest x-ray is used to diagnose changes in chest structure over time.

  □ Nursing Actions

  ▸ Prepare children for the procedure.

  □ Client Education

  ▸ Provide support for families.

  ▸ Assist parents to relieve the child's anxiety during the testing.

Collaborative Care

- Nursing Care

  o Monitor respiratory status including watching for shortness of breath, dyspnea, and audible wheezing. An absence of wheezing may indicate severe constriction of the alveoli.

  o Check ABGs, SaO_2, CBC, and chest x-ray results.

  o Position children to maximize ventilation (high-Fowler's).

  o Administer oxygen therapy as prescribed.

  o Monitor children receiving IV therapy.

  o Maintain a calm and reassuring demeanor.

  o Encourage appropriate immunizations and prompt medical attention for infections.

- Medications
  - Bronchodilators (inhalers)
    - Short-acting beta$_2$-agonists (albuterol [Proventil], terbutaline [Brethine]) provide rapid relief for acute asthma attacks.
    - Cholinergic antagonists (anticholinergic medications), such as ipratropium (Atrovent), block the parasympathetic nervous system, providing relief of acute bronchospasms.

      [handwritten: → check mouth for dryness]
    - Nursing Considerations
      - Instruct children and their families about the proper use of MDI, DPI, or nebulizer.
      - Watch children for tremors and tachycardia when they are taking albuterol.
      - Observe children for dry mouth when they are taking ipratropium.
    - Client Education
      - Encourage older children who are taking ipratropium to suck on hard candies to help with dry mouth.
      - Instruct children to take a bronchodilator inhaler 5 min prior to an anti-inflammatory inhaler to promote bronchodilation and increased absorption of medication.
  - Anti-inflammatory agents
    - Anti-inflammatory agents decrease airway inflammation for long-term management.
    - Corticosteroids (fluticasone [Flovent] and prednisone [Deltasone])
    - Leukotriene modifiers (montelukast [Singulair]), mast cell stabilizers (cromolyn sodium [Intal]), and monoclonal antibodies (omalizumab [Xolair])
    - Nursing Considerations
      - Watch children for decreased immunity function.
      - Monitor children for hyperglycemia. *[handwritten: b/c corticosteroids?]*
      - Advise children to report black, tarry stools.
      - Observe children for fluid retention and weight gain, which may be common.
      - Observe the child's throat and mouth for aphthous (cold sore) lesions.
    - Client Education
      - Encourage children to drink plenty of fluids to promote hydration.
      - Encourage children to take a glucocorticosteroid (prednisone [Deltasone]) with food.
      - Instruct children to rinse mouth or gargle with warm saltwater after the use of an inhaler.
      - Instruct children and their families to watch for redness, sores, or white patches in the mouth, and report them to the provider.

- Interdisciplinary Care

  o Respiratory services for inhalers and breathing treatments

  o Nutritional services for weight loss or gain related to medications or diagnosis

  o Rehabilitation care for children who have prolonged weakness and need assistance with increasing level of activity

- Care After Discharge

  o Client Education

    ■ Instruct children and families how to recognize and avoid triggering agents, such as:

      □ Smoke

      □ Dust

      □ Mold

      □ Sudden weather changes (especially warm to cold)

      □ Seasonal allergens (grass, tree, and weed pollens)

      □ Animal dander

      □ Stress

    ■ Instruct children how to properly self-administer medications (nebulizers and inhalers).

    ■ Educate children and their families regarding infection prevention techniques.

      □ Promote good nutrition.

      □ Reinforce importance of good hand hygiene.

    ■ Encourage prompt medical attention for infections.

    ■ Stress the importance of keeping immunizations, including seasonal influenza and pneumonia vaccines, up to date.

    ■ Encourage regular exercise as part of asthma therapy. Remind children to use medication prior to activity if necessary.

      □ Promotes ventilation and perfusion

      □ Maintains cardiac health

      □ Enhances skeletal muscle strength

    ■ Instruct children how to use relaxation techniques to control anxiety.

- Client Outcomes

  o The child will be able to maintain adequate gas exchange.

  o The child will prevent acute attacks.

  o The child will have relief of symptoms.

  o The child will adhere to the medication regimen.

Complications

- Respiratory failure

  - Persistent hypoxemia related to asthma can lead to respiratory failure.

  - Nursing Actions

    - Monitor oxygenation levels and acid-base balance.

    - Prepare for intubation and mechanical ventilation as indicated.

- Status asthmaticus

  - A life-threatening episode of airway obstruction that is often unresponsive to common treatment

  - Symptoms include wheezing, labored breathing, use of accessory muscles, distended neck veins, and risk for cardiac and/or respiratory arrest.

  - Nursing Actions

    - Assist with emergency intubation.

    - Administer humidified oxygen.

    - Administer three nebulizer treatments of a beta$_2$-agonist, 20 to 30 min apart. Ipratropium may be added to the nebulizer to increase bronchodilation.

    - Monitor IV access, ABGs, and serum electrolytes.

    - Administer corticosteroid (oral, IM). Monitor children receiving a corticosteroid IV bolus.

    - Other therapies may include:

      - Magnesium sulfate via IV bolus or by inhalation, which results in smooth muscle relaxation and decreases inflammation.

      - Heliox via nonrebreathing face mask.

      - Ketamine (Ketalar) via IV bolus.

    - Prepare the child for admission for continued follow-up.

APPLICATION EXERCISES

1. During assessment, which of the following findings may indicate deterioration in a child's respiratory status? (Select all that apply.)

    _____ SaO₂ 95%

    ___✓___ Wheezing

    ___✓___ Substernal retractions

    _____ Pink mucous membranes

    ___✓___ Anxiety

2. A nurse is reviewing the home medications of a child admitted to the pediatric unit for exacerbation of asthma. The nurse recognizes which of the following medications as an anti-inflammatory agent used in long-term management?

    A. Fluticasone (Flovent)

    B. Terbutaline (Brethine)

    C. Ipratropium (Atrovent)

    D. Albuterol (Proventil)

3. A nurse in the pediatric unit is discussing the use of corticosteroid medications with a 12-year-old child and her mother. Which of the following actions should be included in the plan of care? (Select all that apply.)

    ___✓___ Prednisone should be taken with food.

    ___✓___ Check for redness, white patches, and cold sores in the mouth.

    _____ Rinse mouth with an alcohol-based mouthwash after using the inhaler.

    ___✓___ Increase daily oral fluid intake.

    _____ Note weight loss.

4. A nurse is reviewing discharge instructions with the parent of a child who was recently diagnosed with asthma. In a discussion about triggering events, which of the following statements by the parent indicates the need for clarification?

    A. "My child should avoid being outdoors on a windy day when it's dusty."

    B. "The sudden change from cold to warm weather is when asthma can flare up."

    C. "When the pollen count is high, we should keep the doors and windows closed."

    D. "My child should not play in the neighbor's basement since there is mildew on the walls."

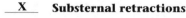

APPLICATION EXERCISES ANSWER KEY

1. During assessment, which of the following findings may indicate deterioration in a child's respiratory status? (Select all that apply.)

_____	SaO$_2$ 95%
__X__	**Wheezing**
__X__	**Substernal retractions**
_____	Pink mucous membranes
__X__	**Anxiety**

Wheezing, substernal retractions, and anxiety are indications of a child's worsening respiratory status. An SaO$_2$ of 95% and pink mucous membranes are signs of normal respiratory function and do not indicate distress.

 NCLEX® Connection: Physiological Adaptations, Alterations in Body Systems

2. A nurse is reviewing the home medications of a child admitted to the pediatric unit for exacerbation of asthma. The nurse recognizes which of the following medications as an anti-inflammatory agent used in long-term management?

A. Fluticasone (Flovent)

B. Terbutaline (Brethine)

C. Ipratropium (Atrovent)

D. Albuterol (Proventil)

Fluticasone is a glucocorticoid used for its long-term anti-inflammatory effects. Terbutaline and albuterol are short-acting beta$_2$ agonists used for acute asthma attacks. Ipratropium is a cholinergic antagonist that provides relief from acute bronchospasm.

 NCLEX® Connection: Pharmacological Therapies, Expected Actions/Outcomes

3. A nurse on the pediatric unit is discussing the use of corticosteroid medications with a 12-year-old child and her mother. Which of the following actions should be included in the plan of care? (Select all that apply.)

__X__ **Prednisone should be taken with food.**

__X__ **Check for redness, white patches, and cold sores in the mouth.**

_____ Rinse mouth with an alcohol-based mouthwash after using the inhaler.

__X__ **Increase daily oral fluid intake.**

_____ Note weight loss.

The child should take prednisone with food to reduce gastric upset. Check the mouth for signs of irritation of the mucous membranes and the presence of aphthous lesions, which may occur due to immunosuppression. Increase fluid intake to promote hydration. Rinse the mouth or gargle with warm saltwater after using the inhaler to prevent irritation of the mucous membranes. Weight gain is common when taking a long-term corticosteroid.

Ⓝ NCLEX® Connection: Pharmacological Therapies, Adverse Effects/ Contraindications/Side Effects/Interactions

4. A nurse is reviewing discharge instructions with the parent of a child who was recently diagnosed with asthma. In a discussion about triggering events, which of the following statements by the parent indicates the need for clarification?

A. "My child should avoid being outdoors on a windy day when it's dusty."

B. "The sudden change from cold to warm weather is when asthma can flare up."

C. "When the pollen count is high, we should keep the doors and windows closed."

D. "My child should not play in the neighbor's basement since there is mildew on the walls."

Asthma triggers include a sudden change in weather, especially warm to cold. Other triggers include smoke, dust, molds, animal dander, stress, and seasonal allergies.

Ⓝ NCLEX® Connection: Physiological Adaptations, Basic Pathophysiology

UNIT 2	NURSING CARE OF CHILDREN WITH SYSTEM DISORDERS
Section:	Respiratory Disorders

Chapter 18   Cystic Fibrosis

Overview

- Cystic fibrosis is a dysfunction of the exocrine glands that causes the glands to produce thick, tenacious mucus.

- Major organs affected are the lungs, pancreas, small intestine, and liver.

- Abnormally thick mucus leads to mechanical obstruction of organs, which alters their functions.

- Sweat and salivary glands excrete excessive electrolytes, specifically sodium and chloride.

Data Collection

- Risk Factors

  ○ Cystic fibrosis is hereditary and transmitted as an autosomal recessive trait. Thus, both parents must be carriers of the gene.

- Subjective Data

  ○ History of chronic respiratory infections, poor weight gain, failure to thrive.

- Objective Data

  ○ Physical Assessment Findings

    ▪ Meconium ileus at birth manifested as distention of the abdomen, vomiting (may be bile-stained), and inability to pass stool

    ▪ Absence of pancreatic enzymes

    ▪ Respiratory findings

      □ Fatigue

      □ Dry, nonproductive cough

      □ Thick, yellow-grey mucus

      □ Positive sputum culture (*Pseudomonas aeruginosa*, *Haemophilus influenzae*)

      □ Fever

      □ Shortness of breath, dyspnea, and wheezing

- □ Cyanosis
- □ Difficulty exhaling air, resulting in hyperinflation of the lungs
- □ Barrel-shaped chest
- □ Clubbing of the fingers and toes
- Gastrointestinal findings
  - □ Stools, known as steatorrhea, which are large, loose, fatty, sticky, foul-smelling stools (due to the presence of protein)
  - □ Rectal prolapse
  - □ Failure to gain weight
  - □ Delayed growth patterns
  - □ Distended abdomen
  - □ Thin arms and legs
  - □ Atrophy of buttocks and thighs
- Integumentary findings
  - □ Sweat, tears, and saliva are abnormally salty
- Endocrine and reproductive system findings
  - □ Delayed puberty
  - □ Viscous cervical mucus
  - □ Decreased or absent sperm
- ○ Laboratory Tests
  - Newborn screening in some states includes the immunoreactive trypsinogen (IRT) analysis which is a heel stick blood test. This is followed by confirmation of the diagnosis by DNA mutant gene identification. More often, in infants, the sweat chloride test is the initial screening test to measure the amount of chloride in skin sweat. A normal chloride concentration of sweat is less than 40 mEq/L. Values of greater than 40 mEq/L in infants are suggestive of cystic fibrosis, and values greater than 60 mEq/L in children indicate a probable diagnosis of cystic fibrosis. The DNA testing follows to confirm the diagnosis.
  - Stool analysis for the presence of pancreatic enzymes; and sputum culture and sensitivity to detect infection.
- ○ Diagnostic Procedures
  - Chest x-ray and pulmonary function testing
    - □ May indicate diffuse atelectasis and obstructive emphysema
    - □ Nursing Actions
      - ‣ Ensure that children are properly positioned for the procedure to avoid the need to repeat the x-ray.

- Abdominal x-ray
  - Detect meconium ileus
  - Nursing Actions
    - Ensure that children are properly positioned for the procedure to avoid the need to repeat the x-ray.

Collaborative Care

- Nursing Care
  - Give respiratory treatments to include aerosol therapy, chest physiotherapy, breathing exercises, and assistance with coughing/expectoration of secretions.
  - Perform CPT 1 hr before meals or 2 hr after meals if possible.
  - Use oxygen with caution to prevent oxygen narcosis.
  - Provide three small meals of high-calorie, high-protein foods with two to three snacks daily.
  - Promote adequate nutritional intake, and provide pancreatic enzymes at all meals and with snacks.
  - Monitor blood glucose levels due to insulin resistance, deficiency, and altered pancreatic excretory function.
  - Encourage adequate fluid and salt intake.
  - Provide meticulous skin care and oral hygiene.
  - Administer antibiotics through a central venous access port.
- Medications
  - Hypoglycemic agents
    - Nursing Considerations
      - Monitor blood glucose levels and administer hypoglycemic agents as prescribed.
  - Bronchodilators (inhalers)
    - Short-acting beta$_2$ agonists, such as albuterol (Proventil), provide rapid relief.
    - Cholinergic antagonists (anticholinergics), such as ipratropium (Atrovent), block the parasympathetic nervous system, providing relief of acute bronchospasms.
    - Nursing Considerations
      - Instruct children and families in the proper use of an MDI, DPI, or nebulizer.
      - Monitor children for tremors and tachycardia when they are taking albuterol.
      - Observe children for dry mouth when taking ipratropium. Perform oral hygiene for young children.

- Client Education
  - Encourage older children to rinse their mouth using ipratropium.
- Antibiotics
  - Antibiotics are used to treat bacterial infections.
  - Nursing Considerations
    - Be aware of allergies.
  - Client Education
    - Advise parents that their children should finish the full course of antibiotics.
- Dornase alfa (Pulmozyme)
  - Decreases the viscosity of mucus and improves lung function
  - Nursing Considerations
    - Monitor children for improvement in PFTs.
  - Client Education
    - Instruct children in the use of a nebulizer.
    - Instruct children to use once daily.
- Pancreatic enzymes – Pancrelipase (Pancrease)
  - Use to treat pancreatic insufficiency associated with cystic fibrosis.
  - Nursing Considerations
    - Give capsules within 30 min of all meals and snacks.
    - Have children swallow capsules whole or sprinkle on food.
- Fat-soluble vitamins (A,D,E,K)
  - A water-miscible form is given due to the altered gastrointestinal absorption of fats.
  - Nursing Considerations
    - Give with meals and snacks.
- Histamine$_2$ receptor antagonist
  - Decreases gastric acidity and promotes GI motility.
  - Nursing Considerations
    - Encourage children to sit upright after meals to reduce reflux.
- Interdisciplinary Care
  - Respiratory therapy, social services, and dieticians may be involved in the care of children who have cystic fibrosis.

- Care After Discharge

  o Ensure that families have information regarding access to medical equipment.

  o Provide information about equipment prior to discharge.

  o Instruct families in ways to provide CPT and breathing exercises. For example, a child can stand on her head by using a large, cushioned chair placed against a wall.

  o Encourage additional salt intake during summer months or if living in hot climates.

  o Promote regular provider visits.

  o Emphasize the need for up-to-date immunizations with the addition of an initial seasonal influenza vaccine at 6 months of age and then yearly.

  o Promote regular physical activity.

  o Encourage the family to participate in a support group and use community resources.

  o Provide information regarding appropriate birth control to adolescents, even though fertility is often reduced or the child is sterile due to blockage of the fallopian tubes or vas deferens by thick mucus.

  o Encourage children and families to participate in career and educational goal setting despite the prognosis of the disease.

- Client Outcomes

  o The child will maintain body system function that supports adequate growth and development for the condition.

  o The child will remain free from infection.

Complications

- Respiratory Complications

  o Children who have cystic fibrosis are at increased risk for hospitalization related to pulmonary and gastrointestinal complications (respiratory infection, rectal prolapse, pancreatic insufficiency, impaired bone health).

  o Nursing Actions

    ▪ Promptly treat respiratory infections with antibiotic therapy.

    ▪ Provide pulmonary hygiene with chest physiotherapy (CPT) (breathing exercises to strengthen thoracic muscles) a minimum of twice a day (in the morning and at bedtime).

    ▪ Have children use a mucus clearance device to assist with mucus removal.

    ▪ Administer bronchodilators through a metered dose inhaler (MDI) or hand-held nebulizer to promote expectoration of excretions.

    ▪ Administer dornase alfa (Pulmozyme) through a nebulizer to decrease viscosity of mucus.

    ▪ Promote physical activity that children enjoy to improve mental well-being, self-esteem, and mucus secretion.

- ○ Client Education

  - ■ Provide instructions regarding the medication regimen, dietary considerations, and infection control precautions.

- Gastrointestinal complications

  - ○ Children who have cystic fibrosis are at an increased risk for hospitalization related to gastrointestinal complications (meconium ileus, pancreatic fibrosis, distal intestinal obstruction syndrome, growth failure).

  - ○ Nursing Actions

    - ■ Administer pancreatic enzymes with meals and snacks.

      - □ The amount of enzyme replacement will vary among children based on each child's deficiency and response to the replacement.

    - ■ Provide supplemental feedings through a gastrostomy tube (G-button).

      View Media Supplement: Gastrostomy (G-button) Tube (Image)

    - ■ Encourage children to select meals and snacks if appropriate.

    - ■ Facilitate high-caloric, high-protein intake through meals and snacks.

    - ■ Administer multiple vitamins and water-soluble forms of vitamins A, D, E, and K.

  - ○ Client Education

    - ■ Encourage the use of stool softeners or laxatives.

    - ■ Instruct children and their families that the capsules may be swallowed whole or opened to sprinkle the contents on a small amount of food.

(A) APPLICATION EXERCISES

1. Which of the following tests is used to confirm a diagnosis of cystic fibrosis?

   A. Sweat chloride
   B. Blood glucose
   C. Arterial blood gases
   D. DNA mutant gene identification

2. A nurse is caring for a newborn in the nursery and suspects that she has cystic fibrosis. Which of the following physical findings supports the nurse's conclusion? (Select all that apply.)

   X ___✓___ Barrel-shaped chest *not in newborn, but in children*
   ___✓___ Failure to pass a meconium stool
   _____ Bile present in regurgitated breast milk
   X ___✓___ Cyanosis → *Not related to newborns (only during transitition) from fetus → birth*
   ___✓___ Large, round distended abdomen

3. Describe how a nurse administers pancrelipase (Pancrease) to pediatric clients.

4. A nurse is reviewing dietary concerns at the home of a child with cystic fibrosis. Which of the following should be included in the diet plan? (Select all that apply.)

   ___✓___ Take water-soluble and multiple vitamins.
   _____ Limit oral fluids.
   ___✓___ Increase calorie and protein intake.
   _____ Decrease salt intake.
   ___✓___ Add between meal snacks.

APPLICATION EXERCISES ANSWER KEY

1. Which of the following tests is used to confirm a diagnosis of cystic fibrosis?

    A. Sweat chloride

    B. Blood glucose

    C. Arterial blood gases

    D. DNA mutant gene identification

    A DNA mutant gene identification test is used to confirm a diagnosis of cystic fibrosis with a very high degree of certainty and is done in early infancy. A sweat chloride test is a screening test that measures the amount of chloride in skin sweat. Abnormally high concentrations of sodium and chloride are unique to cystic fibrosis. Normal chloride concentration of sweat is less than 40 mEq/L. Cystic fibrosis is highly suggestive in infants who have chloride values greater than 40 mEq/L. Values greater than 60 mEq/L indicate a high probability of cystic fibrosis but are not confirmatory. Use the other tests to determine the condition of a client who has cystic fibrosis, but not to diagnose the disorder.

 NCLEX® Connection: Reduction of Risk Potential, Diagnostic Tests

2. A nurse is caring for a newborn in the nursery and suspects that she has cystic fibrosis. Which of the following physical findings supports the nurse's conclusion? (Select all that apply.)

    _____ Barrel-shaped chest

    __X__ **Failure to pass a meconium stool**

    __X__ **Bile present in regurgitated breast milk**

    _____ Cyanosis

    __X__ **Large, round distended abdomen** due to mecomium ileus

    Physical findings of suspected cystic fibrosis in the newborn include failure to pass a meconium stool, bile in vomitus, and abdominal distention due to a meconium ileus. A barrel-shaped chest is seen in children with cystic fibrosis, not a newborn. Cyanosis may be present in the newborn during the transition from fetal to extrauterine life, but is not related to cystic fibrosis. Cyanosis is seen in children with cystic fibrosis.

 NCLEX® Connection: Physiological Adaptations, Basic Pathophysiology

3. Describe how a nurse administers pancrelipase (Pancrease) to pediatric clients.

    This medication is given with all meals and snacks. Capsules can be opened and the contents sprinkled on food, or the capsule can be swallowed whole. The provider will prescribe the dosage based on the needs of the child and the amount of food that the child will consume.

 NCLEX® Connection: Basic Care and Comfort, Nutrition and Oral Hydration

4. A nurse is reviewing dietary concerns at the home of a child with cystic fibrosis. Which of the following should be included in the diet plan? (Select all that apply.)

__X__ **Take water-soluble and multiple vitamins.**

_____ Limit oral fluids.

__X__ **Increase calorie and protein intake.**

_____ Decrease salt intake.

__X__ **Add between meal snacks.**

A child with cystic fibrosis is prescribed multiple vitamins, water-soluble vitamins, and a high-calorie, high-protein diet. Adding snacks between meals is a way to increase calories. Fluid intake should be encouraged to facilitate the thinning of pulmonary secretions. Salt intake should not be decreased due to salt lost in perspiration.

(N) NCLEX® Connection: Basic Care and Comfort, Nutrition and Oral Hydration

UNIT 2: NURSING CARE OF CHILDREN WITH SYSTEM DISORDERS

Section: Cardiovascular and Hematologic Disorders

- Cardiovascular Disorders

- Hematological Disorders

NCLEX® CONNECTIONS

When reviewing the chapters in this section, keep in mind the relevant sections of the NCLEX® outline, in particular:

CLIENT NEEDS: PHARMACOLOGICAL THERAPIES	CLIENT NEEDS: REDUCTION OF RISK POTENTIAL	CLIENT NEEDS: PHYSIOLOGICAL ADAPTATION
Relevant topics/tasks include:	Relevant topics/tasks include:	Relevant topics/tasks include:
• Adverse Effects/ Contraindications/Side Effects/Interactions 　○ Implement procedures to counteract adverse effects of medications. • Dosage Calculation 　○ Use clinical decision making when calculating doses. • Expected Actions/ Outcomes 　○ Reinforce education to client regarding medications.	• Changes/Abnormalities in Vital signs 　○ Check and monitor client vital signs. • Diagnostic Tests 　○ Reinforce client teaching about diagnostic test. • Laboratory Values 　○ Monitor diagnostic or laboratory test results.	• Alterations in Body Systems 　○ Provide care to correct client alteration in body system. • Basic Pathophysiology 　○ Consider general principles of client disease process when providing care. • Fluid and Electrolyte Imbalances 　○ Provide interventions to restore client fluid and/or electrolyte balance.

UNIT 2   NURSING CARE OF CHILDREN WITH SYSTEM DISORDERS

Section: Cardiovascular and Hematologic Disorders

Chapter 19   Cardiovascular Disorders

◎ Overview

- Heart disease may be congenital or it may be acquired, as is the case with rheumatic heart disease.

- Anatomic abnormalities present at birth can lead to congenital heart disease (CHD). These abnormalities result primarily in heart failure and hypoxemia.

- Rheumatic fever is a self-limiting inflammatory disease of the connective tissue. System involvement includes the connective tissue of the heart, joints, central nervous system, skin, and subcutaneous tissue.

    ○ Rheumatic heart disease is the major complication of rheumatic fever, and it results in cardiac valve damage.

CONGENITAL HEART DISEASE (CHD)

◎ Overview

- Anatomic defects of the heart prevent normal blood flow to the pulmonary and/or systemic system.

- Many defects will spontaneously close, but some will require surgical repair.

- Most children with CHD will be diagnosed in the first year of life, but certain children may not exhibit manifestations until later.

- Children with CHD have an increased incidence of other anatomic defects, which may impact their care.

(M) **View Media Supplement:**

- Ventricular Septal Defect (Image)
- Pulmonary Stenosis (Image)
- Coarctation of the Aorta (Image)
- Tetralogy of Fallot (Image)

Data Collection

- Risk Factors

  - Cardiac development occurs very early in fetal life, making it difficult to identify the cause of defects.

  - Maternal factors

    - Rubella in early pregnancy

    - Alcohol and/or other substance abuse during pregnancy

    - Diabetes mellitus

  - Genetic factors

    - History of congenital heart disease in other family members

    - Trisomy 21 (Down syndrome)

    - Presence of other congenital anomalies or syndromes

- Subjective and Objective Data

CONGENITAL HEART DEFECT	MANIFESTATIONS
Ventricular septal defect (VSD) – A hole in the septum between the right and left ventricle that results in increased pulmonary blood flow (left-to-right shunt)	• Loud, harsh murmur that is not usually audible until pulmonary pressures drop at about 4 to 8 weeks of age • Heart failure • Failure to thrive • Small, possibly asymptomatic defects
Atrial septal defect (ASD) – A hole in the septum between the right and left atria that results in increased pulmonary blood flow (left-to-right shunt)	• Loud, harsh murmur • Mild heart failure • Possible enlarged right atrium • Increased oxygen saturations in the right atrium • Asymptomatic (possibly)
Patent ductus arteriosus (PDA) – A condition in which the normal fetal circulation conduit between the pulmonary artery and the aorta fails to close and results in increased pulmonary blood flow (left-to-right shunt)	• Murmur (machine-hum) • Wide pulse pressure • Bounding pulses • Asymptomatic (possibly)
Pulmonary stenosis – A narrowing of the pulmonary valve or pulmonary artery that results in obstruction of blood flow from the ventricles	• Systolic ejection murmur • Right ventricular enlargement • Exercise intolerance • Cyanosis with severe narrowing

CONGENITAL HEART DEFECT	MANIFESTATIONS
Aortic stenosis – A narrowing at, above, or below the aortic valve	• Murmur • Left ventricular enlargement • Chest pain; exercise intolerance; weak, thready pulses; hypotension; dizziness; and syncope
Coarctation of the aorta – A narrowing of the lumen of the aorta, usually at or near the ductus arteriosus, that results in obstruction of blood flow from the ventricles	• Increased blood pressure and oxygen saturation in the upper extremities compared to the lower extremities • Nosebleeds • Headaches, vertigo, leg pain, weak or absent lower extremity pulses (indicate decreased cardiac output)
Transposition of the great arteries – A condition in which the aorta is connected to the right ventricle instead of the left, and the pulmonary artery is connected to the left ventricle instead of the right	• Murmur • Severe cyanosis appearing hours to days after birth (as the PDA closes) • Cardiomegaly • Heart failure
Tricuspid atresia – A complete closure of the tricuspid valve that results in mixed blood flow	• No blood flow from the right atrium to the right ventricle • Severe cyanosis within hours of birth (increased as the PDA closes) • Heart failure • Chronic hypoxemia • Failure to thrive and growth retardation
Tetralogy of Fallot – Four defects that result in mixed blood flow • Pulmonary stenosis • Ventricular septal defect • Overriding aorta • Right ventricular hypertrophy	• Murmur • Cyanosis, severe dyspnea, clubbing of the fingers, hypercyanotic spells, and acidosis • Polycythemia, clot formation • Child frequently assuming a squatting position (decreases venous return) • Failure to thrive and growth retardation

- ○ Manifestations of heart failure (HF)
    - ▪ Impaired myocardial function
        - □ Tachycardia, murmurs, extra heart sounds (S_3 and S_4), diaphoresis, decreased urinary output, fatigue, generalized pallor or mottling, cool extremities, weak peripheral pulses, slow capillary refill, cardiomegaly, anorexia, and failure to thrive

- Pulmonary congestion
  - Tachypnea, dyspnea, crackles heard in lungs, retractions, nasal flaring, use of accessory muscle, stridor, grunting, recurrent respiratory infections, and exercise intolerance
- Systemic venous congestion
  - Hepatomegaly, enlarged spleen, peripheral edema, ascites, and neck vein distention (not seen in infants)
- Manifestations of hypoxemia
  - Cyanosis, poor weight gain, tachypnea, dyspnea, clubbing, and polycythemia

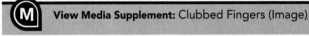

View Media Supplement: Clubbed Fingers (Image)

  - Hypercyanotic spells (blue, or "Tet" spells) are manifested as acute cyanosis and hyperpnea to detect anemia, polycythemia, and electrolyte imbalances.
- Laboratory Tests
  - Hemoglobin (Hgb), hematocrit (Hct), and serum electrolytes
- Diagnostic Procedures
  - ECG monitoring
    - Identifies cardiac dysrhythmias
    - Nursing Actions
      - Assist with the application of electrodes.
      - Assist with maintaining the child in a quiet position.
    - Client Education
      - Tell the child that the test will not be painful.
  - Radiography (chest x-ray)
    - Demonstrates cardiomegaly and increased or decreased pulmonary vascularity associated with congenital anomalies
    - Nursing Actions
      - Assist with positioning the client.
  - Echocardiography
    - Confirms cardiac dysfunction in children without resorting to cardiac catheterization
    - Nursing Actions
      - Assist with positioning the child.

- Cardiac catheterization
  - Cardiac catheterization is an invasive test used for diagnosing, repairing some defects, and evaluating dysrhythmias. A radiopaque catheter is peripherally inserted and threaded into the heart with the use of fluoroscopy. A contrast medium (may be iodine-based) is injected, and images of the blood vessels and heart are taken as the medium is diluted and circulated throughout the body.
  - Nursing Actions
    - Preprocedure
      - Review history and physical examination findings. Signs and symptoms of infections, such as a severe diaper rash, may necessitate canceling the procedure if femoral access is required.
      - Check for allergies to iodine and shellfish.
      - Provide age-appropriate teaching.
      - Describe how long the procedure will take, how the child will feel, and what care will be required after the procedure.
      - Provide for NPO status 4 to 6 hr prior to the procedure. (If the procedure is performed as outpatient, be sure the child and family are given instructions in advance.)
      - Obtain baseline vital signs including oxygen saturation.
      - Inform the child and parents that the child will receive medication for sedation prior to the procedure.
    - Postprocedure
      - Monitor cardiac rhythm and vital signs.
      - Check pulses for equality and symmetry.
      - Observe the temperature and color of the skin. A cool extremity with skin that blanches may indicate arterial obstruction.
      - Monitor insertion site (femoral or antecubital area) for bleeding and/or hematoma.
      - Maintain clean dressing.
      - Monitor I&O to monitor adequate urine output, hypovolemia, or dehydration.
      - Monitor for hypoglycemia. Intravenous fluids with dextrose may be necessary.
      - Prevent bleeding by maintaining the affected extremity in a straight position for 4 to 8 hr.
      - Encourage oral intake, starting with clear liquids.
      - Encourage the child to void to promote excretion of the contrast medium.

□ Client Education

▸ Encourage fluid intake to help with the removal of the dye from the body.

▸ Advise children and their parents to monitor the site for infection and bleeding.

Collaborative Care

- Nursing Care

  ○ General Interventions

    ■ Remain calm when providing care.

    ■ Keep children well-hydrated.

    ■ Conserve the child's energy by providing frequent rest periods; clustering care; providing small, frequent meals; bathing PRN; and keeping crying to a minimum in cyanotic children.

    ■ Perform daily weight and I&O to monitor fluid status and nutritional status.

    ■ Monitor heart rate, blood pressure, serum electrolytes, and renal function to assess for complications.

    ■ Provide support and resources for parents to promote developmental growth in the child.

    ■ Monitor family coping and provide support.

    ■ Improve cardiac function by administering prescribed medications.

    ■ Maintain fluid and electrolyte balance.

      □ Administer potassium supplements if prescribed. These may not be indicated if the child is concurrently taking an ACE inhibitor.

      □ Maintain sodium and fluid restrictions if prescribed.

    ■ Decrease workload of the heart.

      □ Maintain bed rest

      □ Position infants in a car seat or hold them at a 45° angle. Keep safety restraints low and loose on the abdomen.

      □ Allow children to sleep with several pillows and instruct them to maintain a semi-Fowler's or Fowler's position while awake.

    ■ Provide for adequate nutrition.

      □ Plan to feed infants using a feeding schedule of every 3 hr. The infant should be rested, which occurs soon after awakening.

      □ Use a soft preemie nipple or a regular nipple with a slit to provide an enlarged opening.

      □ Hold infants in a semi-upright position.

- Allow infants to rest during feedings, taking approximately 30 min to complete the feeding.

- Gavage feed infants if they are unable to consume enough formula or breast milk.

- Increase caloric density of formula gradually from 20 kcal/oz to 30 kcal/oz.

- Encourage mothers who are breastfeeding to alternate feedings with high-density formula or fortified breast milk.

- Increase tissue oxygenation.

  - Provide cool, humidified oxygen via an oxygen hood (or tent), mask, or nasal cannula.

  - Suction the airway as indicated.

  - Monitor oxygen saturation every 2 to 4 hr.

- Medications

  - Digoxin (Lanoxin)

    - Improves myocardial contractility

    - Nursing Actions

      - Monitor the pulse and withhold the medication as ordered. Generally if an infant's pulse is less than 90/min, the medication should be withheld. In children, the medication should be withheld if the pulse is less than 70/min.

      - Monitor for toxicity as evidenced by bradycardia, dysrhythmias, nausea, vomiting, or anorexia.

      - Monitor serum digoxin levels.

  - Captopril (Capoten) or enalapril (Vasotec)

    - Angiotensin-converting enzyme (ACE) inhibitors reduce afterload by causing vasodilation, resulting in decreased pulmonary and systemic vascular resistance.

    - Nursing Considerations

      - Monitor blood pressure before and after the medication is administered.

      - Monitor for signs of hyperkalemia.

    - Client Education

      - Instruct parents to monitor blood pressure frequently.

  - Furosemide (Lasix) or chlorothiazide (Diuril)

    - Potassium-wasting diuretics rid the body of excess fluid and sodium.

- ■ Nursing Considerations
  - ☐ Monitor intake and output.
  - ☐ Monitor for signs of hypokalemia.
  - ☐ Monitor weight daily.
- Interdisciplinary Care
  - ○ Nutritional Services involvement to further evaluate dietary concerns.
- Care After Discharge
  - ○ Client Education
    - ■ Cardiac catheterization
      - ☐ Reinforce to families how to monitor for possible complications (bleeding, infection, thrombosis).
      - ☐ Limit activity for 24 hr.
      - ☐ Encourage fluids.
    - ■ Digoxin administration
      - ☐ Take apical pulse for 1 min prior to medication administration. Withhold the medication and notify the provider if pulse is lower than specified rate.
      - ☐ Administer digoxin every 12 hr or as prescribed.
      - ☐ Direct oral elixir toward the side and back of mouth when administering.
      - ☐ Give water following administration to prevent tooth decay if the child has teeth.
      - ☐ If a dose is missed, do not give an extra dose or increase the next dose.
      - ☐ If children vomit, do not re-administer the dose.
      - ☐ Observe for signs of digoxin toxicity (decreased heart rate, decreased appetite, nausea, and/or vomiting). Notify the provider if these occur.
      - ☐ Keep the medication in a locked cabinet.
    - ■ Diuretic administration
      - ☐ Mix the oral elixir in a small amount of juice to disguise the bitter taste and prevent intestinal irritation.
      - ☐ Observe for side effects of diuretics, which may include nausea, vomiting, and diarrhea.
      - ☐ Observe for signs and symptoms of serum potassium imbalances (muscle weakness, irritability, excessive drowsiness, increased or decreased heart rate).
    - ■ Encourage children to eat foods high in potassium, such as bran cereals, potatoes, tomatoes, bananas, melons, oranges, and orange juice.

- Instruct families to monitor weight daily.
- Instruct families to report signs and symptoms of worsening heart failure, such as increased sweating and decreased urinary output (fewer wet diapers or less frequent toileting).

- Client Outcomes

  o The child will maintain an adequate cardiac output to maintain activities of daily living.

  o The child will maintain appropriate weight.

Complications

- Potential cardiac catheterization complications and interventions

  o Nausea, vomiting

  o Low-grade fever

  o Loss of pulse in the catheterized extremity

  o Transient dysrhythmias

  o Acute hemorrhage from entry site

  o Nursing Actions

    - Apply direct continuous pressure at 2.5 cm (1 in) above the catheter entry site to center pressure over the location of the vessel puncture.
    - Position children flat to reduce the gravitational effect on the rate of bleeding.
    - Notify the provider immediately.
    - Prepare for the possible administration of replacement fluids and/or medication to control emesis.

  o Client Education

    - Instruct families to monitor for signs of infection and bleeding.

- Hypoxemia

  o A hypercyanotic spell can result in severe hypoxemia, which leads to cerebral hypoxemia, and should be treated as an emergency.

  o Nursing Actions

    - Immediately place children in the knee-chest position, attempt to calm them, and call for help.

- Bacterial endocarditis or subacute bacterial endocarditis (SBE)

    ○ Children with congenital or acquired heart disease are at increased risk for infection of the valves or lining of the heart.

    ○ Children should follow the American Heart Association's recommendations for bacterial endocarditis prophylaxis. These include receiving prophylactic antibiotic therapy prior to dental and surgical procedures (dental extractions, endodontic surgery, surgical procedures that involve the respiratory or gastrointestinal mucosa).

    ○ Causative organisms include *Streptococcus viridians* and *Staphylococcus aureus*.

    ○ Nursing Actions

        ▪ Tell children and their families that intravenous antibiotics will be necessary for approximately 8 weeks.

    ○ Client Education

        ▪ Counsel families about the need for prophylactic antibiotics prior to dental extractions (endodontic surgery, surgical procedures that involve the respiratory or gastrointestinal mucosa).

- Heart failure requiring transplant

    ○ Cardiomyopathy and congenital heart disease are causes of heart failure.

    ○ Nursing Actions

        ▪ Maintain pharmacological support as ordered (oxygen, diuretics, digoxin, afterload reducers such as ACE inhibitors).

        ▪ Provide family and child support.

    ○ Client Education

        ▪ Reinforce regarding the importance of adhering to the medication regimen.

        ▪ Inform children and their families about infection control precautions.

RHEUMATIC FEVER

 Overview

- Rheumatic fever is an inflammatory disease that occurs as a reaction to Group A β-hemolytic streptococcus (GABHS) infection of the throat.

Data Collection

- Risk Factors

    ○ Rheumatic fever usually occurs within 2 to 6 weeks following an untreated or partially treated upper respiratory infection (strep throat) with GABHS.

- Subjective and Objective Data

  o History of recent upper respiratory infection

  o Fever

  o Fatigue

  o Sore throat

  o Activity intolerance

  o Poor appetite

  o Tachycardia, cardiomegaly, prolonged PR interval, new or changed heart murmur, muffled heart sounds, pericardial friction rub, and reports of chest pain, which may indicate carditis

  o Nontender, subcutaneous nodules over bony prominences

  o Large joints (knees, elbows, ankles, wrists, shoulders) that have painful swelling indicating polyarthritis

    ▪ Symptoms last a few days and then disappear without treatment, frequently returning in another joint.

  o Pink, nonpruritic macular rash on the trunk and inner surfaces of extremities that appears and disappears rapidly, indicating erythema marginatum.

  o CNS involvement (chorea) including involuntary, purposeless muscle movements; muscle weakness; involuntary facial movements; difficulty performing fine motor activities; labile emotions; and random, uncoordinated movements of the extremities

  o Irritability, poor concentration, and behavioral problems

  o Laboratory Tests

    ▪ Throat culture for GABHS

    ▪ Blood samples

      □ Elevated or rising serum antistreptolysin-O (ASO) titer – Most reliable

      □ Elevated C-reactive protein (CRP) or erythrocyte sedimentation rate (ESR) – In response to an inflammatory reaction

  o Diagnostic Procedures

    ▪ Cardiac function

      □ ECG to reveal the presence of conduction disturbances and to evaluate the function of the heart and valves

      □ Nursing Actions

        ‣ Position children correctly for the procedure.

      □ Client Education

        ‣ Explain the need for decreased movement during the procedure.

- The diagnosis of rheumatic fever is made on the basis of modified Jones criteria. The child should demonstrate the presence of two major criteria or the presence of one major and two minor criteria following an acute infection with GABHS infection.
  - □ Major criteria
    - ▸ Carditis
    - ▸ Subcutaneous nodules
    - ▸ Polyarthritis
    - ▸ Rash (erythema marginatum)
    - ▸ Chorea
  - □ Minor criteria
    - ▸ Fever
    - ▸ Arthralgia

Collaborative Care

- Medications
  - ○ Penicillin (Pen V) or erythromycin (EryPed)
    - Administer antibiotics as prescribed to eliminate the streptococcal infection.
    - Nursing Considerations
      - □ Observe children for signs of an allergic response (anaphylaxis, hives, rashes). Monitor for side effects such as nausea, vomiting, or diarrhea.
    - Client Education
      - □ Stress the importance of finishing the entire course of the medication.
- Care After Discharge
  - ○ Client Education
    - Reinforce with children and their families the importance of completing the entire 10- to 14-day course of antibiotics as prescribed, even if the child starts to feel better after a few doses.
    - Promote rest and adequate nutrition.
    - Provide information and reassurance related to the development of chorea and its self-limiting nature.
    - Follow the provider's prescribed prophylactic treatment regimen, which may include one of the following: two daily oral doses of 200,000 units of penicillin, a monthly intramuscular injection of 1.2 million units of penicillin G, or a daily oral dose of 1 g of sulfadiazine (Microsulfon). The length of prophylaxis treatment may vary but may be a minimum of 5 years or until 18 years of age.

o   Follow-up

- Seek medical care if infection recurrence is suspected.

- Obtain antibiotic prophylaxis therapy for all dental work and invasive procedures.

- Arrange for medical follow-up every 5 years.

Complications

- Rheumatic heart disease

  o   Nursing Actions

  - Monitor for cardiac rate, rhythm, and presence of murmurs.

  - Prepare children for valve replacement.

  o   Client Education

  - Encourage children and their families to adhere to medical follow-up care.

(A) APPLICATION EXERCISES

1. A nurse is collecting data on an infant with congenital heart disease. Which of the following should the nurse recognize as a manifestation of heart failure? (Select all that apply.)

    _____ Bradycardia

    _____ Cool extremities

    _____ Peripheral edema

    _____ Increased urinary output

    _____ Nasal flaring

2. A nurse is reinforcing instructions given to the mother of a 10-year-old who received a prescription for captopril (Capoten). Which of the following information about this medication should the nurse review with the child's mother?

    A. "Do not allow your child to drink anything for 30 min after the captopril is administered."

    B. "This medication increases heart rate to improve the pumping action of the heart."

    C. "It is important to check your child's blood pressure frequently."

    D. "It is necessary to take and record your child's weight daily."

3. A nurse is caring for a 2-year-old child who is to undergo a diagnostic cardiac catheterization for cardiac defects. Which of the following is an appropriate nursing action when providing care for the child?

    A. Maintain NPO status for 12 hr prior to the procedure.

    B. Obtain oxygen saturation level as part of vital signs.

    C. Check for specific allergies to penicillin.

    D. Insert an indwelling urinary catheter.

4. Match each of the following diagnostic tests performed on a child who has a cardiac disorder with the purpose of the test.

_____	Electrocardiogram (ECG)	A. Identify causative organism.
_____	Echocardiography	B. Identify altered pulmonary or cardiac structures.
_____	Chest x-ray	C. Confirm cardiac dysfunction.
_____	Throat culture	D. Identify heart dysrhythmias.

5. Rheumatic fever is an inflammatory disease that occurs as a reaction to _____.

6. The medications commonly used to treat rheumatic fever are _____.

7. Describe the position that children with Tetralogy of Fallot assume that improves blood flow to the upper body.

APPLICATION EXERCISES ANSWER KEY

1. A nurse is collecting data on an infant with congenital heart disease. Which of the following should the nurse recognize as a manifestation of heart failure? (Select all that apply.)

	Bradycardia
X	**Cool extremities**
X	**Peripheral edema**
	Increased urinary output
X	**Nasal flaring**

   Impaired cardiac function may manifest as cool extremities, tachycardia, and decreased urinary output. Systemic venous congestion may manifest as pulmonary edema, and pulmonary congestion may manifest as nasal flaring.

    NCLEX® Connection: Physiological Adaptations, Basic Pathophysiology

2. A nurse is reinforcing instructions given to the mother of a 10-year-old who received a prescription for captopril (Capoten). Which of the following information about this medication should the nurse review with the child's mother?

   A. "Do not allow your child to drink anything for 30 min after the captopril is administered."

   B. "This medication increases heart rate to improve the pumping action of the heart."

   C. "It is important to check your child's blood pressure frequently."

   D. "It is necessary to take and record your child's weight daily."

   Captopril (Capoten) is an angiotensin-converting enzyme (ACE) inhibitor which reduces afterload, thus decreasing pulmonary and systemic resistance. Instruct parents to monitor their child's blood pressure frequently. Giving the medication with food and fluids and monitoring weight is not a priority.

    NCLEX® Connection: Pharmacological Therapies, Expected Actions/Outcomes

3. A nurse is caring for a 2-year-old child who is to undergo a diagnostic cardiac catheterization for cardiac defects. Which of the following is an appropriate nursing action when providing care for the child?

   A. Maintain NPO status for 12 hr prior to the procedure.

   B. Obtain oxygen saturation level as part of vital signs.

   C. Check for specific allergies to penicillin.

   D. Insert an indwelling urinary catheter.

   Obtaining oxygen saturation is included when obtaining vital signs prior to the procedure. The nurse should maintain NPO status for 4 to 6 hr, check for specific allergies to shellfish and iodine, observe for signs and symptoms of infections, and reinforce teaching that has been done. It is not necessary to insert an indwelling urinary catheter for this procedure.

 NCLEX® Connection: Reduction of Risk Potential, Potential for Complications of Diagnostic Tests/Treatments/Procedures

4. Match each of the following diagnostic tests performed on a child who has a cardiac disorder with the purpose of the test.

__D__	Electrocardiogram (ECG)	A. Identify causative organism.
__C__	Echocardiography	B. Identify altered pulmonary or cardiac structures.
__B__	Chest x-ray	C. Confirm cardiac dysfunction.
__A__	Throat culture	D. Identify heart dysrhythmias.

 NCLEX® Connection: Reduction of Risk Potential, Diagnostic Tests

5. Rheumatic fever is an inflammatory disease that occurs as a reaction to group A beta hemolytic streptococcus (GABHS) of the throat.

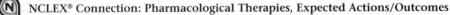 NCLEX® Connection: Physiological Adaptation, Basic Pathophysiology

6. The medications commonly used to treat rheumatic fever are penicillin (Pen V) and erythromycin (Ery-Ped).

NCLEX® Connection: Pharmacological Therapies, Expected Actions/Outcomes

7. Describe the position that children with Tetralogy of Fallot assume that improves blood flow to the upper body.

   Children will squat or draw their knees up tightly to their chest reducing blood flow to the lower extremities.

NCLEX® Connection: Reduction of Risk Potential, Potential for Alterations in Body Systems

UNIT 2	NURSING CARE OF CHILDREN WITH SYSTEM DISORDERS
Section:	Cardiovascular and Hematologic Disorders
Chapter 20	Hematologic Disorders

Overview

- Blood disorders that may affect children include:

  - Epistaxis

  - Iron deficiency anemia

  - Sickle cell anemia

  - Hemophilia

EPISTAXIS

Overview

- Epistaxis is common in childhood.

- Epistaxis may be spontaneous or induced by trauma to the nose.

- Epistaxis may produce anxiety for the child and parents.

- Epistaxis is rarely an emergency.

Data Collection

- Risk Factors

  - Trauma, such as picking or rubbing the nose, may cause mucous membranes in the nose, which are vascular and fragile, to tear and bleed.

  - Low humidity, allergic rhinitis, an upper respiratory virus, blunt injury, or a foreign body in the nose may all precipitate a nosebleed.

  - Medications, such as antihistamines that dry mucous membranes, may increase the number of nosebleeds.

  - Medications that affect clotting factors, such as warfarin (Coumadin), may increase bleeding.

  - Epistaxis may be the result of underlying diseases (Von Willebrand's disease, hemophilia, idiopathic thrombocytopenia purpura [ITP], leukemia).

- Subjective Data

  - History of bleeding gums or blood in body fluids and/or stool

  - History of trauma, illness, allergies, or placing foreign bodies in the nose

- Objective Data

  - Physical Assessment Findings

    - Active bleeding from nose

    - Restlessness and agitation

Collaborative Care

- Nursing Care

  - Maintain a calm demeanor with children and their families.

  - Have children sit up with the head tilted slightly forward to promote draining of blood out of the nose instead of down the back of the throat. Swallowing blood can promote coughing and lead to nausea, vomiting, and diarrhea.

  - Apply pressure to the lower nose, or instruct children to use the thumb and forefinger to press the nares together for 5 to 10 min.

  - If needed, cotton or tissue can be packed into the side of the nose that is bleeding.

  - Encourage children to breathe through the mouth while the nose is bleeding.

  - Apply ice across the bridge of the nose if possible.

  - Keep children from rubbing or picking their nose after bleeding is stopped.

- Care After Discharge

  - Client Education

    - Remind parents to keep young children's fingernails short.

    - Recommend use of a humidifier during the dry winter months.

    - Instruct children to open their mouth when sneezing.

    - For recurrences, remind children to sit up and slightly forward so blood does not flow down the throat and cause coughing.

    - Inform families that bleeding may last 20 to 30 min.

- Client Outcomes

  - The child will have decreased episodes of epistaxis.

Complications

- Excessive Bleeding

  - Nursing Actions

    - Provide support to children during cauterization or packing.

  - Client Education

    - Instruct families to seek medical care if bleeding lasts longer than 30 min or is caused by an injury/trauma.

IRON DEFICIENCY ANEMIA

Overview

- Iron deficiency anemia is the most common anemia in children ages 6 months to 2 years. It is also commonly diagnosed in adolescents 12 to 20 years of age.

- Iron deficiency anemia usually results from an inadequate dietary supply of iron.

- Manifestations are related to the degree of anemia and the result of decreased oxygen to the tissues.

- Prolonged anemia can lead to:

  - Growth retardation

  - Developmental delays, fatigue, tachycardia and irritability

Data Collection

- Risk Factors

  - Premature birth resulting in decreased iron stores

  - Use of non-iron-fortified infant formula

  - Excessive intake of cows' milk in toddlers

    - Milk is not a good source of iron.

    - Milk takes the place of iron-rich solid foods.

  - Malabsorption disorders due to prolonged diarrhea

  - Poor dietary intake of iron

  - Periods of rapid growth, such as adolescence

  - Increased iron requirements (blood loss)

  - Infection

  - Chronic disorders (folate deficiency, sickle cell anemia, hemophilia)

- Subjective and Objective Data

  o Shortness of breath

  o Tachycardia

  o Dizziness or fainting with exertion

  o Pallor

  o Nail bed deformities (concave or "spoon" fingernails)

  o Fatigue, irritability, and muscle weakness

  o Impaired healing, loss of skin elasticity, and thinning of hair

  o Abdominal pain, nausea, vomiting, and loss of appetite

  o Low-grade fever

  o Systolic heart murmur and/or heart failure

  o Laboratory Tests

NORMAL VALUES		
AGE	HGB	HCT
2 months	9.0 to 14.0 g/dL	28% to 42%
6 to 12 years	11.5 to 15.5 g/dL	35% to 45%
12 to 18 years	13.0 to 16.0 g/dL (male) 12.0 to 16.0 g/dL (female)	37% to 49% (male) 36% to 46% (female)

  - CBC – Decreased RBC count, decreased Hgb, and decreased Hct

  - RBC indices – Decreased, indicating microcytic/hypochromic RBCs

    □ Mean corpuscular volume (MVC) – Average size of RBC

    □ Mean corpuscular Hgb (MCH) – Average weight of RBC

    □ Mean corpuscular hemoglobin concentration (MCHC) – Amount of Hgb relative to size of cell

  - Reticulocyte count – May be decreased (indicates bone marrow production of RBCs)

Collaborative Care

- Nursing Care

  o Encourage breastfeeding for infants for first 12 months of life.

  o Recommend iron-fortified formula for infants who are not being breastfed.

  o Modify the infant's diet to include high iron, vitamin C, and protein content.

- ○ Restrict milk intake in toddlers.
  - ▪ Limit milk intake to 32 oz (950 mL) per day.
  - ▪ Avoid giving milk until after a meal.
  - ▪ Do not allow toddlers to carry bottles or cups of milk.
- ○ Allow for frequent rest periods.
- • Medications
  - ○ Iron Supplements
    - ▪ Nursing Considerations
      - □ Give 1 hr before or 2 hr after milk or antacid to prevent decreased absorption.
      - □ Inform children and parents that gastrointestinal side effects (diarrhea, constipation, nausea) are common at the start of therapy and that these will decrease over time.
      - □ Administer iron supplements on an empty stomach. However, administration may not be tolerated during initial treatment and may be given after meals.
      - □ Give vitamin C to help increase absorption.
      - □ Mix liquid iron preparation with a small amount of juice or water.
      - □ Use a straw with liquid preparation to prevent staining of teeth. After administration, children should rinse their mouths with water.
      - □ Remind parents not to crush sustained-release tablets.
      - □ Remind children not to chew sustained-release tablets.
      - □ Evenly distribute doses throughout the day to maximize RBC production by providing bone marrow with a continuous supply of iron.
      - □ Use a Z-track into deep muscle for parenteral injections. Do not massage after injection.
    - ▪ Client Education
      - □ Educate children and families to expect stools to be black.
- • Care After Discharge
  - ○ Client Education
    - ▪ Advise families that diarrhea, constipation, or nausea may occur at the start of therapy, but these side effects are usually self-limiting.
    - ▪ Provide information regarding appropriate iron administration
    - ▪ Encourage adequate intake of fiber and fluids to prevent constipation.

- Encourage foods high in iron
  - ☐ Infants – Cereal and iron-fortified formula
  - ☐ Older children – Dried legumes; dried fruits; nuts; green, leafy vegetables; iron-fortified breads; iron-fortified flour; poultry; and red meat
- Instruct parents to store iron in a child-proof bottle out of the reach of children to help prevent accidental overdose. Suggest parents keep only a one-month supply of iron in the house as a precautionary measure against accidental overdose.
- Encourage parents to allow children to rest.
- Inform parents that the length of treatment will be determined by response to the treatment. Hgb levels can take up to 3 months to increase.
- Instruct parents to return for follow-up laboratory tests to determine the effectiveness of treatment.

- Client Outcomes
  - ○ The child's RBC count will be within the expected reference range.
  - ○ The child will have increased energy and demonstrate the ability to perform ADLs.

Complications

- Heart failure
  - ○ Heart failure can develop due to the increased demand on the heart to increase oxygen to tissues.
  - ○ Nursing Actions
    - Monitor cardiac rhythm.
    - Give cardiac medications as prescribed.
  - ○ Client Education
    - Inform families about the signs and symptoms of heart failure.
    - Reinforce how to monitor pulse rates.

SICKLE CELL ANEMIA

 Overview

- Sickle cell disease (SCD) is a group of diseases in which there is abnormal sickle hemoglobin S (HbS).

- Manifestations and complications of sickle cell anemia are the result of RBC sickling, which leads to increased blood viscosity, obstruction of blood flow, and tissue hypoxia.

  ○ Manifestations of sickle cell anemia are not usually apparent before 4 to 6 months of age, due to the presence of fetal Hgb in infants.

    ■ The RBCs have the ability to develop a sickled shape. This is usually precipitated by increased oxygen demands (infection, emotional stress, pain) or decreased levels of oxygen (pulmonary infections, high altitude, cold stress in winter months).

- Tissue hypoxia causes tissue ischemia, which results in pain.

- Increased destruction of RBCs also occurs.

- Sickle cell crisis is the exacerbation of sickle cell anemia.

- Sickle cell anemia is usually diagnosed soon after birth. If not, toddlers or preschoolers will present in crisis following an infection of the respiratory or GI tract.

 View Media Supplement: Sickle Cell Anemia (Image)

Data Collection

- Risk Factors

  ○ Sickle cell anemia (SCA) is the most common type of this group and is found primarily in African-Americans. Other forms of SCD may affect individuals of Mediterranean, Indian, or Middle Eastern descent.

  ○ SCA is an autosomal recessive genetic disorder in which normal hemoglobin A (HbA) is partially or completely replaced with HbS.

  ○ Children with sickle cell trait do not manifest the disease but can pass the trait to their offspring.

- Subjective and Objective Data

  ○ Family history of sickle cell anemia or sickle cell trait

  ○ Reports of pain, crisis, and management

  ○ Shortness of breath/fatigue

  ○ Tachycardia

  ○ Pallor or jaundice

  ○ Nail bed deformities

  ○ Lethargy, irritability, and muscle weakness

  ○ Impaired healing, loss of skin elasticity, and thinning of hair

  ○ Abdominal pain, nausea, vomiting, and loss of appetite

CRISIS	MANIFESTATIONS

Vaso-occlusive (painful episode resulting from ischemia)
• Usually lasts 4 to 6 days
	• Acute
	  ○ Severe abdominal pain
	  ○ Swollen, extremely painful joints, hands, and feet
	  ○ Anorexia, vomiting, and fever
	  ○ Hematuria
	  ○ Obstructive jaundice and hepatic coma
	  ○ Visual disturbances
	  ○ Priapism in males
	• Chronic
	  ○ Increased risk of respiratory infections and/or osteomyelitis
	  ○ Retinal detachment and blindness
	  ○ Systolic murmurs
	  ○ Renal failure and enuresis
	  ○ Liver failure
	  ○ Seizures
	  ○ Deformities of the skeleton

Sequestration	• Excessive pooling of blood in the liver (hepatomegaly) and spleen (splenomegaly) • Tachycardia, dyspnea, weakness, pallor, leading to circulatory collapse
Aplastic	• Extreme anemia as a result of decreased RBC production
Hyperhemolytic	• Increased rate of RBC destruction leading to anemia, jaundice, and/or reticulocytosis

- ○ Laboratory Tests
  - ▪ CBC to detect anemia
  - ▪ Sickledex (sickle solubility test) – A screening tool that will detect the presence of HbS but will not differentiate the trait from the disease
  - ▪ Hgb electrophoresis – Separates the various forms of Hgb and is the definitive diagnosis of sickle cell anemia
- ○ Diagnostic Procedures
  - ▪ Transcranial Doppler (TCD) test
    - ▫ Use to assess intracranial vascular flow and detect the risk for cerebrovascular accident (CVA).
    - ▫ Perform this test annually for children ages 2 to 16 who have SCA.

Collaborative Care

- Nursing Care

  - Promote rest to decrease oxygen consumption of the tissue.

  - Administer oxygen as prescribed if hypoxia is present.

  - Maintain fluid and electrolyte balance.

    - Monitor I&O.

    - Give oral fluids.

    - Monitor IV fluids with electrolyte replacement.

  - Pain Management

    - Use an interdisciplinary approach.

    - Treat mild to moderate pain with acetaminophen (Tylenol) or ibuprofen (Advil). Manage severe pain with opioid analgesics.

    - Apply comfort measures, such as warm packs to painful joints.

  - Assist in monitoring clients who are receiving blood.

  - Treat and prevent infection.

    - Administer antibiotics.

    - Perform frequent hand hygiene.

    - Give oral prophylactic penicillin.

    - Administer immunizations to include pneumococcal vaccine (PVC), meningococcal vaccine (MCV4), and yearly seasonal influenza vaccine.

  - Monitor and report laboratory results – RBCs, Hgb, Hct, and liver function

  - Encourage passive range-of-motion exercises to prevent venous stasis.

- Medications

  - Opioids – Codeine, morphine sulfate, oxycodone, hydrocodone (Dilaudid), and methadone (Dolophine)

    - Opioids provide analgesia for pain management.

    - Nursing Considerations

      - Administer orally (immediate or sustained release) or by IV route.

      - Administer on a regular schedule to maintain good pain control.

      - Assist with clients who are receiving patient-controlled analgesia.

    - Client Education

      - Reinforce the need to avoid activities that require mental alertness.

- Interdisciplinary Care

  o Participate in interdisciplinary care with the provider, physical therapist, and social worker.

  o Provide information about genetic counseling.

- Care After Discharge

  o Client Education

    - Instruct families to identify signs and symptoms of crisis and infection.

    - Advise families of the importance of promoting rest and adequate nutrition for children.

    - Encourage children and families to maintain good hand hygiene and avoid individuals with colds/infection/viruses.

    - Give specific directions regarding fluid intake requirements, such as how many bottles or glasses of fluid should be consumed daily.

    - Encourage maintenance of up-to-date immunizations.

    - Advise children to wear a medical identification wristband or medical identification tags.

- Client Outcomes

  o The child will have a decrease in the number of crisis occurrences.

  o The child will have good pain control.

Complications

- CVA

  o Nursing Actions

    - Observe for and report signs and symptoms, which include:

      □ Seizures

      □ Abnormal behavior

      □ Weak extremity and/or inability to move an extremity

      □ Slurred speech

      □ Changes in vision

      □ Vomiting

      □ Severe headache

  o Client Education

    - Inform families that blood transfusions should be performed every 3 to 4 weeks following a CVA.

- Acute chest syndrome

    ○ May be life threatening

    ○ Nursing Actions

        ▪ Observe for and report signs and symptoms, which include:

            ☐ Chest pain

            ☐ Fever of 38.9° C (102° F) or higher

            ☐ Congested cough

            ☐ Tachycardia

            ☐ Dyspnea

            ☐ Retractions

            ☐ Decreased oxygen saturations

HEMOPHILIA

Overview

- Hemophilia is a disorder that results in an impaired ability to control bleeding.

- Bleeding time is extended due to lack of clotting factors. Bleeding may be internal or external.

- Manifestations may be present early in infancy but may not be evident until infant begins teething, sitting up, or crawling.

- Parents may observe excessive bruising with minor falls or contact.

- Hemophilia has different levels of severity depending on the percentage of clotting factor a child's body contains. For example, a child with mild hemophilia may have up to 49% of the normal factor VIII in his body, while a person with severe hemophilia has very little factor VIII.

- Both hemophilia A and B are X-linked recessive disorders.

TYPES OF HEMOPHILIA	
HEMOPHILIA A	HEMOPHILIA B
• Deficiency of factor VIII • Also referred to as classic hemophilia • Accounts for 80% of cases	• Deficiency of factor IX • Also referred to as Christmas disease

Data Collection

- Subjective Data

  - Episodes of bleeding, excessive bleeding, reports of joint pain and stiffness, impaired mobility, and activity intolerance

- Objective Data

  - Physical Assessment Findings

    - Active bleeding, which includes bleeding gums, epistaxis, hematuria, and/or tarry stools

    - Hematomas and/or bruising

    - Hemarthrosis as evidenced by joint pain, stiffness, warmth, swelling, redness, loss of range of motion, and deformities

    - Headache, slurred speech, and a decreased level of consciousness

  - Laboratory Tests

    - Prolonged partial thromboplastin time (PPT)

    - Factor-specific assays to determine deficiency

  - Diagnostic Procedures

    - DNA testing

      - Detects classic hemophilia trait in females

Collaborative Care

- Nursing Care

  - Management of bleeding in the hospital

    - Avoid taking temperature rectally.

    - Avoid unnecessary skin punctures and use surgical aseptic technique.

    - Apply pressure for 5 min after injections, venipuncture, or needle sticks.

    - Monitor urine, stool, and nasogastric fluid for occult blood.

    - Control localized bleeding.

      - Administer factor replacement.

      - Observe for side effects, which include headache, flushing, low sodium, and alterations in heart rate and blood pressure.

      - Encourage children to rest and immobilize the affected joints.

      - Elevate and apply ice to the affected joints.

- Medications
  - 1-deamino-8-Δ-arginine vasopressin (DDAVP) is a synthetic form of vasopressin that increases plasma factor VIII (antihemophilic factor [AHF])
    - Effective for mild, but not severe, hemophilia
    - Nursing Considerations
      - May be given prior to dental or surgical procedures
  - Factor VIII, products that contain factor VIII, pooled plasma, and recombinant products
    - Used to prevent and treat hemorrhage
    - Nursing Considerations
      - Assist with the care of children who are receiving an IV infusion.
    - Client Education
      - Instruct children and families that treatment may require numerous doses.
  - Corticosteroids
    - Used to treat hematuria, acute episodes of hemarthrosis, and chronic synovitis
    - Nursing Considerations
      - Monitor for infection and bleeding.
    - Client Education
      - Encourage children and families to maintain good hand hygiene and avoid individuals with colds/infection/viruses.
  - Nonsteroidal anti-inflammatory agents
    - Used to treat chronic synovitis
    - Nursing considerations
      - Monitor for infection.
    - Client Education
      - Encourage children to take the medication with food.
- Interdisciplinary Care
  - Participate in interdisciplinary care with the provider, physical therapist, and social worker.
  - Provide information about genetic counseling.

- Care After Discharge

  - Client Education

    - Reinforce to parents ways to prevent bleeding at home.

      - Place infants or children in a padded crib.

      - Provide a safe home and a play environment that is free of clutter. Place padding on corners of furniture.

      - Dress toddlers in extra layers of clothing to provide additional padding.

      - Set activity restrictions to avoid injury. Acceptable activities include low-contact sports (tennis, swimming, golf). While participating in these activities, children should wear protective equipment.

      - Use soft-bristled toothbrushes.

    - Encourage regular exercise and physical therapy after active bleeding is controlled.

    - Encourage families to maintain up-to-date immunizations.

    - Reinforce the importance of wearing a medical identification wristband or necklace.

    - Reinforce how to identify signs and symptoms of internal bleeding and hemarthrosis.

    - Encourage the family to participate in a support group.

- Client Outcomes

  - The child will have decreased bleeding episodes.

  - The child will be free from injury.

Complications

- Joint deformity (most often elbows, knees, and ankles)

  - Repeated episodes of hemarthrosis (bleeding into joint spaces) lead to impaired range of motion, pain, tenderness, and swelling, which can develop into joint deformities.

  - Nursing Actions

    - Take appropriate measures to rest, immobilize, elevate, and apply ice to the affected joints during active bleeding.

    - Encourage active range of motion after active bleeding is controlled.

    - Encourage maintenance of ideal weight to minimize stress on joints.

    - Encourage maintenance of regular exercise and physical therapy.

(A) APPLICATION EXERCISES

1. A nurse is reinforcing instructions given to a child and his family about epistaxis. Which of the following positions should the nurse remind the child to take when experiencing a nosebleed?

    A. Sit up and lean forward.

    B. Sit up and tilt the head back.

    C. Lie down supine.

    D. Lie in prone position.

2. A nurse is reinforcing teaching to the mother of a child who is being discharged following an episode of epistaxis. Which of the following statements by the mother indicates the need for further teaching?

    A. "I'll keep my son's fingernails short."

    B. "I'll remind my son to keep his mouth closed when he sneezes."

    C. "I will add a humidifier to my shopping list."

    D. "An episode of bleeding could last 20 to 30 minutes."

3. Describe the risk factors for epistaxis.

4. A nurse is discussing the new prescription for liquid oral iron, which was given to the parent of a child who is to begin taking this supplement. Which of the following statements by the parent indicates the need for further teaching?

    A. I should call the doctor if my child has a tarry stool.

    B. I will give my child a glass of citrus juice with the iron to increase the absorption of iron.

    C. I will have the child use a straw when taking this medication to prevent staining the teeth.

    D. I should give the medication between meals to increase iron absorption.

5. A nurse is discussing foods that are a good source of iron with a group of parents. The nurse asks the parents to select luncheon menus that are appropriate. Which of the following menus has the greatest iron content?

LUNCH A	LUNCH B	LUNCH C
• Chili made with ground beef and dried kidney beans • 8 oz trail mix with dried apricots, raisins, and almonds • 8 oz (240 mL) orange drink	• Macaroni and cheese • Iceberg lettuce with dressing • Fresh pear • 8 oz (240 mL) 2% milk	• Peanut butter on white bread • Carrot and celery sticks • 4 graham crackers • 8 oz (240 mL) lemonade

6. Match the following laboratory tests with the condition for which they are a screening or testing method.

_____ Transcranial Doppler Test	1. Presence of HbS
_____ Sickledex	2. Anemia
_____ Hemoglobin electrophoresis	3. CVA
_____ CBC	4. Sickle cell disease

7. A nurse is caring for a child who has acute sickle cell crisis. Identify pharmacological interventions for pain management. (Select all that apply.)

_____ Oxycodone (OxyContin)

_____ A patient-controlled access (PCA) pump

_____ Methadone (Dolophine)

_____ Warm packs

_____ Range-of-motion of extremities

8. Hemophilia A is a disorder characterized by a deficiency of _____.

APPLICATION EXERCISES ANSWER KEY

1. A nurse is reinforcing instructions given to a child and his family about epistaxis. Which of the following positions should the nurse remind the child to take when experiencing a nosebleed?

   A. Sit up and lean forward.

   B. Sit up and tilt the head back.

   C. Lie down supine.

   D. Lie in prone position.

   Sitting up with the head tilted slightly forward promotes drainage of blood out of the nose instead of down the back of the throat. Swallowing blood can promote coughing and lead to nausea, vomiting, and diarrhea. The other positions listed are not effective.

    NCLEX® Connection: Reduction of Risk Potential, Potential for Alterations in Body Systems

2. A nurse is reinforcing teaching to the mother of a child who is being discharged following an episode of epistaxis. Which of the following statements by the mother indicates the need for further teaching?

   A. "I'll keep my son's fingernails short."

   B. "I'll remind my son to keep his mouth closed when he sneezes."

   C. "I will add a humidifier to my shopping list."

   D. "An episode of bleeding could last 20 to 30 minutes."

   Discharge teaching should include keeping the child's fingernails short, use of a humidifier especially during winter months, and a nosebleed episode can last 20 to 30 minutes. The mother should encourage her son to keep his mouth open when sneezing to decrease air pressure within the nasal cavity.

   NCLEX® Connection: Reduction of Risk Potential, Potential for Alterations in Body Systems

3. Describe the risk factors for epistaxis.

   Risk factors for nosebleeds include trauma, which can be due to the child picking or rubbing his nose, fragile nasal tissues that are prone to bleeding, low humidity, allergies, blunt trauma, foreign body, medications such as antihistamines that dry mucous membranes, anticoagulant medications, and underlying bleeding disorders such as leukemia.

   NCLEX® Connection: Physiological Adaptation, Basic Pathophysiology

4. A nurse is discussing the new prescription for liquid oral iron, which was given to the parent of a child who is to begin taking this supplement. Which of the following statements by the parent indicates the need for further teaching?

    A. I should call the doctor if my child has a tarry stool.

    B. I will give my child a glass of citrus juice with the iron to increase the absorption of iron.

    C. I will have the child use a straw when taking this medication to prevent staining the teeth.

    D. I should give the medication between meals to increase iron absorption.

    A tarry stool indicates the dosage of iron is appropriate and the parents do not need to notify the provider about this finding. Instructions related to oral iron administration include giving the medication with orange or citrus juice and between meals to increase the iron absorption. Use of a straw when taking the medication will prevent staining of the teeth.

     NCLEX® Connection: Pharmacological Therapies, Adverse Effects/Contraindications/Side Effects/Interactions

5. A nurse is discussing foods that are a good source of iron with a group of parents. The nurse asks the parents to select luncheon menus that are appropriate. Which of the following menus has the greatest iron content?

LUNCH A	LUNCH B	LUNCH C
• Chili made with ground beef and dried kidney beans • 8 oz trail mix with dried apricots, raisins, and almonds • 8 oz (240 mL) orange drink	• Macaroni and cheese • Iceberg lettuce with dressing • Fresh pear • 8 oz (240 mL) 2% milk	• Peanut butter on white bread • Carrot and celery sticks • 4 graham crackers • 8 oz (240 mL) lemonade

    Lunch A contains the highest iron content because it includes ground beef, kidney beans, dried raisins, apricots, and nuts. Rich sources of iron include dried fruits and legumes, nuts, green, leafy vegetables, chicken, cereals, iron-fortified flour, breads and infant formula, and ground beef. Macaroni and cheese, iceberg lettuce, fresh fruits, carrot and celery sticks, and vanilla wafers are not iron-containing foods. Peanut butter contains some iron, the orange drink and lemonade contain no iron, and milk is calcium-fortified.

     NCLEX® Connection: Basic Care and Comfort, Nutrition and Oral Hydration

6. Match the following laboratory tests with the condition for which they are a screening or testing method.

__3__	Transcranial Doppler Test	1. Presence of HbS
__1__	Sickledex	2. Anemia
__4__	Hemoglobin electrophoresis	3. CVA
__2__	CBC	4. Sickle cell disease

Transcranial Doppler (TCD) is used to diagnose the presence of a cerebrovascular accident (CVA). The Sickledex test is a screening test for sickle cell anemia and trait. Hgb electrophoresis is the definitive test for sickle cell anemia and differentiates it from sickle cell trait. The CBC tests for a variety of general problems, such as anemia.

Ⓝ **NCLEX® Connection: Reduction of Risk Potential, Diagnostic Tests**

7. A nurse is caring for a child who has acute sickle cell crisis. Identify pharmacological interventions for pain management. (Select all that apply.)

__X__	**Oxycodone (OxyContin)**
__X__	**A patient-controlled access (PCA) pump**
__X__	**Methadone (Dolophine)**
__X__	**Warm packs**
_____	Range-of-motion of extremities

Interventions to manage pain should include the use of opioids (oxycodone, methadone) for severe pain. Use a patient-controlled access (PCA) pump if indicated. In addition, warm packs offer comfort to painful joints. Range-of-motion is not appropriate due to the painful, swollen joints of acute sickle cell crisis.

Ⓝ **NCLEX® Connection: Pharmacological Therapies, Pharmacological Pain Management**

8. Hemophilia A is a disorder characterized by a deficiency of **factor VIII**.

Ⓝ **NCLEX® Connection: Physiological Adaptations, Basic Pathophysiology**

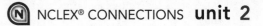

UNIT 2: NURSING CARE OF CHILDREN WITH SYSTEM DISORDERS

Section: Gastrointestinal Disorders

- Acute Infectious Gastrointestinal Disorders

- Gastrointestinal Structural and Inflammatory Disorders

NCLEX® CONNECTIONS

When reviewing the chapters in this section, keep in mind the relevant sections of the NCLEX® outline, in particular:

CLIENT NEEDS: BASIC CARE AND COMFORT

Relevant topics/tasks include:
- Elimination
  - Identify client at risk for impaired elimination.
- Nutrition and Oral Hydration
  - Monitor and provide for nutritional needs of client.

CLIENT NEEDS: REDUCTION OF RISK POTENTIAL

Relevant topics/tasks include:
- Potential for Alterations in Body Systems
  - Reinforce client teaching on methods to prevent complications associated with activity level/diagnosed illness/disease.
- Potential for Complications of Diagnostic Tests/Treatments/Procedures
  - Reinforce teaching to prevent complications due to client diagnostic tests/treatments/procedures.
- Potential for Complications from Surgical Procedures and Health Alterations
  - Identify client response to surgery or health alterations.

CLIENT NEEDS: PHYSIOLOGICAL ADAPTATION

Relevant topics/tasks include:
- Alterations in Body Systems
  - Identify signs and symptoms of infections.
- Fluid and Electrolyte Imbalances
  - Monitor client response to interventions to correct fluid and/or electrolyte imbalance.
- Medical Emergencies
  - Notify primary health care provider about client unexpected response/emergency situation.

UNIT 2	NURSING CARE OF CHILDREN WITH SYSTEM DISORDERS
Section:	Gastrointestinal Disorders

Chapter 21 Acute Infectious Gastrointestinal Disorders

Overview

- Diarrhea may be mild to severe and it may be acute or chronic. It may result in mild to severe dehydration.

  - Acute diarrhea may follow secondary to an upper respiratory or urinary tract infection or antibiotic use.

  - Acute infectious diarrhea (infectious gastroenteritis) is a result of various bacterial, viral, and/or parasitic infections. The onset of gastroenteritis is often abrupt with rapid loss of fluids and electrolytes from persistent vomiting and diarrhea.

  - Chronic diarrhea is related to chronic conditions (malabsorption syndrome, lactose intolerance, food allergies, inflammatory bowel disease).

Data Collection

- Risk Factors

  - Exposure to causative agent, recent travel

  - Risk factors for *Enterobius vermicularis* (pinworm) include crowded places (school, day care) or crowded living spaces (such as more than one family living together).

- Subjective and Objective Data

  - Reports of fatigue, malaise, change in behavior, change in stool pattern, poor appetite, weight loss, and pain

  - Monitor for signs and symptoms of dehydration.

    - Dry, pale skin

    - Cool lips

    - Dry mucous membranes

    - Decreased skin turgor

    - Diminished urinary output

    - Concentrated urine

    - Thirst

- Rapid pulse
- Sunken fontanels
- Decreased blood pressure

SIGNS AND SYMPTOMS OF SPECIFIC PATHOGENS		
PATHOGEN	MANIFESTATIONS	TRANSMISSION/INCUBATION
Rotavirus	• Commonly causes diarrhea in young children • Induces fever and vomiting for 2 days • Produces watery diarrhea for 5 to 7 days	• Transmission is fecal-oral. • The incubation period is 48 hr.
Escherichia coli (E. coli)	• Causes watery diarrhea for 1 to 2 days, followed by abdominal cramping and bloody diarrhea • Could lead to hemolytic uremic syndrome (HUS)	• Transmission depends on the strain of *E. coli*. • The incubation period is 3 to 4 days.
Salmonella nontyphoidal groups	• Causes nausea, vomiting, abdominal cramping, bloody diarrhea, and fever (may be afebrile in infants) • Causes headache, confusion, drowsiness, and seizures • May lead to meningitis or septicemia	• Transmission occurs from person to person, but also from undercooked meats and poultry. • The incubation period is 6 to 72 hr.
Clostridium difficile (C. difficile)	• Causes mild, watery diarrhea for a few days • May cause less severe symptoms in children than adults • May cause leukocytosis, hypoalbuminemia, and high fever in certain children • May lead to pseudomembranous colitis	• Transmission occurs through contact with colonized spores, and it is commonly transmitted in health care settings. • There is a nonspecified incubation period.
Clostridium botulinum (C. botulinum)	• Causes abdominal pain, cramping, and diarrhea • May cause respiratory compromise or CNS symptoms	• Transmission occurs through contaminated food products. • The incubation period is 12 to 26 hr.

SIGNS AND SYMPTOMS OF SPECIFIC PATHOGENS		
PATHOGEN	MANIFESTATIONS	TRANSMISSION/INCUBATION
Staphylococcus	• Causes food poisoning resulting in severe diarrhea, nausea, and vomiting	• Transmission occurs through food that is inadequately cooked or refrigerated. • The incubation period is 1 to 8 hr.
Enterobius vermicularis (pinworm) is a parasitic worm that is white, threadlike, and approximately ⅓ to ½ inch long.	• Causes perianal itching, enuresis, sleeplessness, restlessness, and irritability due to itching	• Transmission is fecal-oral with infestation beginning when eggs are inhaled or swallowed.

Giardia lamblia	• Causes the following in children 5 years of age or younger:
	  o Diarrhea
	  o Vomiting
	  o Anorexia
	• Causes the following in older children:
	  o Abdominal cramps
	  o Intermittent loose, malodorous, pale, greasy stools
		• Transmission occurs from person to person.
		• The nonmotile stage of protozoa may survive in the environment for months.

- o Laboratory Tests
  - ▪ Perform a CBC with differential to determine anemia and/or infection.
  - ▪ Hct, Hgb, BUN, creatinine, and urine specific gravity levels are usually elevated with dehydration.
  - ▪ Stool test for occult blood.
  - ▪ Perform a urinalysis.
- o Diagnostic Procedures
  - ▪ Tape test
    - □ A tape test should be performed to check for *Enterobius vermicularis*.
    - □ Nursing Actions
      - ▸ Provide instructions to the parents.

□ Client Education

▸ Tell the parents to place transparent tape over the child's anus at night. The tape should be removed the following morning prior to the child toileting or bathing. If possible, have the parent apply the tape after the child has gone to sleep and remove it before the child awakens.

▸ Inform the parents that the specimen should be brought to the laboratory for microscopic evaluation.

▸ Teach the parents to use good hand hygiene during this procedure.

■ Infectious gastroenteritis

□ Rotavirus – Enzyme immunoassay (stool sample)

□ *E. coli* – Sorbitol-MacConkey agar (stool sample)

□ Salmonella – Gram-stained stool culture

□ *C. difficile* – Stool culture

□ *C. botulinum* – Blood and stool culture

□ Staphylococcus – Identification of organism in stool, blood, food, or aspirate

□ *G. lamblia* – Enzyme immunoassay (stool sample)

Collaborative Care

● Nursing Care

○ Obtain baseline height and weight.

○ Obtain daily weights at the same time each day.

○ Avoid taking a rectal temperature.

○ Assess and monitor I&O (urine and stool).

○ Monitor children receiving IV replacement fluids.

○ Monitor children receiving IV antibiotics.

○ Administer oral rehydration therapy (ORT).

■ Start replacement with an oral replacement solution (ORS) of 75 to 90 mEq of Na$^+$/L at 40 to 50 mL/kg over 4 hr.

■ Determine the need for further rehydration after initial replacement.

□ Initiate maintenance therapy with ORS of 40 to 60 mEq of Na$^+$/L and limit to 150 mL/kg/day.

▸ Give ORS alternately with appropriate intake.

▷ Give infants water, breast milk, or lactose-free formula if supplementary fluid is needed.

▷ Older children may resume their regular diets for additional intake.

▸ Replace each diarrheal stool with 10 mL/kg of ORS for ongoing diarrhea. If stool volume is known, use a 1:1 replacement of ORS.

- Medications

  - Metronidazole (Flagyl) and tinidazole (Tindamax)

    - Indicated for *C. difficile* and *G. lamblia*

    - Nursing Considerations

      - Monitor for allergies.

      - Monitor for GI upset.

    - Client Education

      - Instruct children and their families to take the medication as prescribed and to report any GI disturbances.

  - Mebendazole (Vermox), albendazole (Albenza), and pyrantel pamoate (Pin-Rid, Antiminth)

    - Indicated for *Enterobius vermicularis*

    - Nursing Considerations

      - Administer in a single dose that may need to be repeated in 2 weeks.

      - Administer mebendazole for children older than 2 years of age.

    - Client Education

      - Instruct families that the medication may need to be repeated within 3 weeks.

- Care After Discharge

  - Client Education

    - Have the parents inform the child's school or day care center of the infection/ infestation. The child should stay home during the incubation period.

    - Reinforce to families to use commercially prepared ORS when the child experiences diarrhea. Foods and fluids to avoid include:

      - Fruit juices, carbonated sodas, and gelatin, which all have high carbohydrate content, low electrolyte content, and a high osmolality

      - Caffeine, due to its mild diuretic effect

      - Chicken or beef broth, which has too much sodium and not enough carbohydrates

      - Bananas, rice, applesauce, and toast (BRAT diet)

        ‣ This diet has low nutritional value, high carbohydrate content, and low electrolytes.

    - Provide frequent skin care to prevent skin breakdown.

    - Teach families how to avoid the spread of infectious diseases.

      - Change bed linens and underwear daily for several days.

      - Cleanse toys and child care areas thoroughly to prevent further spread or reinfestation.

- ◻ Keep toys separate and avoid shaking linens to prevent the spread of disease.

- ◻ Shower frequently.

- ◻ Avoid undercooked or under-refrigerated food.

- ◻ Perform proper hand hygiene after toileting and after changing diapers.

- ◻ Do not share dishes and utensils. Wash them in hot, soapy water or in the dishwasher.

- ◻ Clip nails and discourage nail biting and thumb sucking.

- ◻ Clean toilet areas.

- • Client Outcomes

  - ○ The child will remain free of infection.

  - ○ The child will maintain adequate hydration.

Complications

- • Dehydration

TYPE OF DEHYDRATION	MANIFESTATIONS
Isotonic	• Water and sodium are lost in nearly equal amounts. • Major loss from extracellular fluid leads to a reduced volume of circulating fluid. • Hypovolemic shock may result. • Serum sodium is within the expected reference range (130 to 150 mEq/L).
Hypotonic	• Electrolyte loss is greater than water loss. • Water changes from extracellular fluid to intracellular fluid. • Physical manifestations are more severe with smaller fluid loss. • Serum sodium is less than 130 mEq/L.
Hypertonic	• Water loss is greater than electrolyte loss. • Fluid shifts from intracellular to extracellular. • Shock is less likely. • Neurologic changes (change in level of consciousness, irritability, hyperreflexia) may occur. • Serum sodium concentration is greater than 150 mEq/L.

LEVEL OF DEHYDRATION	WEIGHT LOSS	MANIFESTATIONS
Mild	5% in infants 3% to 4% in children	• Behavior, mucous membranes, anterior fontanel, pulse, and blood pressure are all within the expected reference range. • Capillary refill is greater than 2 seconds. • Slight thirst may be experienced. • Urine-specific gravity is greater than 1.020.
Moderate	10% in infants 6 to 8% in children	• Capillary refill is between 2 and 4 seconds. • Thirst and irritability may be experienced. • Pulse is slightly increased with normal to orthostatic blood pressure. • Mucous membranes are dry and tears and skin turgor are decreased. • Urine-specific gravity is greater than 1.020 (oliguria).
Severe	15% in infants 10% in children	• Capillary refill is greater than 4 seconds. • Tachycardia is present and orthostatic blood pressure may progress to shock. • Extreme thirst is present. • Mucous membranes are very dry and skin is tented. • The anterior fontanel is sunken. • Oliguria or anuria is present.

- ○ Nursing Actions
  - ■ Monitor the administration of IV fluids as prescribed (usually dextrose 5% in a saline solution).
  - ■ Fluid replacement should be rapid for isotonic and hypotonic dehydration, but fluid replacement should take for 24 to 48 hr for hypertonic dehydration to prevent cerebral edema.
  - ■ Avoid antiemetics because vomiting usually resolves with treatment of dehydration.
  - ■ Determine the cause of diarrhea. Antibiotics are usually reserved for children who are immunocompromised.
- ○ Client Education
  - ■ Instruct the parents to monitor weight daily.
  - ■ Tell the children and their families that the child should consume small amounts of liquids several times a day to prevent vomiting.

Ⓐ APPLICATION EXERCISES

1. A nurse is reviewing the tape test with a parent who phoned the clinic for assistance. Explain how this test is done?

2. Which of the following data confirms that a 12-year-old child has severe dehydration?

   A. Weight dropped from 40 kg (88 lb) to 36 kg (79.2 kg).

   B. Capillary refill is 2 to 3 seconds.

   C. Slight thirst is present.

   D. Urine specific gravity 1.025.

3. A nurse in an urgent care clinic is reviewing routes of transmission of salmonella (non-typhoidal) with the parents of a child brought to the clinic with diarrhea. Which of the following routes should be discussed? (Select all that apply.)

   _____ Undercooked chicken

   _____ Inadequate hand hygiene

   _____ Contact with infected pets

   _____ Puncture wound

   _____ Mosquito bites

4. The mother of a 3-year-old child who has been identified as having rotavirus asks how her child got the disease. How should the nurse respond?

5. A nurse is reviewing the use of mebendazole (Vermox) with the mother of a child who is to be treated for pinworms. Which of the following is included in this discussion? (Select all that apply.)

   _____ Apply the medication to the rectal area.

   _____ Bring in a stool sample for analysis in 1 to 2 weeks.

   _____ Administer an initial dose.

   _____ Repeat the dose in 2 weeks if indicated.

   _____ Do not treat other family members.

6. A nurse is caring for a child who has *Giardia lamblia*. Which of the following findings should the nurse expect to find?

   A. Bloody emesis

   B. Malodorous, greasy stools

   C. Respiratory distress

   D. Headache

APPLICATION EXERCISES ANSWER KEY

1. A nurse is reviewing the tape test with a parent who phoned the clinic for assistance. Explain how this test is done?

   The parent places a strip of transparent tape over the child's anus at bedtime. The tape is removed the following morning before toileting or bathing and taken to the designated laboratory or clinic for evaluation. It is best if the tape is applied while the child is asleep and removed before awakening. Parents should be instructed to thoroughly wash their hands after the procedure.

 NCLEX® Connection: Reduction of Risk Potential, Laboratory Values

2. Which of the following data confirms that a 12-year-old child has severe dehydration?

   A. Weight dropped from 40 kg (88 lb) to 36 kg (79.2 kg).

   B. Capillary refill is 2 to 3 seconds.

   C. Slight thirst is present.

   D. Urine specific gravity 1.025.

   The child with severe dehydration has lost about 10% body weight, has a capillary refill greater than 4 seconds, presents with extreme thirst, and oliguria or anuria is present. Other findings should include tachycardia, orthostatic blood pressure, possibly shock, dry mucous membranes, and tenting of the skin. A capillary refill of 2 to 3 seconds and urine-specific gravity greater than 1.020 indicates moderate dehydration. Slight thirst may be experienced in mild dehydration.

 NCLEX® Connection: Physiological Adaptation, Fluid and Electrolyte Imbalances

3. A nurse in an urgent care clinic is reviewing routes of transmission of salmonella (non-typhoidal) with the parents of a child brought to the clinic with diarrhea. Which of the following routes should be discussed? (Select all that apply.)

X	**Undercooked chicken**
X	**Inadequate hand hygiene**
X	**Contact with infected pets**
____	Puncture wound
____	Mosquito bites

   Routes of transmission of salmonella include undercooked meats and poultry products, fecal-oral route by inadequate hand hygiene, and contact with infected pets. Blood exposure from puncture wounds or mosquito bites is not a route of transmission.

 NCLEX® Connection: Safety and Infection Control, Standard/Transmission-Based/Other Precautions/Surgical Asepsis

4. The mother of a 3-year-old child who has been identified as having rotavirus asks how her child got the disease. How should the nurse respond?

Rotavirus is **usually transmitted by fecal-oral contamination, thus inadequate hand hygiene can be a major source of contamination. The child could have contracted it in a day care center from improper hand hygiene by other children and staff, toys, eating utensils or equipment that were not thoroughly disinfected, and contact with contaminated bed linens or clothing worn by other children.**

 NCLEX® Connection: Safety and Infection Control, Standard/Transmission-Based/Other Precautions/Surgical Asepsis

5. A nurse is reviewing the use of mebendazole (Vermox) with the mother of a child who is to be treated for pinworms. Which of the following is included in this discussion? (Select all that apply.)

	Apply the medication to the rectal area.
X	**Bring in a stool sample for analysis in 1 to 2 weeks.**
X	**Administer an initial dose.**
X	**Repeat the dose in 2 weeks if indicated.**
	Do not treat other family members.

Mebendazole is an anthelmintic which is administered orally in a single dose to treat pinworms. The mother should bring in a stool sample for analysis in 1 to 2 weeks. If needed, a repeat dose of medication is given at 2 weeks. Pinworms are easily transmitted, so all household members should be treated.

 NCLEX® Connection: Pharmacological Therapies, Expected Actions/Outcomes

6. A nurse is caring for a child who has *Giardia lamblia*. Which of the following findings should the nurse expect to find?

A. Bloody emesis

B. Malodorous, greasy stools

C. Respiratory distress

D. Headache

A child with *Giardia lamblia* manifests malodorous, pale, watery, greasy stools as well as abdominal cramping, diarrhea, anorexia, vomiting, and constipation. Bloody emesis, respiratory distress, and headache are not related findings.

 NCLEX® Connection: Safety and Infection Control, Standard/Transmission-Based/Other Precautions/Surgical Asepsis

UNIT 2   NURSING CARE OF CHILDREN WITH SYSTEM DISORDERS

Section: Gastrointestinal Disorders

Chapter 22   Gastrointestinal Structural and Inflammatory Disorders

Overview

- Gastrointestinal structural disorders include:

  - Gastroesophageal reflux disease (GERD)

  - Hypertropic pyloric stenosis

  - Hirschsprung's disease

  - Intussusception

  - Appendicitis and Meckel's diverticulum

    - These affect structures in the gastrointestinal tract, but they are inflammatory disorders.

  - Cleft lip and palate

    - These are considered structural disorders, but they have different assessment findings and management.

GASTROINTESTINAL STRUCTURAL AND INFLAMMATORY DISORDERS

Overview

- Gastroesophageal reflux (GER) occurs when the gastric contents reflux back up into the esophagus, making esophageal mucosa vulnerable to injury from gastric acid and resulting in gastroesophageal reflux disease (GERD). GER in infants is usually self-limiting and resolves by the end of the first year of life.

  - GERD may result in failure to thrive, bleeding, and difficulty with swallowing.

- Hypertropic pyloric stenosis is the thickening of the pyloric sphincter, which creates an obstruction.

- Hirschsprung's disease, or congenital aganglionic megacolon, is a structural anomaly of the gastrointestinal (GI) tract that is caused by lack of ganglionic cells in segments of the colon and results in mechanical obstruction.

  - Stool accumulates due to lack of peristalsis in the non-innervated area of the bowel (usually rectosigmoid), causing the bowel to dilate.

  - Hirschsprung's disease is usually diagnosed in infants, but chronic milder symptoms may occur in late childhood.

- Meckel's diverticulum is a complication resulting from failure of the omphalomesenteric duct to fuse during embryonic development.

  o The diverticulum may be up to 4 inches in length and is found in the small intestine.

- Intussusception is the telescoping of the intestine over itself. This usually occurs in infants and young children up to 5 years of age, but it is most common between 3 and 9 months of age.

- Appendicitis is inflammation of the appendix caused by an obstruction of the opening of the appendix, possibly due to fecal matter, swollen lymphoid tissue, or (in rare cases) a parasite.

- Consequences from peritonitis can lead to electrolyte imbalances and shock.

Data Collection

- Risk Factors

  o GERD is more likely to occur in premature infants and infants born with congenital defects (neurologic disorders, esophageal disorders, hiatal hernia, cystic fibrosis, cerebral palsy).

  o Hypertrophic pyloric stenosis has a genetic component.

  o Hirschsprung's disease may be either an acute or chronic disorder.

  o Intussusception is more common in children who have cystic fibrosis.

- Subjective and Objective Data

STRUCTURAL DISORDER	FINDINGS
GERD	<ul><li>Infants</li><ul><li>Excessive spitting up or forceful vomiting, irritability, excessive crying, blood in stool or vomitus, arching of back and stiffening</li><li>Apnea or apparent life-threatening event</li></ul><li>Older children</li><ul><li>Reports of heartburn, abdominal pain, difficulty swallowing, chronic cough, and Sandifer syndrome (in which there is repetitive stretching and arching of head and neck that may mimic seizure activity)</li></ul></ul>
Hypertrophic pyloric stenosis	<ul><li>Vomiting that often occurs 30 to 60 min after a meal and becomes projectile as obstruction worsens</li><li>Constant hunger</li><li>Olive-shaped mass in the right upper quadrant of the abdomen and possible peristaltic wave that moves from left to right when lying supine</li><li>Failure to gain weight and signs of dehydration, such as skin that is dry and/or pale, cool lips, dry mucous membranes, decreased skin turgor, diminished urinary output, concentrated urine, thirst, rapid pulse, sunken eyes, and decreased blood pressure</li></ul>

STRUCTURAL DISORDER	FINDINGS

Hirschsprung's disease	• Newborns
	  ○ Failure to pass meconium within 24 to 48 hr, refusal to eat, episodes of vomiting bile, and abdominal distention
	• Infants
	  ○ Failure to thrive, constipation, abdominal distention, episodes of vomiting and diarrhea
	• Older children
	  ○ Constipation, abdominal distention, visible peristalsis, ribbon-like stool, palpable fecal mass, and a malnourished appearance

Intussusception	• Normal comfort interrupted by periods of sudden and acute pain • Palpable, sausage-shaped mass in the right upper quadrant of the abdomen and/or a tender, distended abdomen • Stools that are mixed with blood and mucus that resemble the consistency of red currant jelly
Appendicitis	• Abdominal pain; generalized pain that typically begins at the peri-umbilical area and localizes to the right lower quadrant (pain may be most intense at McBurney's point, located about halfway between the anterior superior iliac crest and the umbilicus); pain that increases with movement; rigid abdomen • Fever, tachycardia, possible vomiting, constipation and/or diarrhea, anorexia, pallor, lethargy, and/or irritability
Meckel's diverticulum	• Abdominal pain, bloody stools without pain, bright red mucus in infant stools

- ○ Laboratory Tests
  - ■ Serum electrolyte levels will be consistent, with changes occurring due to vomiting and resulting in:
    - □ Decreased sodium and potassium levels
    - □ Increased pH and bicarbonate caused by metabolic alkalosis
  - ■ An elevated BUN indicates dehydration.
  - ■ A CBC may show an elevated WBC count greater than 10,000/mm³ with a shift to left (increased immature neutrophils, referred to as bands), as well as an elevated C-reactive protein, but this may not be specific to the diagnosis.
- ○ Diagnostic Procedures
  - ■ Hypertrophic pyloric stenosis
    - □ Ultrasound of the abdomen
      - ▸ An ultrasound will reveal an elongated, sausage-shaped mass and an elongated pyloric area.

- GERD
  - □ Upper GI series to detect GI structural abnormalities
  - □ 24-hr intraesophageal pH monitoring study
    - ▸ Measures the amount of gastric acid reflux into the esophagus
  - □ Endoscopy with biopsy to detect esophagitis and strictures
  - □ Scintigraphy
    - ▸ Identifies cause of gastric content aspiration
- Hirschsprung's disease
  - □ Rectal biopsy
    - ▸ Full-thickness biopsies will reveal the absence of ganglion cells.
- Intussusception
  - □ Ultrasound, barium enema
- Appendicitis
  - □ CT scan of the abdomen
    - ▸ The CT scan will show an enlarged diameter of appendix, as well as thickening of the appendiceal wall.
- Meckel's diverticulum
  - □ Radionucleotide scan
    - ▸ This scan will show the presence of gastric mucosa.
- Nursing Actions
  - □ Assist with positioning.
  - □ Administer contrast medium if prescribed.
  - □ Monitor for signs of bleeding following biopsies.
- Client Education
  - □ Instruct client about the need to remain still.

Collaborative Care

- Nursing Care
  - ○ Vomiting
    - Position children on their side or with the head elevated to prevent aspiration.
    - Document the amount and characteristics of vomitus, and describe vomiting behavior to aid in diagnosis of etiology.
    - Monitor fluid and electrolyte balance to assess for deficits.
    - Provide oral care after children vomit to prevent damage to teeth from hydrochloric acid contact.

○ GER –Treatment for infants/children is based on the severity of symptoms:

- Offer small, frequent feedings of thickened formula.

- Position children with the head elevated at 30° after they have eaten.

- Place infants in a prone position for sleep, which can prevent aspiration of stomach contents. This is only recommended for infants with severe GERD.

- Administer a proton pump inhibitor, such as omeprazole (Prilosec), or an H_2-receptor antagonist, such as ranitidine (Zantac).

- Therapeutic Procedures

STRUCTURAL DISORDER	PROCEDURE
GERD	Surgical manipulation or Nissen fundoplication (wraps the fundus of the stomach around the distal esophagus to decrease the chance of reflux)
Hypertrophic pyloric stenosis	Surgical incision into the pyloric sphincter (pylorotomy)
Hirschsprung's disease	Surgical removal of the aganglionic section (may require temporary colostomy)
Intussusception	Surgical reduction if inflating the bowel with air or administering a barium enema is not successful
Appendicitis	Surgical removal of appendix via laparoscopic or open method
Meckel's diverticulum	Surgical removal of diverticulum

- Nursing Actions

  □ Preoperative

    ‣ Prepare children and their families for the surgical or therapeutic procedure.

    ‣ Maintain good hydration by administering electrolytes and fluid replacement.

  □ Postoperative

    ‣ Institute incremental feedings beginning with a solution of clear liquid/glucose/electrolytes and assessing for readiness to progress back to breast milk or formula. The infant may continue to vomit for 24 to 48 hr after surgery.

    ‣ Position infants with their heads slightly elevated to prevent reflux. Infants usually progress well and are discharged on the second or third postoperative day.

- Client Education
  - Instruct the parents about signs/ symptoms of dehydration.
  - Instruct the parents to observe the incision and monitor for signs of infection.
  - Demonstrate proper hand hygiene techniques.
  - Encourage the parents to be active in the care of their children.
  - Show the parents of a child who has a temporary colostomy for Hirschsprung's disease how to perform colostomy care before discharge.

- Client Outcomes
  - The child will remain free from infection.
  - The child will remain hydrated.
  - The child will maintain adequate nutrition.
  - The child will maintain adequate elimination.

Complications

- GERD
  - Recurrent pneumonia, weight loss, and failure to thrive
    - Repeated reflux of stomach contents can lead to erosion of the esophagus or pneumonia if stomach contents are aspirated. Esophageal damage can lead to the inability to eat.
    - Nursing Actions
      - Monitor for signs and symptoms of pneumonia and failure to thrive.
      - Thicken feedings as prescribed.
      - Sit children upright and feed small, frequent meals.
    - Client Education
      - Reinforce information with the parents about feeding techniques to promote gastric emptying, proper positioning, and use of medication.

- Appendicitis
  - Peritonitis
    - Occurs when the intestinal lining and/or peritoneum is perforated, allowing intestinal contents to enter the peritoneal cavity. Peritonitis may result from a ruptured appendix. Peritonitis often occurs within 48 hr of onset of appendicitis.
    - Nursing Actions
      - Observe for signs and symptoms of peritonitis.
        - Rigid, board-like abdomen
        - Absent bowel sounds

- ▸ Severe pain

- ▸ Fever

- ▸ Increased WBCs

- ▸ Possible shock and death

- □ Pain management

  - ▸ Determine level of pain using a developmentally appropriate tool.

  - ▸ Administer analgesics as prescribed.

- □ Monitor IV fluid therapy.

- □ Monitor response to IV antibiotics for infection.

- □ Manage nasogastric tube suction.

- □ Provide preoperative and postoperative nursing care.

- □ Provide surgical wound care with wound irrigation and/or dressings if delayed wound closure is necessary.

- □ Provide psychosocial support for the child and family.

- ■ Client Education

  - □ Reinforce instructions to children and their families about preoperative care, such as the need to maintain NPO status and the need for pain medication.

  - □ Reinforce instructions to children and their families about postoperative care, such as early ambulation, advancement of diet, wound care, and monitoring for infection.

- • Hirschsprung's disease

  - ○ Enterocolitis

    - ■ Enterocolitis is inflammation of the bowel resulting in fever and explosive diarrhea with the child appearing very ill.

    - ■ Treatment is aimed at resolving enterocolitis, preventing bowel perforation, maintaining hydration, initiating antibiotic therapy, and performing surgery for colostomy or ileostomy if there is extensive bowel involvement.

    - ■ Nursing Actions

      - □ Monitor abdominal girth.

        - ▸ Measure abdominal girth with a paper tape measure at the level of the umbilicus or at the widest point of the abdomen.

        - ▸ Mark the area with a pen to assure continuity of future measurements.

      - □ Monitor for signs of sepsis, peritonitis, or shock caused by enterocolitis.

      - □ Monitor and manage fluid, electrolyte, and blood product replacement.

      - □ Administer antibiotics as prescribed.

- Meckel's diverticulum

  ○ GI hemorrhage and bowel obstruction

    ■ Hemorrhage may occur with ruptured Meckel's diverticulum.

    ■ Nursing Actions

      □ Monitor for signs of gastric distention and/or vomiting.

      □ Monitor for signs of bleeding.

      □ Test stools for occult blood.

      □ Monitor complete blood counts for signs of anemia

      □ Provide general preoperative care.

      □ Encourage bed rest.

    ■ Client Education

      □ Inform the parents about signs and symptoms of obstruction.

      □ Inform the parents about signs and symptoms of hemorrhage.

CLEFT LIP AND PALATE

Overview

- Cleft lip (CL) results from the incomplete fusion of the oral cavity during intrauterine life. Cleft palate (CP) results from the incomplete fusion of the palatine plates during intrauterine life.

 View Media Supplement: Cleft Palate (Image)

- Although a cleft lip and palate may occur together, either defect may also appear alone. The defects can be unilateral (one sided) or bilateral (two sided)

- Cleft palate repair (palatoplasty) traditionally takes place after the palate has developed, but new surgical techniques may allow repair to take place earlier.

- Surgery may be done in stages throughout several years.

- Nursing interventions include preoperative instructions, postoperative care, and family support.

Data Collection

- Risk Factors

  ○ May be multifactorial, including:

    ■ Heredity (as the incidence of cleft palate is higher in relatives of people with the defect)

    ■ Teratogens (especially maternal intake of phenytoin [Dilantin]), maternal smoking, and family tendency)

- Objective Data

  - Physical Assessment Findings

    - CL defect is visible, but CP alone may only be visible when examining the mouth.

Collaborative Care

- Nursing Care

  - Support and encourage the parents in the general care of their child preoperatively and postoperatively.

  - Promote parent-infant bonding.

  - Promote healthy self-esteem throughout the child's development.

- Interdisciplinary Care

  - Care of children with CL and CP requires care from members of various disciplines (plastic surgeon, orthodontist, ENT specialist, speech and language therapist, occupational therapist, dietary consult, social services worker).

- Surgical Interventions

  - Cheiloplasty (repair of cleft lip early in infancy) and palatoplasty (repair of cleft palate)

    - If both defects are present, cleft lip repair is generally performed first, followed by cleft palate repair at a later date. New techniques in anesthesia and newborn surgery allow closure at an earlier time. Closure of the palate should be done early enough to prevent speech defects.

    - Nursing Actions

      - Preoperative

        - Cleft lip and cleft palate repair

          - Inspect the infant's lip and palate using a gloved finger to palpate the infant's palate.

          - Determine the infant's ability to suck.

          - Obtain the infant's baseline weight.

          - Observe interaction between the family and infant.

          - Determine family coping and support.

          - Refer the parents to appropriate support groups.

          - Contact social services to provide needed services (financial, insurance) for the family and infant.

▫ Postoperative

- ▸ Cleft lip and cleft palate repair

  - ▹ Perform standard postoperative care, including monitoring of vital signs and measuring pain using an age-appropriate tool.

  - ▹ Keep infants pain free postoperatively to decrease crying and stress on repair.

  - ▹ Administer analgesics as prescribed.

  - ▹ Observe the operative sites for signs of crusting and infection. Use saline on a sterile swab to clean the incision site. Apply antibiotic ointment if prescribed.

  - ▹ Determine the infant's ability to eat. Monitor I&O and weigh daily.

  - ▹ Observe the family's interaction with the infant.

  - ▹ Identify family coping and support.

- ▸ Cleft lip repair

  - ▹ Monitor the integrity of the postoperative protective device to ensure proper positioning.

  - ▹ Position infants upright (infant car seat position), on her back, or on her side in the immediate postoperative period to maintain the integrity of the repair.

  - ▹ Apply elbow restraints to keep infants from pulling at the repair site. The cuff of the restraints may be pinned to the infant's clothing. A jacket restraint may be necessary to prevent an older infant from rolling over.

  - ▹ Restraints should be removed periodically to observe skin, allow limb movement, and provide for comfort.

  - ▹ Use saline on a sterile swab to clean the incision site. Apply antibiotic ointment if prescribed.

  - ▹ Gently aspirate secretions of mouth and nasopharynx to prevent respiratory complications.

- ▸ Cleft palate repair

  - ▹ Change the infant's position frequently to facilitate breathing. The infant may be placed on the abdomen in the immediate postoperative period.

  - ▹ Monitor infants receiving intravenous fluids until they are able to eat and drink.

  - ▹ Monitor packing, which is usually removed in 2 to 3 days.

  - ▹ Avoid placing objects (tongue depressor, pacifier) in the infant's mouth after cleft palate repair.

▷ Avoid using objects for feeding (forks, spoons, pacifiers, straws) that could harm the cleft palate repair.

▷ Avoid foods that could damage the palate repair.

▷ The infant may be discharged on a soft diet.

- Client Education

  □ Preoperative

  ▸ Encourage and support the parents as they bond with the infant and provide care.

  ▸ Support the mother's decision to continue breastfeeding her infant. Instruct her to place the breast fully into the newborn's mouth, making a seal. Assist her to be open to alternatives, such as using breast milk placed in special feeding devices, if necessary.

  ▸ Provide instruction to promote feeding. Tell the parents to use an enlarged nipple, stimulate the infant's suck reflex, and ensure that the infant swallows appropriately. To prevent choking and coughing, steady gentle pressure should be held on the bottom of the bottle.

  ▸ Tell the parents to limit feedings to 20 to 30 min to prevent fatigue. Also tell parents to allow infants to rest frequently after each feeding.

  ▸ Identify alternate feeding devices (special nipples for bottles).

   View Media Supplement: Cleft Palate Feeder (Image)

  ▸ Tell the parents to feed infants in an upright position.

  ▸ Instruct parents to burp infants more frequently due to the amount of air swallowed. This will help prevent aspiration and abdominal distention.

  ▸ Show parents how to use bulb suction as needed.

  ▸ Prepare parents for impending surgery.

  □ Postoperative

  ▸ Inform the parents that infants may require elbow restraints for 4 to 6 weeks. Instruct the parents in the proper use of the restraints and to periodically remove them one at a time to allow for exercise.

  ▸ Assist the parents with proper feeding techniques.

  ▸ Instruct the parents in proper care of operative site.

- Client Outcomes

  ○ The child will remain free from infection.

  ○ The child's suture line will remain intact.

  ○ The child will maintain nutrition.

Complications

- Aspiration

  o Aspiration is the result of fluids entering the structural defect.

  o Nursing Actions

    ▪ Feed infants in an upright position.

    ▪ Burp infants often.

    ▪ Use a bulb syringe to suction oral and nasopharyngeal secretions.

  o Client Education

    ▪ Instruct the parents about the proper position for feeding.

    ▪ Instruct the parents to learn CPR.

- Ear infections and hearing loss

  o Related to altered structure and recurrent infections

  o Nursing Actions

    ▪ Feed infants in an upright position. Monitor temperature.

  o Client Education

    ▪ Instruct the parents about signs/symptoms of ear infections.

    ▪ Encourage early intervention.

- Speech and language delay

  o More common with cleft palate

  o Client Education

    ▪ Encourage the parents to contact provider at first signs of infection.

    ▪ Discuss involvement of a speech therapist for care.

- Dental problems

  o Teeth may not erupt normally and orthodontia is usually necessary later in life.

  o Client Education

    ▪ Instruct the parents and children (if age appropriate) to promote healthy dental hygiene.

    ▪ Encourage the parents to seek early dental care.

Ⓐ APPLICATION EXERCISES

1. Match the following structural defects with the correct assessment data.

   _____ Hirschsprung's disease

   _____ Intussusception

   _____ Hypertrophic pyloric stenosis

   _____ GERD

   _____ Meckel's diverticulum

   1. Olive-shaped mass in right upper quadrant
   2. Painless, bloody stools
   3. Severe constipation with bouts of diarrhea; failure to pass meconium in newborns
   4. Stool of currant jelly consistency
   5. Excess spitting up or forceful vomiting

2. A nurse is reviewing discharge instructions with the parent of an infant newly diagnosed with GERD. Which of the following statements by the parent indicates a need for further teaching?

   A. "I will add rice cereal to the formula to thicken it."

   B. "Feeding him two large meals a day will work well for his schedule."

   C. "I'll make sure we sit him up in the infant seat when he eats."

   D. "Giving him his Prilosec with the syringe is so easy."

Scenario: A nurse is caring for an infant who has undergone a palatoplasty (cleft palate repair) and is admitted to the pediatric unit.

3. Which of the following nursing actions should the nurse take when caring for the infant? (Select all that apply.)

   _____ Change positions frequently between abdomen and side-lying.

   _____ Check placement of packing.

   _____ Offer pacifier as needed.

   _____ Use spoon for feeding.

   _____ Remove any drainage from incision with sterile swabs.

4. Describe instructions the parents will receive related to care of the infant upon discharge.

5. A child is admitted to the pediatric unit with appendicitis and laparoscopic surgery will be performed later in the afternoon. The child's mother asks for a nurse to check on her daughter because she thinks something has happened. Which of the following data suggests the appendix has ruptured? (Select all that apply.)

   _____ Abdomen is rigid, board-like

   _____ Child rates pain as 10 on scale of 0 to 10

   _____ Hyperactive bowel sounds

   _____ WBCs are 7,000/mm³

   _____ Temperature is 103.2 F (39.6 C)

6. Data collection findings for an infant who has intussusception include _____.

7. Intussusception is diagnosed using the radiologic procedure of _____.

8. Therapeutic procedures to treat intussusception include _____.

APPLICATION EXERCISES ANSWER KEY

1. Match the following structural defects with the correct assessment data.

   __3__ Hirschsprung's disease
   __4__ Intussusception
   __1__ Hypertrophic pyloric stenosis
   __5__ GERD
   __2__ Meckel's diverticulum

   1. Olive-shaped mass in right upper quadrant
   2. Painless, bloody stools
   3. Severe constipation with bouts of diarrhea; failure to pass meconium in newborns
   4. Stool of currant jelly consistency
   5. Excess spitting up or forceful vomiting

   NCLEX® Connection: Physiological Adaptations, Basic Pathophysiology

2. A nurse is reviewing discharge instructions with the parent of an infant newly diagnosed with GERD. Which of the following statements by the parent indicates a need for further teaching?

   A. "I will add rice cereal to the formula to thicken it."

   B. "Feeding him two large meals a day will work well for his schedule."

   C. "I'll make sure we sit him up in the infant seat when he eats."

   D. "Giving him his Prilosec with the syringe is so easy."

   Feeding the infant two large meals a day does not promote effective gastric emptying in an infant with GERD. Discharge instructions should include thickening the infant formula, feeding in an upright position, offering small, frequent meals, and correctly administering medications. Parents should also be instructed to monitor for signs of respiratory infection and weight loss.

   NCLEX® Connection: Basic Care and Comfort, Nutrition and Oral Hydration

Scenario: A nurse is caring for an infant who has undergone a palatoplasty (cleft palate repair) and is admitted to the pediatric unit.

3. Which of the following nursing actions should the nurse take when caring for the infant? (Select all that apply.)

   __X__ **Change positions frequently between abdomen and side-lying.**

   __X__ **Check placement of packing.**

   _____ Offer pacifier as needed.

   _____ Use spoon for feeding.

   _____ Remove any drainage from incision with sterile swabs.

   Place the infant on the abdomen or side and change positions frequently to facilitate effective breathing and drainage of secretions. Check placement of the packing in the palate. Do not place any objects in the infant's mouth, including pacifiers, spoons, or swabs to avoid interrupting the incision and packing.

    NCLEX® Connection: Reduction of Risk Potential, Potential for Complications from Surgical Procedures and Health Alterations

4. Describe instructions the parents will receive related to care of the infant upon discharge.

   Review care of the incision. Instruct parents on the correct use of elbow restraints and their periodic removal so the infant will not suck his thumb or place any objects in his mouth. Discuss feeding techniques related to special feeding. Include feeding the infant in an upright position, burping frequently, and using the bulb syringe as well as signs of ear infections and monitoring the infant's temperature. Discuss use of medications, follow-up appointments, and referrals for CPR training.

   NCLEX® Connection: Reduction of Risk Potential, Potential for Complications from Surgical Procedures and Health Alterations

5. A child is admitted to the pediatric unit with appendicitis and laparoscopic surgery will be performed later in the afternoon. The child's mother asks for a nurse to check on her daughter because she thinks something has happened. Which of the following data suggests the appendix has ruptured? (Select all that apply.)

__X__	**Abdomen is rigid, board-like**
__X__	**Child rates pain as 10 on scale of 0 to 10**
_____	Hyperactive bowel sounds
_____	WBCs are 7,000/mm³
__X__	**Temperature is 103.2 F (39.6 C)**

Signs and symptoms of peritonitis due to a ruptured appendix include a rigid, board-like abdomen, absent bowel sounds, severe pain, fever, elevated WBCs, and signs of shock. Bowel sounds would not be hyperactive. WBC of 7,000/mm3 is within the expected range of findings.

(N) NCLEX® Connection: Physiological Adaptations, Basic Pathophysiology

6. Data collection findings for an infant who has intussusception include **a palpable, sausage-shaped mass in the right, upper quadrant of the abdomen.**

(N) NCLEX® Connection: Physiological Adaptations, Alterations in Body Systems

7. Intussusception is diagnosed using the radiologic procedure of **barium enema or ultrasound.**

(N) NCLEX® Connection: Reduction of Risk Potential, Diagnostic Tests

8. Therapeutic procedures to treat intussusception include **surgical reduction, inflating air into the bowel, or barium enema.**

(N) NCLEX® Connection: Reduction of Risk Potential, Therapeutic Procedures

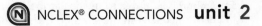

UNIT 2: NURSING CARE OF CHILDREN WITH SYSTEM DISORDERS

Section: Genitourinary and Reproductive Disorders

- Enuresis and Urinary Tract Infections

- Structural Disorders of the Genitourinary Tract and Reproductive System

- Renal Disorders

NCLEX® CONNECTIONS

When reviewing the chapters in this section, keep in mind the relevant sections of the NCLEX® outline, in particular:

CLIENT NEEDS: BASIC CARE AND COMFORT

Relevant topics/tasks include:
- Elimination
  - Identify client at risk for impaired elimination.
- Non-Pharmacological Comfort Interventions
  - Apply therapies for comfort and treatment of inflammation/swelling.
- Nutrition and Oral Hydration
  - Reinforce client teaching on special diets based on client diagnosis/nutritional needs and cultural considerations.

CLIENT NEEDS: REDUCTION OF RISK POTENTIAL

Relevant topics/tasks include:
- Changes/Abnormalities in Vital signs
  - Compare vital signs to client baseline vital signs.
- Laboratory Values
  - Reinforce client teaching on purposes of laboratory tests.
- Potential for Alterations in Body Systems
  - Compare current client clinical data to baseline information.

CLIENT NEEDS: PHYSIOLOGICAL ADAPTATION

Relevant topics/tasks include:
- Alterations in Body Systems
  - Perform care for client after surgical procedure.
- Fluid and Electrolyte Imbalances
  - Provide interventions to restore client fluid and/or electrolyte balance.

UNIT 2	NURSING CARE OF CHILDREN WITH SYSTEM DISORDERS
Section:	Genitourinary and Reproductive Disorders
Chapter 23	Enuresis and Urinary Tract Infections

Overview

- Enuresis is defined as uncontrolled or unintentional urination that occurs after a child is beyond an age at which bladder control is achieved.

- A urinary tract infection (UTI) is an infection in any portion of the urinary tract (cystitis, urethritis, pyelonephritis).

ENURESIS

Overview

- Inappropriate urination must occur at least twice a week for at least 3 months and the child must be at least 5 years of age before a diagnosis of enuresis is considered.

- Enuresis is more commonly seen in males.

- Organic causes related to genitourinary dysfunction must be ruled out prior to diagnosis of enuresis.

Data Collection

- Risk Factors

  o Enuresis has no clear etiology, but it may be related to:

    ▪ Family history of enuresis

    ▪ Disorders associated with bladder dysfunction

    ▪ Emotional factors

- Subjective Data

  o History of toilet training, voiding behaviors, and bowel movement patterns

  o History of chronic or acute illness (urinary tract infection, diabetes mellitus, sickle cell disease, neurologic deficits)

  o History of family disruptions or other emotional stressors o   Family history of enuresis

    o   Fluid intake, especially in the evening

Collaborative Care

- Nursing Care

  - Evaluate the child's and family's understanding of enuresis.

  - Educate children and families regarding the management of enuresis (fluid restriction prior to bedtime, bladder training, medications).

  - Evaluate the child's self-esteem.

  - Evaluate the child's coping strategies and available support systems.

  - Evaluate the family's coping.

  - Evaluate peer and family support groups.

- Medications

  - Antidiuretics – Desmopressin acetate (DDAVP)

    - Used to reduce the volume of urine in the bladder

    - Nursing Considerations

      - Inform families of possible side effects (headache, nausea, flushing, mild abdominal cramps, fluid retention)

    - Client Education

      - Encourage families to restrict the child's fluid intake after dinner.

      - Instruct families to administer the medication at bedtime.

      - Instruct families to keep nasal medications in the refrigerator.

  - Tricyclic antidepressants – Imipramine hydrochloride (Tofranil)

    - Nursing Considerations

      - Inform families of possible side effects (dry mouth, constipation, insomnia, anxiety).

    - Client Education

      - Instruct families to administer the mediation 1 hr before bedtime.

  - Anticholinergics – Oxybutynin chloride (Ditropan)

    - Reduces bladder contractions

    - Nursing Considerations

      - Monitor for effectiveness of therapy.

- Client Education
  - Instruct children and their families to watch for side effects (dry mouth, drowsiness, nausea, allergic reaction).

- Therapeutic Procedures
  - Bladder stretching exercises
    - Children should drink fluid and hold the urine as long as possible, which may increase the functional size of the bladder. Pelvic muscle exercises should be practiced throughout the day to help with bladder control.
    - Client Education
      - Instruct children about holding urine for as long as possible.
      - Tell children how to perform pelvic muscle exercises to improve bladder control.

- Care After Discharge
  - Client Education
    - Explain to families that enuresis is not a behavioral problem and should not be punished.
    - Help the parents identify ways to improve the child's self-image related to enuresis.
    - Advise children and their families that therapies for enuresis may be helpful for a short time, but they may not provide a cure. Support the child and parents in their decisions.

- Client Outcomes
  - The child will eliminate nighttime wetness.
  - The child will maintain positive self-esteem.

Complications

- Emotional problems (poor self-esteem, altered body image, social isolation, fears)
  - Nursing Actions
    - Support children and their families by listening to concerns and correcting misperceptions.
    - Recommend use of appropriate resources (support groups, counseling) as needed.
  - Client Education
    - Assist children and their families to understand the emotional aspects of the disorder. Early interventions can alleviate long-term emotional issues.
    - Suggest that children and their families participate in a support group.

URINARY TRACT INFECTIONS

Overview

- An upper urinary tract infection (UTI) is a condition such as pyelonephritis. Urinary reflux from the bladder into the ureters may contribute to pyelonephritis.

- Untreated UTIs may lead to renal damage/failure or urosepsis.

- Organisms that cause UTIs include Escherichia coli (most common), Proteus, Pseudomonas, Klebsiella, and Staphylococcus aureus.

- Diagnosis is made by detection of bacteria in the urine.

Data Collection

- Risk Factors

  o Urinary stasis

  o Urinary tract anomalies

  o Reflux within the urinary tract system

  o Constipation

  o Onset of toilet training

  o Female gender (due to short urethra in close proximity to the rectum)

  o Synthetic, tight underwear and wet bathing suits

  o Sexual activity

- Subjective Data

  o Presenting symptoms vary depending on age.

    ▪ Urinary frequency with voiding of small amounts, urgency, and nocturia

    ▪ Dysuria, bladder cramping, or spasms

    ▪ Discomfort or pain in back or abdomen

    ▪ Urinary incontinence in a child already toilet trained

    ▪ Infants

      □ Irritability/fussiness

      □ Crying upon urination

      □ Poor feeding

      □ Nausea, vomiting, and diarrhea

- Objective Data
    - Physical Assessment Findings
        - Fever
        - Diaper rash, perineal itching, and a reddened perineal area
    - Laboratory Tests
        - Urinalysis and urine culture and sensitivity
            - Sterile catheterization and/or suprapubic aspiration is the most accurate method for obtaining urine for urinalysis and culture in children less than 2 years of age.
            - Obtain a clean-catch urine sample from children who are able to cooperate.
            - Nursing Actions
                - If a suprapubic aspiration is to be performed, confirm that consent has been obtained.
                - To prevent a falsely low bacterial count, avoid having the child drink a large amount of oral fluids prior to obtaining a urine specimen.
                - Take the specimen for culture to the laboratory without delay.
                - Expected findings
                    - Urine culture – Positive for infecting organisms
                    - Urinalysis – Positive for bacteria and protein, cloudy, foul-smelling, bright red, and tea- or cola-colored with a pH greater than 7
                    - Microscopic exam of urine – RBC and WBC reveal greater than 100,000 organisms/mL
            - Client Education
                - Educate children and their families about the procedure for collecting a suprapubic aspiration, urine catheterization, or clean-voided specimen.
    - Diagnostic Procedures
        - Cystoscopy, voiding cystoureterography, intravenous pyelograms (IVP), and urodynamic tests
            - Use these tests after the resolution of a UTI to assess for anatomic or physical defects.
                - Nursing Actions
                    - Provide information to children and their families about the procedure for the diagnostic test prescribed.
                    - Ask if the child is allergic to iodine/shellfish, if a contrast medium is to be used.

▷ Sedate infants and young children if required. Assist the older child to remain quiet during the examinations.

▷ Maintain children on NPO status after midnight in preparation for a cystoscopy and IVP. IVP requires bowel preparation.

▷ Prepare children if catheterization is necessary.

▷ Monitor children after the procedure, according to facility protocol.

Collaborative Care

- Nursing Care

  o Encourage frequent voiding and complete emptying of the bladder.

  o Encourage fluids.

  o Monitor urine output.

  o Prepare children for diagnostic tests.

  o Administer a mild analgesic (acetaminophen [Tylenol]) for pain management.

  o Encourage sitz baths PRN.

- Medications

  o Antibiotics – Sulfamethoxazole and trimethoprim (Septra)

    ▪ Penicillins, cephalosporins, and nitrofurantoin (Macrobid)

    ▪ Nursing Considerations

      ☐ Monitor for potential allergic response.

    ▪ Client Education

      ☐ Instruct parents to have their children complete all prescribed antibiotics, even if symptoms are no longer present.

- Care After Discharge

  o Client Education

    ▪ Instruct the family to watch for signs and symptoms of recurrence of UTIs (dysuria, frequency, urgency).

    ▪ Provide instruction to prevent recurrence.

      ☐ Instruct females and parents of young children to wipe the perineal area from front to back.

      ☐ Instruct parents to retract and clean the foreskin of male infants.

      ☐ Instruct children and their families to keep underwear dry.

      ☐ Suggest the use of cotton underwear.

      ☐ Tell children to maintain adequate hydration.

- □ Instruct parents to avoid providing caffeinated or carbonated beverages. Recommend clear liquids.

- □ Instruct avoidance of bubble baths.

- □ Encourage frequent voiding.

- □ Encourage complete emptying of bladder using double voiding.

- □ Advise children and their families to avoid constipation and straining with bowel movements.

- □ Encourage adolescents who are sexually active to void immediately after intercourse.

- Client Outcomes

  o The child will be free from urinary tract infection.

  o The child will have preserved renal function.

Complications

- Progressive kidney injury

- Urosepsis

  o Nursing Actions

    ■ Monitor for signs and symptoms of UTIs.

  o Client Education

    ■ Reinforce teaching about prevention, early identification, and treatment of UTIs.

Ⓐ APPLICATION EXERCISES

Scenario: A nurse is caring for a school-age child with a UTI and a history of recurrent UTIs.

1. What findings related to the child's urine should the nurse expect to find?

2. The nurse is reinforcing discharge teaching with the child and her mother regarding the prevention of subsequent UTIs. Which of the following should be included in the teaching? (Select all that apply.)

    _____ Avoid bubble baths.

    _____ Have the child change her bathing suit immediately after swimming.

    _____ Encourage the child to go to the bathroom every 6 hr.

    _____ Have the child wear cotton underpants.

    _____ Instruct the child to wipe from front to back after voiding.

3. A nurse is assisting with the admission of a child who is having a cystoscopy with IVP to the pre-procedure area. Which of the following questions should the nurse ask the mother in data collection? (Select all that apply.)

    _____ "What were the results of the laxatives and enema?"

    _____ "Is your child allergic to iodine or shellfish?"

    _____ "Have other family members had these procedures?"

    _____ "What was his bedtime last night?"

    _____ "Does he need a night light when sleeping?"

4. A nurse in the pediatric clinic is reviewing the medication desmopressin acetate (DDAVP) with the mother of a child being treated for enuresis. Which of the following statements by the mother indicates a need for teaching?

    A. "I will give the medication in the evening."

    B. "It is important to limit how much he drinks after dinner."

    C. "The medication is applied to clean skin."

    D. "The bottle should be kept refrigerated."

(A) APPLICATION EXERCISES ANSWER KEY

Scenario: A nurse is caring for a school-age child with a UTI and a history of recurrent UTIs.

1. What findings related to the child's urine should the nurse expect to find?

   The child's urine may be cloudy and foul-smelling due to the presence of protein and bacteria. The color may range from bright red to tea or cola-colored due to the presence of red blood cells and the concentration of the urine. It may be foamy due to protein. The volume varies depending upon the age of the child but quantity is often reduced.

    NCLEX® Connection: Basic Care and Comfort, Elimination

2. The nurse is reinforcing discharge teaching with the child and her mother regarding the prevention of subsequent UTIs. Which of the following should be included in the teaching? (Select all that apply.)

X	**Avoid bubble baths.**
X	**Have the child change her bathing suit immediately after swimming.**
	Encourage the child to go to the bathroom every 6 hr.
X	**Have the child wear cotton underpants.**
X	**Instruct the child to wipe from front to back after voiding.**

   Bubble baths should not be taken by a child who is prone to UTIs. The wet lining of a bathing suit can foster bacterial growth, therefore, wet clothing should be changed as soon as possible. Cotton underwear keeps the perineal area drier than nylon preventing bacterial growth. The mother should encourage the child to go to the bathroom every 2 to 4 hr to prevent urine stasis. The perineal area should be wiped from front to back, otherwise, bacteria is introduced into the urinary meatus.

    NCLEX® Connection: Basic Care and Comfort, Elimination

3. A nurse is assisting with the admission of a child who is having a cystoscopy with IVP to the pre-procedure area. Which of the following questions should the nurse ask the mother in data collection? (Select all that apply.)

    __X__   **"What were the results of the laxatives and enema?"**

    __X__   **"Is your child allergic to iodine or shellfish?"**

    _____   "Have other family members had these procedures?"

    _____   "What was his bedtime last night?"

    _____   "Does he need a night light when sleeping?"

Questions to be included in data collection should be about the results of the laxatives and enema used for preoperative preparation. During an IVP, the bowel must be empty of stool in order to visualize the structures of the urinary tract. The IVP requires an injection of contrast medium which is contraindicated if there is an iodine or shellfish allergy. The other questions do not clarify whether the procedure can proceed. Asking about other family members having the procedure should clarify prior knowledge of the mother. Asking about the child's sleep patterns is part of developmental assessment but not relevant to the procedure.

Ⓝ NCLEX® Connection: Reduction of Risk Potential, Diagnostic Tests

4. A nurse in the pediatric clinic is reviewing the medication desmopressin acetate (DDAVP) with the mother of a child being treated for enuresis. Which of the following statements by the mother indicates a need for teaching?

A. "I will give the medication in the evening."

B. "It is important to limit how much he drinks after dinner."

C. "The medication is applied to clean skin."

D. "The bottle should be kept refrigerated."

Give the medication in the evening, restrict fluids after the evening meal, and keep the medication in the refrigerator. The medication is given as a nasal spray.

Ⓝ NCLEX® Connection: Pharmacological Therapies, Medication Administration

UNIT 2	NURSING CARE OF CHILDREN WITH SYSTEM DISORDERS
Section:	Genitourinary and Reproductive Disorders

Chapter 24   Structural Disorders of the Genitourinary Tract and Reproductive System

Overview

- Various structural disorders may be evident at birth and may affect normal genitourinary and reproductive function. These disorders include bladder exstrophy, hypospadias, epispadias, phimosis, cryptorchidism, and hydrocele.

- Children become aware of and are very interested in the genital area, normality of genital function, and gender differences between the ages of 3 and 6 years of age. Due to this, repair of structural defects should be done ideally between 6 to 15 months of age, but before age 3, to minimize impact on body image and to promote healthy development.

Data Collection

- Risk Factors

  o Hypospadias and epispadias may have a genetic link.

  o Ambiguous genitalia may be associated with congenital adrenal hyperplasia.

- Objective Data

  o Physical Assessment Findings

    ▪ Defect may or may not be visible.

    ▪ Bladder exstrophy is the protrusion of the bladder through an abdominal opening resulting from failure of the abdominal wall and other underlying structures to fuse in utero.

    ▪ Hypospadias occurs when the location of the urethral meatus is either on the bottom or on the ventral surface of the penis. Hypospadias may be accompanied by a chordee, which is a fibrous band on the ventral side of the penis resulting in a ventral curvature of the penis.

    ▪ Epispadias occurs when the location of the urethral meatus is on the dorsal side of the penis.

 View Media Supplement: Hypospadias, Epispadias, Chordee (Image)

    ▪ Phimosis is the narrowing of the preputial opening of the foreskin that prevents the foreskin from retracting over the penis.

- Cryptorchidism is the failure of one or both testicles to descend through the inguinal canal.

- Hydrocele is an abnormal collection of fluid in the scrotum.

- Ambiguous genitalia are congenital malformations that prevent visual identification of a child's sex.

  o Diagnostic Procedures

  - Ambiguous genitalia – Chromosome analysis is used to determine genetic karyotype.

    □ Ultrasonography is useful in assessing the presence or absence of genital and urinary structures.

    □ Biochemical tests may detect adrenal cortical syndromes.

    □ Nursing Actions

      ‣ Provide support for parents during the diagnosis.

      ‣ Administer sedation and assist with the procedure as needed.

    □ Client Education

      ‣ Advise the family and/or child about the procedure and what to expect.

      ‣ If NPO status is necessary, explain the parameters to the family and/or child.

Collaborative Care

- Nursing Care

  o Nursing care should focus on education and support of children and their families.

  - Evaluate the family's perception of the child's defect, family support, and coping.

  - Assist parents to identify ways to help children maintain a good self-image.

- Surgical Interventions

  - Structural defects will be treated with surgical intervention. The goal of most structural defect repairs is to preserve or create normal urinary and sexual function. Early intervention will minimize emotional trauma.

  - Nursing Actions

    □ Preoperative

      o Provide education to children and their families related to the procedure and expectations for postoperative care.

      ‣ Provide emotional support to children and their families.

      ‣ Encourage the parents to express concerns and fears related to the surgical procedure and outcomes.

☐ Postoperative

▸ Determine level of pain using an appropriate pain assessment tool.

▸ Administer pain medication as prescribed. An antispasmodic, such as oxybutynin (Ditropan), may be prescribed to treat painful bladder spasms.

▸ Monitor intake and output.

▸ Monitor urinary catheters, drains, or stents.

▸ Provide wound and/or dressing care.

▸ Monitor for signs of infection, such as redness, warmth, drainage, or edema at surgical site. Monitor for fever, lethargy, and foul-smelling urine.

▸ Do not provide tub baths for at least 1 week.

▸ Limit activity as prescribed.

■ Client Education

☐ Explain procedures at the appropriate level for children and their families.

☐ Use age-appropriate interventions to allay fears and anxiety.

☐ Help children understand that surgery is not a punishment, and it will not mutilate the body.

• Client Outcomes

○ The child will be free from infection.

○ The child will recover from surgical procedure without complications.

Complications

• Infection

○ Nursing Action

■ Observe for signs of infection including fever, skin inflammation, foul urine odor, cloudy urine, and/or urinary frequency.

○ Client Education

■ Instruct families to observe for signs of infection.

■ Tell families to report any signs of infection immediately.

• Emotional problems (poor self-esteem, altered body image, social isolation, fears)

○ Nursing Actions

■ Support children and their families by listening to concerns and correcting misperceptions.

■ Use play therapy for toddlers and preschoolers.

○ Client Education

■ Recommend children and their families attend a support group.

(A) APPLICATION EXERCISES

1. Match the area of the body a nurse should examine with the associated genitourinary structural defect.

_____ Dorsal surface of the penis	1. Exstrophy of the bladder
_____ Foreskin	2. Cryptorchidism
_____ Lower abdomen	3. Phimosis
_____ Scrotal sac	4. Epispadius
_____ Inguinal canal	5. Hypospadias
_____ Bottom or ventral surface of penis	6. Hydrocele

2. A nurse is discussing preoperative care with the parent of a child who will undergo surgery to correct hypospadias and a chordee. The parent states, "My son is only 8-months-old, why doesn't the surgeon wait to do the surgery until he is older?" Which of the following is the appropriate response by the nurse?

   A. "Children typically become aware of genitalia and gender between ages three and six. It's preferable to do the surgery when they are younger to minimize the impact on their self-image."

   B. "The surgery needs to be done at a young age before the constriction of the foreskin worsens and your son starts having urinary tract infections."

   C. "You're probably worried about this being painful, but I assure you that your son will receive pain medication after the surgery."

   D. "Your son will recover quickly and he's healthy, which is probably why the surgeon wants your son to have the surgery done now."

APPLICATION EXERCISES ANSWER KEY

1. Match the area of the body a nurse should examine with the associated genitourinary structural defect.

__4__	Dorsal surface of the penis	1. Exstrophy of the bladder
__3__	Foreskin	2. Cryptorchidism
__1__	Lower abdomen	3. Phimosis
__6__	Scrotal sac	4. Epispadius
__2__	Inguinal canal	5. Hypospadias
__5__	Bottom or ventral surface of penis	6. Hydrocele

NCLEX® Connection: Physiological Adaptations, Basic Pathophysiology

2. A nurse is discussing preoperative care with the parent of a child who will undergo surgery to correct hypospadias and a chordee. The parent states, "My son is only 8-months-old, why doesn't the surgeon wait to do the surgery until he is older?" Which of the following is the appropriate response by the nurse?

   A. "Children typically become aware of genitalia and gender between ages three and six. It's preferable to do the surgery when they are younger to minimize the impact on their self-image."

   B. "The surgery needs to be done at a young age before the constriction of the foreskin worsens and your son starts having urinary tract infections."

   C. "You're probably worried about this being painful, but I assure you that your son will receive pain medication after the surgery."

   D. "Your son will recover quickly and he's healthy, which is probably why the surgeon wants your son to have the surgery done now."

   A child's awareness of their genitalia, its function, and gender differences occurs between three and six years of age, therefore repair of defects is ideally done between six and 15 months of age to minimize the impact on body image and to promote healthy development. Repair of hypospadias and chordee does not involve constriction of the foreskin, which is typical of a phimosis defect. Assuming the parent is worried about pain is inappropriate and does not address the parent's question. While the child may be healthy, the nurse should not give false reassurance related to the child's rapid recovery.

NCLEX® Connection: Reduction of Risk Potential, Potential for Complications from Surgical Procedures and Health Alterations

UNIT 2	NURSING CARE OF CHILDREN WITH SYSTEM DISORDERS
Section:	Genitourinary and Reproductive Disorders

Chapter 25   Renal Disorders

Overview

- Acute glomerulonephritis (AGN)

    o   Acute glomerulonephritis may occur as a single episode or may be the result of a disease, usually following an infectious process. The most common types are pneumococcal, streptococcal, and viral infections.

    o   Oliguria, edema, hypertension, circulatory congestion, hematuria, and proteinuria are common findings associated with AGN.

- Nephrotic syndrome is a group of symptoms, not a disease. It is the most common presentation of glomerular injury in children. Three forms of the syndrome include primary, congenital, and secondary nephrotic syndrome. The most common form of disease in children is minimal change nephrotic syndrome and accounts for 80% of all cases.

ACUTE GLOMERULONEPHRITIS (AGN)

Overview

- Acute poststreptococcal glomerulonephritis (APSGN) is the most common of the postinfectious renal diseases.

    o   APSGN is an antibody-antigen disease that occurs as a result of certain strains of the Group A ß-hemolytic streptococcal infection and is most commonly seen in children between the ages of 6 and 7.

    o   The exact mechanism of the pathophysiology for APSGN is not certain. It is believed that immune complexes develop and become trapped in the glomerular capillary loop at the basement membrane. This produces swelling and occlusion of the capillary lumen and results in alterations in the glomerular filtration rate.

    o   Renal manifestations usually occur 10 to 21 days post infection.

    o   Prognosis varies depending upon the specific cause, but spontaneous recovery generally occurs after the acute illness. Recurrence is not common.

Data Collection

- Risk Factors

  - Infection with pneumococcal, streptococcal, or viral agent

- Subjective Data

  - Recent upper respiratory infection or streptococcal infection

  - Lack of specific reports (Older children may report abdominal discomfort, headaches, painful urination, and anorexia/nausea.)

- Objective Data

  - Physical Assessment Findings

    - Decreased glomerular filtration rate leading to decreased urine output

    - Anorexia

    - Pallor

    - Vague reports of discomfort (headache, abdominal pain, dysuria)

    - Dyspnea

    - Orthopnea

    - Moist crackles on auscultation

    - Distended neck veins

    - Periorbital edema

    - Facial edema that is worse in the morning but then spreads to extremities and abdomen with progression of the day

    - Mild to severe hypertension

    - Pale appearance, irritability, and lethargy (The child seems ill.)

  - Laboratory Tests

    - Throat culture to identify possible streptococcus infection (usually negative by the time of diagnosis)

    - Urinalysis – Proteinuria, smoky or tea-colored urine, hematuria, cell debris (red cells and casts), elevated specific gravity

    - Renal function – Elevated BUN and creatinine

    - Antistreptolysin-O (ASO) titer – Positive indicator for the presence of streptococcal antibodies

    - Antihyaluronidase (AHase), antideoxyribonuclease B (ADNase-B), and streptozyme antibodies may be present.

    - Serum complement (C3) – Decreased initially; increases as recovery takes place; returns to normal at 8 to 10 weeks post-glomerulonephritis

- ○ Diagnostic Procedures
    - ■ Chest x-ray
        - □ Use to identify pulmonary complications, especially during the edematous phase
            - ‣ Pulmonary edema
            - ‣ Cardiac enlargement
            - ‣ Pleural effusions
        - □ Nursing Actions
            - ‣ Ensure that adolescents are not pregnant.
            - ‣ Assist with proper positioning.
        - □ Client Education
            - ‣ Explain the procedure to children and their families.

Collaborative Care

- • Nursing Care
    - ○ Monitor I&O.
    - ○ Monitor daily weights; weigh children on the same scale with the same amount of clothing daily.
    - ○ Monitor vital signs.
    - ○ Monitor neurologic status and observe for behavior changes, especially in children who have edema, hypertension, and gross hematuria. Implement seizure precautions if condition indicates.
    - ○ Encourage adequate nutritional intake within restriction guidelines. A regular diet with elimination of high sodium foods will be appropriate for most.
        - ■ Restrict foods high in potassium during periods of oliguria.
        - ■ Provide small, frequent meals of favorite foods due to a decrease in appetite.
    - ○ Manage fluid restrictions as prescribed. Fluids may be restricted during periods of edema and hypertension.
    - ○ Monitor skin for breakdown areas and prevent pressure sores.
        - ■ Encourage frequent turning and repositioning.
        - ■ Keep skin dry.
        - ■ Pad bony prominences and use a specialty mattress.
        - ■ Elevate edematous body parts.
    - ○ Observe tolerance for activity. Provide for frequent rest periods.
    - ○ Provide for age-appropriate diversional activities.

- ○ Cluster care to facilitate rest and tolerance of activity.

- ○ Monitor and prevent infection.

  - Advise children to turn, cough, and deep breathe to prevent pulmonary involvement.

  - Monitor vital signs, especially temperature, for changes secondary to infection.

  - Maintain good hand hygiene.

  - Administer antibiotic therapy as prescribed.

- ○ Provide emotional support.

- Medications

  - ○ Diuretics and antihypertensives

    - Use to remove accumulated fluid and manage hypertension

    - Nursing Considerations

      - ☐ Monitor blood pressure.

      - ☐ Monitor intake and output.

      - ☐ Monitor for electrolyte imbalances, such as hypokalemia.

      - ☐ Observe for side effects of medications.

    - Client Education

      - ☐ Encourage children to eat food high in potassium if potassium-sparing diuretics are not used.

      - ☐ Inform children and their families that dizziness can occur with the use of antihypertensives.

      - ☐ Instruct children and their families to take the medication as prescribed and notify the provider if side effects occur. Give instructions to continue the medication unless instructed otherwise.

- Interdisciplinary Care

  - ○ Nutrition services can offer dietary support.

- Care After Discharge

  - ○ Client Education

    - Encourage children to verbalize feelings related to body image.

    - Educate children and their families regarding appropriate dietary management.

    - Encourage adequate rest.

    - Inform families about the need for follow-up care. The child should be seen by the provider weekly for several weeks and then monthly until the disease is fully resolved.

    - Show families how to monitor blood pressure and daily weight.

- ■ Instruct families about administration and side effects of diuretics and antihypertensive medications.

- ■ Encourage children and their families to avoid contact with others who may be ill.

- • Client Outcomes

  - ○ The child will maintain optimal renal function.

  - ○ The child will maintain blood pressure within the expected reference range.

  - ○ The child and family will have adequate support.

NEPHROTIC SYNDROME

Overview

- • Nephrotic syndrome

  - ○ In nephrotic syndrome, alterations in the glomerular membrane allow proteins (especially albumin) to pass into the urine, resulting in decreased serum osmotic pressure. The exact cause of glomerular alteration is not well understood and is thought to be due to metabolic, biochemical, physiochemical, or immune-mediated causes.

  - ○ Nephrotic syndrome is characterized by hyperlipidemia, proteinuria, hypoalbuminemia, and edema.

  - ○ Management of nephrotic syndrome is aimed at reducing the excretion of protein, reducing fluid retention, preventing infection, and preventing complications.

Data Collection

- • Risk Factors

  - ○ Minimal change nephrotic syndrome (MCNS)

    - ■ Peak incidence is between 2 and 7 years of age.

    - ■ Cause is unknown, but it may have a multifactorial etiology (immune-mediated, biochemical).

  - ○ Secondary nephrotic syndrome (occurs after or is associated with glomerular damage due to a known cause)

  - ○ Congenital nephrotic syndrome (an inherited disorder)

- • Subjective Data

  - ○ Weight gain over a short period of days or weeks

  - ○ Poor appetite, possibly anorexia, nausea and vomiting, and diarrhea

  - ○ Decreased activity levels

  - ○ Irritability

- Objective Data
  - Physical Assessment Findings
    - Weight gain
    - Edema (facial/periorbital) is worse in morning and decreases as the day progresses.
    - Ascites and dependent edema (especially in the labia, scrotum, legs, and ankles)
    - Dark, frothy urine, decreased urine output, and oliguria
    - Normal or slightly elevated blood pressure
  - Laboratory Tests
    - Urinalysis/24-hr urine collection
      - Proteinuria – Protein greater than 3+ or 4+ (greater than 3.5 g in 24 hr)
      - Hyaline casts
      - Increased specific gravity
      - Color change
    - Serum chemistry
      - Hypoalbuminemia – Reduced serum protein and albumin
      - Hyperlipidemia – Elevated serum lipid levels
      - Hemoconcentration – Elevated Hgb, Hct, and platelets
  - Diagnostic Procedures
    - Kidney biopsy is indicated only if nephrotic syndrome is unresponsive to steroid therapy.
      - Biopsy will show damage to the epithelial cells lining the basement membrane of the kidney.

Collaborative Care

- Nursing Care
  - Provide rest.
  - Monitor I&O. Monitor urine for specific gravity and protein.
  - Monitor daily weights; weigh children on the same scale, with the same amount of clothing, at the same time of day.
  - Monitor edema and measure abdominal girth daily. Measure at the widest area, usually at or above the umbilicus. Monitor degree of pitting, color, and texture of skin.

- ○ Monitor and prevent infection.

  - ■ Assist children to turn, cough, and deep breathe to prevent pulmonary involvement.

  - ■ Monitor vital signs, especially temperature, for changes secondary to infection.

  - ■ Maintain good hand hygiene.

  - ■ Administer antibiotic therapy as prescribed.

- ○ Encourage nutritional intake within restriction guidelines. Salt and fluids may be restricted during the edematous phase. Increase protein in diet to replace protein losses.

- ○ Cluster care to provide for rest periods.

- ○ Check skin for breakdown areas. Prevent pressure sores.

  - ■ Avoid use of urinary collection bags in very young children.

  - ■ Pad bony prominences or use a specialty mattress to prevent breakdown of skin.

  - ■ Encourage frequent turning and repositioning of children.

  - ■ Keep the child's skin dry.

  - ■ Elevate edematous body parts.

- • Medications

  - ○ Corticosteroid – Prednisone (Deltasone)

  - ○ Nursing Considerations

    - ■ Administer for 7 to 21 days (based on response) and then taper over several months with decreasing doses until discontinued.

    - ■ Monitor for infection.

  - ○ Client Education

    - ■ Educate children and their families to avoid large crowds (to decrease the risk of infection).

    - ■ Instruct families to administer the medication on alternate days after the first 4 weeks of therapy.

    - ■ Inform children and their families that using corticosteroids can increase appetite, cause weight gain (especially in the face), and cause mood swings.

  - ○ Diuretic – Furosemide (Lasix)

    - ■ Eliminates excess fluid from the body

    - ■ Nursing Considerations

      - □ Encourage children to eat foods that are high in potassium.

      - □ Monitor serum electrolyte levels periodically.

- ○ 25% albumin
    - ▪ Increases plasma volume and decreases edema
    - ▪ Nursing Considerations
        - □ Monitor children receiving IV infusion.
        - □ Monitor I&O.
        - □ Watch for anaphylaxis.
  - ○ Cyclophosphamide (Cytoxan)
    - ▪ Monitor children who cannot tolerate prednisone or who have repeated relapses of MCNS.
- Interdisciplinary Care
  - ○ Nutrition services can offer suggestions for dietary management.
- Care After Discharge
  - ○ Client Education
    - ▪ Encourage children to verbalize feelings related to body image.
    - ▪ Reinforce teaching to children regarding appropriate dietary management.
    - ▪ Encourage adequate rest.
    - ▪ Reinforce instructions to families about the need for follow-up care. Children should be seen by the provider weekly for several weeks and then monthly until the disease is fully resolved.
    - ▪ Inform families of strategies to decrease the risk of infection (good hand hygiene, up-to-date immunizations, avoidance of infected people).
    - ▪ Show families how to monitor blood pressure, daily weight, and protein in urine. Instruct the family to notify the provider if symptoms worsen, which indicates relapse.
    - ▪ Reinforce to families about administration and side effects of medication.
    - ▪ Provide support to families and offer health and community services as needed. Relapses can cause physical, emotional, and financial stress for the child and family.
  - ○ Client Outcomes
    - ▪ The child will be free of infection.
    - ▪ The child will maintain optimal renal function.
    - ▪ The child will maintain a blood pressure that is within a normal reference range.
    - ▪ The child and family will have adequate support.

Complications

- Sepsis/Infection

    o Steroid therapy increases the risk for infection.

        ■ Common infections seen in children with nephrotic syndrome include pneumonia, peritonitis, and cellulitis.

    o Nursing Actions

        ■ Keep children away from potential infection sources.

        ■ Monitor for signs of infection.

    o Client Education

        ■ Reinforce to families the importance of completing the full dose of antibiotic.

        ■ Reinforce to families about the need for performing frequent hand hygiene.

        ■ Reinforce to families about signs and symptoms of infection and when to contact the provider.

        ■ Reinforce to families about potential infection sources (live plants, sick family members).

Ⓐ APPLICATION EXERCISES

Scenario: A nurse is caring for a school-age child with acute glomerulonephritis who is taking potassium-sparing diuretics.

1. The nurse anticipates discussing the diet with the child and his parents. The diet should include

   A. potassium-rich foods.

   B. foods low in cholesterol.

   C. an increase in calories.

   D. a sodium restriction.

2. The nurse is reviewing discharge instructions with the child and his parent. Which of the following should the nurse include? (Select all that apply.)

   _____ Weigh the child daily.

   _____ Check the child's apical pulse daily.

   _____ Resume usual physical activity.

   _____ Continue the prescribed antibiotics.

   _____ Elevate edematous body parts.

Scenario: A nurse is assisting with the admission of a toddler who has nephrotic syndrome.

3. Which of the following objective data should the nurse anticipate collecting from the child?

   A. Elevated blood pressure

   B. Facial edema noticeable in the evening

   C. 3+ to 4+ protein in the urine

   D. Arms and legs appear thin with loose skin

4. The child is to start a prescription for prednisone (Deltasone). Describe how the medication will be administered and the possible effects the medication can have on the child.

Ⓐ APPLICATION EXERCISES ANSWER KEY

Scenario: A nurse is caring for a school-age child with acute glomerulonephritis who is taking potassium-sparing diuretics.

1. The nurse anticipates discussing the diet with the child and his parents. The diet should include

   A. potassium-rich foods.

   B. foods low in cholesterol.

   C. an increase in calories.

   D. a sodium restriction.

   The diet for a client with glomerulonephritis who is taking potassium-sparing diuretics will have a sodium restriction identified by the provider. Encouraging potassium-rich foods could lead to hyperkalemia. There are no restrictions related to cholesterol or the need for increased calories.

   Ⓝ **NCLEX® Connection: Basic Care and Comfort, Nutrition and Oral Hydration**

2. The nurse is reviewing discharge instructions with the child and his parent. Which of the following should the nurse include? (Select all that apply.)

X	**Weigh the child daily.**
X	**Check the child's apical pulse daily.**
	Resume usual physical activity.
X	**Continue the prescribed antibiotics.**
X	**Elevate edematous body parts.**

   Discharge instructions for the school-age child with acute glomerulonephritis should include checking weight and blood pressure daily, continuing the prescribed antibiotics and elevating edematous body parts. In addition, the child should limit activity to provide for adequate rest, follow a sodium-restricted diet, return to the provider as identified, take diuretics and antihypertensive medications as prescribed, and avoid contact with persons who are ill.

   Ⓝ **NCLEX® Connection: Reduction of Risk Potential, Potential for Alterations in Body Systems**

Scenario: A nurse is assisting with the admission of a toddler who has nephrotic syndrome.

3. Which of the following objective data should the nurse anticipate collecting from the child?

    A. Elevated blood pressure

    B. Facial edema noticeable in the evening

    C. 3+ to 4+ protein in the urine

    D. Arms and legs appear thin with loose skin

    The child with nephrotic syndrome will have large amounts of protein in the urine and hematuria may be present. Blood pressure will be low to normal. Facial edema will be worse in the morning and decrease throughout the day. Ascites with dependent edema is present and more pronounced in the legs, ankles, labia, and scrotum.

    (N) NCLEX® Connection: Reduction of Risk Potential, System Specific Assessment

4. The child is to start a prescription for prednisone (Deltasone). Describe how the medication will be administered and the possible effects the medication can have on the child.

    The child will start to take large doses which are tapered over time. Review the administration schedule after discharge with the parents. Effects of this medication can include increased appetite, weight gain which may be more apparent in the face, and mood swings. The child is at increased risk for infection while on the medication.

    (N) NCLEX® Connection: Pharmacological Therapies, Adverse Effects/ Contraindications/Side Effects/Interactions

UNIT 2: NURSING CARE OF CHILDREN WITH SYSTEM DISORDERS

Section: Musculoskeletal Disorders

- Fractures

- Musculoskeletal Congenital Disorders

- Chronic Neuromusculoskeletal Disorders

NCLEX® CONNECTIONS

When reviewing the chapters in this section, keep in mind the relevant sections of the NCLEX® outline, in particular:

CLIENT NEEDS: BASIC CARE AND COMFORT

Relevant topics/tasks include:
- Mobility/Immobility
  - Provide care to client in traction.
- Nonpharmacologic Comfort Interventions
  - Apply therapies for comfort and treatment of inflammation/swelling.
- Rest and Sleep
  - Provide measures to promote sleep/rest.

CLIENT NEEDS: PHARMACOLOGICAL THERAPIES

Relevant topics/tasks include:
- Adverse Effects/Contraindications/Side Effects/Interactions
  - Monitor anticipated interactions among client prescribed medications and fluids.
- Expected Actions/Outcomes
  - Evaluate client response to medication.
- Pharmacological Pain Management
  - Identify client need for pain medication.

CLIENT NEEDS: REDUCTION OF RISK POTENTIAL

Relevant topics/tasks include:
- Potential for Alterations in Body Systems
  - Perform circulatory checks.
- Potential for Complications of Diagnostic Tests/Treatments/Procedures
  - Implement measures to prevent complication of client condition or procedure.
- Therapeutic Procedures
  - Assist with performance of a diagnostic or invasive procedure.

UNIT 2	NURSING CARE OF CHILDREN WITH SYSTEM DISORDERS
Section:	Musculoskeletal Disorders

Chapter 26   Fractures

Overview

- A fracture occurs when the resistance between a bone and an applied stress yields to the applied stress, resulting in a disruption to the integrity of the bone.

- Bone healing and remodeling is faster in children than in adults, due to a thicker periosteum and good blood supply.

- Epiphyseal plate injuries may result in altered bone growth.

- Radiographic evidence of previous fractures in various stages of healing or in infants may be the result of physical abuse or osteogenesis imperfecta.

Data Collection

- Risk Factors

  o Developmental characteristics, ordinary play, activities, and recreation place children at risk for injury (falls from climbing or running; trauma to bones from skateboarding, skiing, playing soccer, or playing basketball).

- Subjective Data

  o Pain

  o Muscle spasms (occur from the pulling forces of the bone when not aligned)

  o Loss of function

  o Report of children refusing to ambulate or crawl

- Objective Data

  o Physical Assessment Findings

  ▪ Common types of fractures in children

  □ Plastic deformation (bend) – The bone is bent no more than 45°.

  □ Buckle (torus) – A bulge or raised area is present at the fracture site.

□ Greenstick – A fracture occurs in only one cortex of the bone.

□ Spiral fracture – occurs from twisting motion (may be due to physical abuse)

View Media Supplement: Fractures (Image)

□ Complete – Divides the fragments, these fragments may remain attached by a periosteal hinge.

□ Incomplete – Bone fragments are still attached.

▸ The fracture line can be transverse, oblique, or spiral.

□ Simple or closed – The fracture occurs without a break in the skin

□ Open or compound – The fracture occurs with an open wound and bone protruding.

□ Complicated fracture – The fracture results in injury to other organs and tissues.

- Crepitus – A grating sound created by the rubbing together of bone fragments

- Deformity – May observe internal rotation of extremity, shortened extremity, and visible bone with open fracture

- Visible muscle spasms – Occur from the pulling forces of the bone when not aligned

- Edema – Swelling from trauma

- Ecchymosis – Bleeding into underlying soft tissues from trauma

- Neurovascular Check

□ Pain – Determine the child's pain level, location, and frequency. Use an age-appropriate pain rating scale and have the child describe the pain.

□ Sensation – Check children for numbness or a tingling sensation of the extremity. Loss of sensation may indicate nerve damage.

□ Skin temperature – Check the extremity for temperature. The extremity should be warm, not cool, to touch.

□ Skin color – Observe the color of the affected extremity. Check distal to the injury and look for changes in pigmentation.

□ Capillary refill – Press the nail beds of the affected extremity until blanching occurs. Blood return should be within 3 seconds.

□ Pulses – Pulses should be palpable and strong. Pulses should also be equal to the pulses of the unaffected extremity.

□ Movement – Children should be able to move the affected extremity in passive motion.

- ○ Diagnostic Procedures
    - ■ Radiographic assessment
        - □ Radiographic films are the most common diagnostic tool used for fractures.
        - □ Nursing Actions
            - ‣ Instruct and assist children to remain still during the procedure.
            - ‣ Sedate children if prescribed.
        - □ Client Education
            - ‣ Educate children and their parents about what to expect during the procedure.
            - ‣ Provide emotional support.

Collaborative Care

- ● Nursing Care
    - ○ Provide emergency care at the time of injury.
        - ■ Maintain ABCs.
        - ■ Monitor vital signs, pain, and neurologic status.
        - ■ Check the neurovascular status of the injured extremity.
        - ■ Position children in a supine position.
        - ■ Stabilize the injured area, avoiding unnecessary movement.
        - ■ Elevate the affected limb and apply ice packs.
        - ■ Administer analgesics as prescribed.
        - ■ Keep children warm.
    - ○ General nursing interventions
        - ■ Check pain frequently using an age-appropriate pain tool and use appropriate pain management, both pharmacological and nonpharmacological.
        - ■ Monitor neurovascular status on a regular schedule. Report any change in status.
        - ■ Maintain proper alignment.
        - ■ Promote range of motion of fingers, toes, and unaffected extremities.
        - ■ Instruct children and their families regarding activity restrictions.

- Medications

  - Analgesics

    - Administer analgesics for pain.

    - Nursing Considerations (for use of opioid analgesia)

      - When using opioid analgesia, monitor for respiratory depression and constipation.

    - Client Education

      - Reinforce the need for adequate pain relief.

      - Reinforce the need for proper nutrition and hydration.

- Interdisciplinary Care

  - Orthopedic specialists are generally consulted for fracture care in children.

  - Notify social services in situations in which abuse is suspected.

- Therapeutic Procedures

  - Casting

    - Plaster of Paris casts are heavy, are not water resistant, and can take 10 to 72 hr to dry. Synthetic fiberglass casts are light, are water resistant, and dry very quickly (in 5 to 30 min).

    - Prior to casting, the skin area should be observed for integrity, cleaned, and dried. Bony prominences should be padded to prevent skin breakdown. The casting material is then applied by the provider.

    - Nursing Actions

      - Position child on a firm mattress. Use an over-bed trapeze for an older child.

      - Elevate the cast above the level of the heart during the first 24 to 48 hr to prevent swelling.

      - Apply ice for the first 24 hr to decrease swelling.

      - Turn and position child every 2 hr so that dry air circulates around and under the cast for faster drying. This will also prevent pressure from changing the shape of the cast.

        ▸ Do not use heat lamps or warm hair dryers.

      - Turn children frequently while supporting all extremities and joints.

      - Instruct child to keep the affected extremity supported (with a sling) or elevated when sitting.

      - Check for increased warmth or hot spots on the cast surface, which could indicate infection.

      - If a wound is present, monitor the skin through the window that has been placed in an area of the cast to allow for skin inspection.

- □ Monitor for drainage on the cast. Outline any drainage on the outside of the cast with a marker (and note date and time) so it can be monitored for any additional drainage.

- □ Check the general skin condition and the area around the cast edges.

- □ Provide routine skin care and thorough perineal care to maintain skin integrity.

- □ Use moleskin over any rough area of the cast that may rub against the child's skin.

- □ Cover areas of the cast with plastic to avoid soiling from urine or feces.

- □ Assist with proper crutch fitting and reinforce proper use.

- ■ Client Education

  - □ Tell children and their families that when the cast is applied it will feel warm, but it will not cause a burn.

  - □ Tell children to report pain that is extremely severe or is not relieved 1 hr after the administration of pain medication.

  - □ Show child and their family how to perform neurovascular checks and when to contact the provider.

  - □ Give instructions for the proper use of crutches for lower extremity casts.

  - □ Reinforce skin and perineal care with a spica cast.

  - □ Instruct children not to place any foreign objects under the cast to avoid trauma to the skin.

  - □ Reinforce use of proper restraints when transporting children in any vehicle.

  - □ Tell children and their families about cast removal and cast cutter.

  - □ Instruct children to soak the extremity in warm water and then apply lotion after the cast has been removed

- ○ Traction care – Traction, countertraction, and friction are the three components used to align, immobilize, and reduce muscle spasms associated with certain fractures. Through the use of a forward-pulling force and a backward force, adding or removing weight controls the degree of force applied to maintain traction and alignment. The type of traction used will vary depending on the fracture, age of the child, and associated injuries.

  - ■ Skin traction uses a pulling force that is applied by weights (may be used intermittently). Using tape and straps applied to the skin along with boots and/ or cuffs, weights are attached by a rope to the extremity (Buck's traction, Russell's traction).

  - ■ Skeletal traction uses a continuous pulling force that is applied directly to the skeletal structure and/or specific bone. A pin or rod is inserted through or into the bone. Force is applied through the use of weights attached by rope. Skeletal traction (90°/90° traction) allows child to change positions without interfering with the pull of the traction and decreases complications associated with immobility and traction.

- Halo traction is another type of skeletal traction that uses a halo-type bar that encircles the head. Screws are inserted into the outer table of the skull. The halo is attached to either bed traction or rods that are secured to a vest worn by the child.

 View Media Supplement: Halo Traction (Image)

- Nursing Actions
  - Maintain body alignment and realign if children seem uncomfortable or report pain.
  - Provide pharmacological and nonpharmacological interventions for the management of pain and muscle spasms.
  - Notify the provider if children experience severe pain from muscle spasms that is unrelieved with medications and/or repositioning.
  - Monitor neurovascular status.
  - Routinely monitor the child's skin integrity and document findings.
  - Check pin sites for pain, redness, swelling, drainage, or odor. Provide pin care per facility protocol.
  - Check for changes in elimination and maintain usual patterns of elimination.
  - Check that all the hardware is tight and that the bed is in the correct position.
  - Maintain weights so that they hang freely and the ropes are free of knots. Do not lift or remove weights unless prescribed and supervised by the provider or physical therapist.
  - Assure that the wrench to release the rods is attached to the vest when using halo traction in the event that CPR is necessary.
  - Move children in halo traction as a unit without applying pressure to the rods. This will prevent loosening of the pins and pain.
  - Consult with the provider for an over-bed trapeze to assist child to move in bed.
  - Provide range of motion and encourage activity of non-immobilized extremities to maintain mobility and prevent contractures.
  - Promote frequent position changing within restrictions of traction.
  - Remove sheets from the head of the bed to the foot of the bed, and remake the bed in the same manner.
- Client Education
  - Instruct about the need for adequate hydration and nutrition while in traction.
  - Reinforce about the use and need for stool softeners.
  - Tell child and parents to report signs of infection.

- Surgical Interventions

  - Depending on the type of fracture, surgical intervention may be required. The most common fractures requiring surgery include supracondylar fractures and fractures of the humerus and femur.

  - Surgical reduction is achieved by either a closed (no incision) or open (with incision) reduction with or without pinning.

    - Nursing Actions

      - Monitor for signs of infection at the incision site.

      - Encourage mobilization as soon as prescribed.

      - Medicate for pain as needed.

    - Client Education

      - Teach and reinforce to children and their families what to expect before and after the procedure, including NPO status.

      - Instruct about the need for pain medication.

- Care After Discharge

  - Client Education

    - Reinforce proper cast care, as well as pin care if indicated.

    - Reinforce how to perform neurovascular checks and when to call or return to the provider.

    - Reinforce about the need for and use of antipruritic medications if prescribed by the provider.

    - Instruct the parents to maintain physical restrictions as prescribed.

    - Instruct the parents in appropriate pain management.

    - Instruct the parents to report signs and symptoms of increasing pain, redness, inflammation and/or fever to the health care provider.

    - Instruct the parents regarding the importance of follow-up care as instructed by the provider.

- Client Outcomes

  - The child will heal without complications.

  - The child will maintain normal bowel function.

  - The child will remain free of infection.

Complications

- Compartment syndrome

  - Compartment syndrome occurs when pressure within one or more of the muscle compartments of the extremity compromises circulation resulting in an ischemia-edema cycle with compromised neurovascular status.

  - Pressure can result from external sources, such as a tight cast or a constrictive, bulky dressing. Internal sources, such as an accumulation of blood or fluid within the muscle compartment, can also cause pressure.

  - If untreated, tissue necrosis can result. Neuromuscular damage occurs within 4 to 6 hr.

  - Findings

    - Increased pain that is unrelieved with elevation

    - Intense pain when passively moved

    - Paresthesia or numbness

    - Pallor

  - Nursing Actions

    - Monitor the extremity at frequent intervals. Notify the provider if compartment syndrome is suspected so that the cast may be cut.

    - Prevention

      - Loosen the constrictive dressing or cut the bandage or tape.

      - Elevate the extremity and apply ice. If compartment syndrome is suspected, to ensure adequate perfusion, the arm should not be elevated above the level of the heart.

    - Prepare children for fasciotomy.

  - Client Education

    - Instruct children to report pain that is not relieved by analgesics, pain that continues to increase in intensity, numbness or tingling, or a change in color of the extremity.

- Osteomyelitis

  - Infection within the bone secondary to a bacterial infection from an outside source, such as with an open fracture (endogenous) or from a bloodborne bacterial source (hematogenous)

  - Signs and symptoms

    - Children will appear ill.

    - Children will not want to use the affected extremity.

    - The site of infection will be tender, and bone pain will worsen with movement.

    - Warmth, erythema, edema, and fever may occur.

- o Nursing Actions
  - Assist in diagnostic procedures, such as obtaining skin, blood, and bone cultures.
  - Assist with joint or bone biopsy.
  - Monitor children receiving IV fluids and antibiotic therapy.
  - Assist with proper positioning to promote comfort.
  - Administer pain medication as prescribed.
  - Consult with the parents and provider regarding home care needs.
- o Client Education
  - Educate children and their families about the length of treatment that may be needed.
  - Remind children to avoid bearing any weight until cleared by the provider.
  - Advise the parents to provide for diversional activities consistent with the child's level of development.
  - Educate children about the need for proper nutrition.

Ⓐ APPLICATION EXERCISES

Scenario: A nurse is caring for a school-age child who has sustained a cervical fracture while diving into a swimming pool. After surgery, the child is placed in halo traction attached to rods and a vest to stabilize the fracture.

1. When collecting data about the halo traction, which of the following should the nurse include? (Select all that apply.)

    _____ Condition of the skin under the vest

    _____ Availability of the rod-release wrench

    _____ Condition of the pin sites

    _____ Position of the weights on the ropes

    _____ Condition of the tape and straps on the skin

2. Describe the appropriate pin site care that should be included in the nurse's plan of care.

3. A nurse is caring for a child following surgical repair of a fractured femur. Which of the following nursing actions prevents the development of compartment syndrome?

    A. Apply heat to the extremity.

    B. Place the child in Fowler's position.

    C. Elevate the extremity.

    D. Check the dorsalis pedis pulse.

4. A nurse is reviewing discharge teaching with the parent of a child who has osteomyelitis. Which of the following statements by the parent indicates the need for further teaching?

    A. "I know he will be on antibiotics for a long time."

    B. "I'm happy he will be able to walk on his injured leg."

    C. "I will make sure he gets increased protein in his diet as well as vitamin C for healing."

    D. "Having his friends over again for board games will be good for my son."

5. The sound that can be heard when bone fragments rub together is known as _crepitus_.

6. A fracture without a break in the skin is a _closed or simple_ fracture.

7. In cases of physical abuse, a _spiral_ fracture often occurs due to a twisting motion.

APPLICATION EXERCISES ANSWER KEY

> **Scenario:** A nurse is caring for a school-age child who has sustained a cervical fracture while diving into a swimming pool. After surgery, the child is placed in halo traction attached to rods and a vest to stabilize the fracture.

1. When collecting data about the halo traction, which of the following should the nurse include? (Select all that apply.)

X	**Condition of the skin under the vest**
X	**Availability of the rod-release wrench**
X	**Condition of the pin sites**
_____	Position of the weights on the ropes
_____	Condition of the tape and straps on the skin

   Data collection regarding halo traction includes condition of the skin under the vest and at the pin sites, and the location of the wrench to release the rods attached to the vest. The nurse should also verify that all connections on the halo and rods are tight. Halo traction with rods and a vest does not have weights on ropes attached to the traction and there is no tape or strap on the child's skin. These should be checked with skeletal and skin traction.

    NCLEX® Connection: Basic Care and Comfort, Mobility/Immobility

2. Describe the appropriate pin site care that should be included in the nurse's plan of care.

   The nurse should check the pin sites for pain, redness, swelling, drainage, or odor. Care of the pin sites should follow facility protocol and should include cleaning with sterile water or other prescribed solution, and the application of antibacterial ointment and sterile gauze. Some orthopedic surgeons may prefer the sites to remain undisturbed.

    NCLEX® Connection: Basic Care and Comfort, Mobility/Immobility

3. A nurse is caring for a child following surgical repair of a fractured femur. Which of the following nursing actions prevents the development of compartment syndrome?

   A. Apply heat to the extremity.

   B. Place the child in Fowler's position.

   C. Elevate the extremity.

   D. Check the dorsalis pedis pulse.

   Elevation of the extremity and the application of ice are nursing actions that prevent the development of compartment syndrome. Placing the child in Fowler's position is not indicated and may constrict blood flow to the lower extremity. Checking the pedal pulse monitors circulation to the extremity but is not a preventative action.

 NCLEX® Connection: Basic Care and Comfort, Mobility/Immobility

4. A nurse is reviewing discharge teaching with the parent of a child who has osteomyelitis. Which of the following statements by the parent indicates the need for further teaching?

   A. "I know he will be on antibiotics for a long time."

   B. "I'm happy he will be able to walk on his injured leg."

   C. "I will make sure he gets increased protein in his diet as well as vitamin C for healing."

   D. "Having his friends over again for board games will be good for my son."

   Weight bearing or use of the affected body part is avoided unless prescribed by the provider and would require further teaching. The child is often on long-term antibiotic therapy. Added protein and vitamin C for healing should be included in teaching about proper nutrition. Diversional activities consistent with the child's age and physical limitations are important after discharge.

 NCLEX® Connection: Basic Care and Comfort, Mobility/Immobility

5. The sound that can be heard when bone fragments rub together is known as **crepitus**.

   Crepitus may be heard at the site of a complete or incomplete fracture.

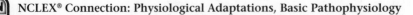 NCLEX® Connection: Physiological Adaptations, Basic Pathophysiology

6. A fracture without a break in the skin is a **closed or simple** fracture.

   A closed or simple fracture does not involve a break in the skin. An open or compound fracture will involve injury to the skin.

NCLEX® Connection: Physiological Adaptations, Basic Pathophysiology

7. In cases of physical abuse, a **spiral** fracture often occurs due to a twisting motion.

   Spiral fractures are typically seen in cases of physical abuse where twisting of the extremity has occurred.

NCLEX® Connection: Physiological Adaptations, Basic Pathophysiology

UNIT 2	NURSING CARE OF CHILDREN WITH SYSTEM DISORDERS
Section:	Musculoskeletal Disorders

Chapter 27   Musculoskeletal Congenital Disorders

Overview

- Congenital clubfoot is a complex deformity of the ankle and foot. Description of the deformity will be dependent upon the position of the ankle and foot. The most common deformity is talipes equinovarus (inward and downward position), and it may be bilateral.

  - Congenital clubfoot occurs as an isolated defect or is diagnosed in association with other disorders, including cerebral palsy and spina bifida.

- Developmental dysplasia of the hip (DDH) is a broad term that is used to describe a variety of disorders resulting in abnormal development of the hip structures.

  - DDH may be identified during prenatal or postnatal periods or early in childhood.

- Scoliosis is a complex deformity of the spine that also affects the ribs.

  - Scoliosis is characterized by a lateral curvature of the spine and spinal rotation that causes rib asymmetry.

  - Not all curvatures of the spine are scoliosis. A curve of less than 10° may be a postural variation.

  - Idiopathic or structural scoliosis is the most common form of scoliosis and can be seen in isolation or associated with other conditions.

View Media Supplement:

- Club Foot (Image)
- Developmental Dysplasia of the Hip (Image)
- Brace for Scoliosis (Image)

Data Collection

- Risk Factors

  - Clubfoot

    - The etiology is not known, but it may be related to abnormal embryonic development.

    - Clubfoot is classified as positional (intrauterine crowding), syndromic (associated with other deformities), or congenital (idiopathic).

    - Variations of the deformity and manifestations may be present in one or both feet.

- ○ DDH may be affected by family history, gender, birth order, intrauterine position, and/ or laxity of a joint.

  - Predisposing factors include intrauterine placement, mechanical situations (size of infant, multiple births, breech presentation), and genetic factors.

- ○ Idiopathic scoliosis can be congenital, idiopathic, or acquired (result of neuromuscular disorders).

  - Idiopathic scoliosis may be present at birth or occur in early childhood. Onset usually occurs during the preadolescent growth spurt.

  - Idiopathic scoliosis may have a genetic link.

- Subjective and Objective Data

  - ○ The defect may be visible or the child and/or family may report findings such as a clicking sound with diaper changes (with DDH) or clothing that does not hang correctly (with scoliosis).

  - ○ Clubfoot

DEFORMITY NAME	MANIFESTATION
Talipes equinovarus (most common)	Plantar flexion with feet bending inward
Talipes calcaneus	Dorsiflexion of feet with toes higher than heels
Talipes equinus	Plantar flexion of feet with toes lower than heels
Talipes varus	Inversion of feet (toes pointing toward midline)
Talipes valgus	Eversion of feet (toes pointing laterally)

  - ○ DDH

    - Asymmetrical gluteal and thigh folds

    - Limited abduction of hips

    - One knee that appears shorter when the infant is supine with thighs flexed at 90° towards the abdomen (Allis sign)

    - For infants from birth to 3 months of age, the provider performs the Barlow and Ortolani tests. The hips are taken through adduction (the thighs are brought towards the midline) and abduction, and an audible click or clunk is heard as the head of the femur on the affected hip can be moved from the socket (Barlow test) and then reduced back into the socket (Ortolani test) by manipulation of the joint.

    - For children able to walk, observe postural gait.

      - □ Abnormal downward tilting of pelvis on the unaffected side when bearing weight on the affected side (Trendelenburg sign)

      - □ Waddling gait or abnormal lordosis of spine if bilateral dislocation

  - ○ Scoliosis

    - Asymmetry in scapula, ribs, flanks, shoulders, and hips

    - Improperly fitting clothing (one leg shorter than the other)

- ○ Diagnostic Procedures
  - ■ Clubfoot
    - □ Prenatal ultrasound
      - ▸ Used to identify the deformity
    - □ Radiograph
      - ▸ Used to determine bone placement and tissue involvement for clubfoot
  - ■ DDH
    - □ Ultrasound
      - ▸ An ultrasound should be performed at 2 weeks of age to determine the cartilaginous head of the femur.
    - □ X-ray
      - ▸ An x-ray can diagnose DDH in infants older than 4 months of age.
  - ■ Scoliosis
    - □ Screen during preadolescence for boys and girls.
      - ▸ Observe the child, who should be wearing only underwear, from the back.
      - ▸ Have the child bend over at the waist with arms hanging down and observe for asymmetry of ribs and flank.
    - □ Diagnosis is made using x-rays of the child in a standing position from the neck to the groin and determining the angle of curvature using the Cobb technique with a scoliometer.
    - □ Nursing Actions
      - ▸ Assist with positioning as needed.
      - ▸ Assist with sedation of the child if prescribed.
    - □ Client Education
      - ▸ Reinforce explanation of diagnostic procedures.
      - ▸ Provide emotional support.

Collaborative Care

- • Nursing Care
  - ○ Interventions for the child with clubfoot or DDH
    - ■ Encourage parents to hold and cuddle the child.
    - ■ Encourage parents to meet the developmental needs of the child.
    - ■ Instruct parents to maintain the cast or harness used to treat clubfoot or DDH.
    - ■ Perform neurovascular and skin integrity checks after cast or harness placement.

- Therapeutic Procedures

  o Clubfoot – Management of clubfoot will depend upon the severity of the deformity.

    - Passive exercise should be performed for a minor deformity

    - Serial casting is begun after birth before the newborn is discharged home. Weekly casting to stretch the skin and other structures of the foot is done until maximum correction is accomplished.

    - Surgical intervention should occur if maximum correction is not achieved by 3 months of age.

    - Nursing Actions

      □ If casted, check neurovascular status.

    - Client Education

      □ Educate families about how to perform gentle stretching of the foot as prescribed.

      □ Educate families about the importance of serial casting, cast care, and follow-up appointments.

  o DDH – Pavlik harness

    - A Pavlik harness can be used from birth up to 5 or 6 months of age. It is a noninvasive device for keeping hips in a continually abducted position, which allows for the femoral head to remain in contact with the acetabulum.

    - Infants will wear the harness continuously for 3 to 5 months, until the hip is determined, by radiograph, to be stable. Frequent follow-ups will be needed for strap adjustment.

    - Nursing Actions

      □ Check skin integrity frequently.

      □ Ensure proper positioning at all times.

      □ Determine the family's ability to adjust the harness.

    - Client Education

      □ Instruct families to keep the harness on continuously, except during bathing, if prescribed.

      □ Instruct families to return for follow-up visits weekly at the start of therapy and then as needed.

      □ Reinforce teaching about skin care. Encourage application of a cotton shirt and cotton socks under the harness to prevent irritation and the avoidance of powders and lotions.

○ DDH – Hip spica cast

- A hip spica cast can be used for infants older than 6 months of age. It can also be used in children whose hips were not stabilized by use of the Pavlik harness. A short course of traction is sometimes used prior to the application of a hip spica cast.

- Nursing Actions

  □ Maintain the hip spica cast.

  □ Perform frequent neurovascular checks.

  □ Perform range of motion with the unaffected extremities.

  □ Check skin integrity at frequent intervals, especially in the diaper area.

  □ Use an age-appropriate pain tool to determine management of pain. Administer pain medication as prescribed.

  □ Evaluate hydration status frequently.

  □ Check elimination status daily.

- Client Education

  □ Reinforce teaching regarding positioning, turning, neurovascular assessments, and care of the cast.

    ▸ Position casts on pillows.

    ▸ Keep the casts elevated until dry.

    ▸ Encourage frequent position changes to allow for drying.

    ▸ Handle the casts with the palm of the hand until dry.

  □ Note color and temperature of toes on casted extremity.

  □ Give sponge baths to avoid wetting the cast.

  □ Use a waterproof barrier around the genital opening of spica cast to prevent soiling with urine or feces.

  □ Educate regarding care after discharge with emphasis on using appropriate equipment (stroller, wagon, car seat) for maintaining mobility.

○ Scoliosis – Bracing and exercise

- Mild scoliosis (curvature of 10 to 20°) is treated with bracing and exercise to maintain strength and to maintain muscles of the abdomen and spine.

- Nursing Actions

  □ Monitor for signs of skin breakdown in the child wearing a brace.

  □ Monitor adherence to therapy.

- Client Education

  □ Reinforce that the brace will not correct the curve but will help to stabilize it until growth is completed.

  □ Suggest decorating the brace to encourage acceptance by adolescents.

- □ Instruct children and their families about the importance of adherence. Instruct children to wear the brace 23 out of 24 hr a day.

- □ Reinforce teaching done by a physical therapist.

- □ Reinforce the need to exercise along with the use of the brace.

- □ Reinforce the need to assess skin for breakdown. Educate the child and/or family to have the child wear a cotton t-shirt under the brace and to avoid the use of powders and lotions.

- Surgical Interventions

  - ○ Surgery is generally needed for curves greater than 40°. A type of internal fixation system (Harrington, Dwyer, Zielke) may be used to straighten and realign the spine along with a bony fusion to stabilize the correction.

  - ○ Repair is performed from either an anterior and/or posterior approach. The type of instrumentation selected is based on surgeon preference and client needs.

  - ○ The goal of repair is to achieve maximal correction and maximal mobility with minimal complications.

  - ○ Nursing Actions

    - ■ Preoperative

      - □ Suggest to adolescents and their families to obtain autologous (self-donated) blood donations.

      - □ Obtain routine laboratory studies, including a type and cross match for blood as prescribed.

      - □ Inform the adolescent and/or family about what can be expected during the postoperative period, admission to the intensive care unit, use of monitoring equipment, NG tube, chest tubes, indwelling catheters, and self-administering analgesic pumps.

    - ■ Postoperative

      - □ Perform standard postoperative care to prevent complications.

      - □ Monitor pain using an age-appropriate pain tool.

      - □ Assist with pain management using a patient-controlled analgesic pump as prescribed.

      - □ Turn adolescents frequently by log rolling to prevent damage to the spinal fusion.

      - □ Observe skin for pressure areas, especially if a brace has been prescribed.

      - □ Prevent rubbing and pressure from brace.

      - □ Provide skin care by keeping skin clean and dry.

      - □ Monitor surgical and drain sites for signs of infection. Provide wound care as prescribed.

      - □ Auscultate bowel sounds and check for paralytic ileus.

- □ Monitor for decreases in hemoglobin and hematocrit. Observe for signs of bleeding.

- □ Assist with the monitoring of blood transfusion as prescribed.

- □ Encourage mobility as soon as tolerated.

- □ Perform range of motion on unaffected extremities.

- □ Provide age-appropriate activities and opportunities to visit with friends and family during the hospital stay.

- ○ Client Education

  - ■ Preoperative

    - □ Reinforce teaching (use of incentive spirometer, turning, coughing, deep breathing) to prevent complications.

    - □ Demonstrate the use of a patient-controlled analgesic pump if age appropriate.

    - □ Demonstrate log rolling that will be used after surgery.

    - □ Demonstrate the respiratory therapy techniques that will be used postoperatively to reduce complications of anesthesia.

    - □ Discuss medical terms that are unfamiliar to the adolescent and/or family.

  - ■ Postoperative

    - □ Emphasize the importance of physical therapy and proper positioning of the spine.

    - □ Encourage independence following surgery for the adolescent who has a brace.

    - □ Encourage the adolescent to contact friends when able.

    - □ Emphasize the necessity of follow-up care.

- • Care After Discharge

  - ○ Client Education

    - ■ Reinforce the expected course of treatment and recovery.

    - ■ Suggest that families arrange the environment to facilitate the adolescent's ability to be as independent as possible (keep favorite items within reach).

    - ■ Emphasize the necessity of follow-up care.

- • Client Outcomes

  - ○ The child will maintain a functional foot with minimal complications with clubfoot.

  - ○ The child will remain free from complications of immobility.

  - ○ The child will increase and maintain optimal mobilization.

Complications

- Complications for clubfoot, DDH, and scoliosis will be related to:

  ○ Postoperative complications (atelectasis, ileus, wound infection)

  ○ Effects of immobilization (decreased muscle strength, bone demineralization, decreased metabolic rate, altered bowel motility)

  ○ Effects of casting or bracing (skin breakdown, neurovascular alterations)

- Infection

  ○ Infection may be caused by bacteria, such as *Staphylococcus aureus*.

  ○ Nursing Actions

    ■ Monitor vital signs. Observe changes in temperature that could be associated with complications of infection.

    ■ Keep the cast dry and intact.

    ■ Monitor for changes in neurovascular status (numbness; tingling; decreased mobility, sensation, or capillary refill).

    ■ Reposition the child frequently.

    ■ Maintain a high-fiber diet and promote adequate hydration.

    ■ Monitor bowel and bladder elimination. Report any changes, especially the decrease or absence of bowel sounds or distention.

    ■ Report any foul odor from cast or urine.

    ■ Observe changes in behavior, especially increasing irritability in infants.

  ○ Client Education

    ■ Reinforce expected complications of specific treatment or procedure with the children and their families.

    ■ Reinforce the need to notify the provider with any concerns or signs of complications.

    ■ Educate children and their families about follow-up.

Ⓐ APPLICATION EXERCISES

1. A nurse is caring for a 3-month-old infant who has been placed in a Pavlik harness. The nurse is reviewing discharge teaching to the parents. Which of the following should be included in the review? (Select all that apply.)

   _____ Remove the harness when giving a bath.

   _____ Check the skin under the straps frequently.

   _____ Adjust the straps whenever they seem too loose.

   _____ Apply lotion frequently to the skin under the straps.

   _____ Do not place the straps over articles of clothing.

2. A nurse is reviewing the plan of care for a 9-month-old infant immediately following the application of a left hip spica cast. Which of the following nursing actions should the nurse plan to take? (Select all that apply.)

   _____ Check the condition of the skin under the edges of the cast.

   _____ Perform range of motion of the affected extremity.

   _____ Check capillary refill of the toes frequently.

   _____ Position the left leg on a small pillow.

   _____ Use fingertips when repositioning until the cast is dry.

3. Following surgical instrumentation of the spine for scoliosis, the nurse will reposition the child from side to side by_____.

4. The correct terminology for a clubfoot where the foot bends inward is talipes _____.

5. DDH is an abbreviation for _____.

6. A nurse in the pediatric clinic is talking to a 12-year-old child who is concerned about having to wear a brace following a diagnosis of scoliosis. The client states, "I have a friend who had surgery to fix her scoliosis. Why don't I need surgery?" Which of the following is the correct response by the nurse?

   A. "You will need to wear the brace until you are able to donate adequate blood pre-operatively."

   B. "Your scoliosis is probably mild with a curvature of less than 20 degrees."

   C. "Bracing is done to prevent, not treat scoliosis."

   D. "You are not old enough for a surgical repair."

(A) APPLICATION EXERCISES ANSWER KEY

1. A nurse is caring for a 3-month-old infant who has been placed in a Pavlik harness. The nurse is reviewing discharge teaching to the parents. Which of the following should be included in the review? (Select all that apply.)

   __X__ **Remove the harness when giving a bath.**

   __X__ **Check the skin under the straps frequently.**

   _____ Adjust the straps whenever they seem too loose.

   _____ Apply lotion frequently to the skin under the straps.

   _____ Do not place the straps over articles of clothing.

   Parents of an infant in a Pavlik harness should only remove the harness when bathing the infant. The skin under the straps should be checked frequently for signs of irritation. The straps should be adjusted only when indicated by the provider. Lotions and powder should not be used under the straps. The infant should wear a cotton t-shirt and cotton socks to prevent irritation from the straps.

    NCLEX® Connection: Basic Care and Comfort, Mobility/Immobility

2. A nurse is reviewing the plan of care for a 9-month-old infant immediately following the application of a left hip spica cast. Which of the following nursing actions should the nurse plan to take? (Select all that apply.)

   __X__ **Check the condition of the skin under the edges of the cast.**

   _____ Perform range of motion of the affected extremity.

   __X__ **Check capillary refill of the toes frequently.**

   __X__ **Position the left leg on a small pillow.**

   _____ Use fingertips when repositioning until the cast is dry.

   The nursing care plan for an infant with a spica cast includes checking the condition of the skin under the edges of the cast for signs of irritation, checking capillary refill of the toes frequently, and using pillows to position the affected extremity. Range of motion exercises should be done on the unaffected extremity and upper body. Only the palms are used when repositioning the child until the cast is dry.

    NCLEX® Connection: Basic Care and Comfort, Mobility/Immobility

3. Following surgical instrumentation of the spine for scoliosis, the nurse will reposition the child from side to side by **logrolling**.

   (N) NCLEX® Connection: Basic Care and Comfort, Mobility/Immobility

4. The correct terminology for a clubfoot where the foot bends inward is talipes **equinovarus**.

   (N) NCLEX® Connection: Basic Care and Comfort, Mobility/Immobility

5. DDH is an abbreviation for **developmental dysplasia of the hip**.

Ⓝ NCLEX® Connection: Basic Care and Comfort, Mobility/Immobility

6. A nurse in the pediatric clinic is talking to a 12-year-old child who is concerned about having to wear a brace following a diagnosis of scoliosis. The client states, "I have a friend who had surgery to fix her scoliosis. Why don't I need surgery?" Which of the following is the correct response by the nurse?

   A. "You will need to wear the brace until you are able to donate adequate blood pre-operatively."

   B. "Your scoliosis is probably mild with a curvature of less than 20 degrees."

   C. "Bracing is done to prevent, not treat scoliosis."

   D. "You are not old enough for a surgical repair."

   Mild scoliosis is treated by bracing and exercise when the curvature is 10 to 20 degrees. A brace is not worn because autologous blood donation is being done. Bracing is used to treat, not prevent scoliosis. Surgical repair is based on the need for maximal correction and mobility, the surgeon's preference, and the client's needs. It is not based on the child's age.

Ⓝ NCLEX® Connection: Basic Care and Comfort, Mobility/Immobility

UNIT 2	NURSING CARE OF CHILDREN WITH SYSTEM DISORDERS
Section:	Musculoskeletal Disorders
Chapter 28	**Chronic Neuromusculoskeletal Disorders**

Overview

- Chronic neuromusculoskeletal disorders affect the brain, muscles, joints, and skeletal structures of the body.

- Cerebral palsy (CP) is a nonprogressive impairment of motor function, especially that of muscle control, coordination, and posture.

- Spina bifida refers to defects in intrauterine closure of the bony spine. Spina bifida is further classified as spina bifida occulta and spina bifida cystica (meningocele or myelomeningocele, which are visible defects in the spine with a saclike protrusion at any level of the spinal column at the midline of the back).

  o In meningocele, the sac contains meninges and spinal fluid. Myelomeningocele contains meninges, spinal fluid, and nerves

- Down syndrome is a chromosomal abnormality.

- Juvenile idiopathic arthritis (JIA) is a group of chronic autoimmune inflammatory diseases affecting joints and other tissues. There is chronic inflammation of the synovium of the joints with effusion that leads to wearing down and damage to the articular cartilage.

- Muscular dystrophy (MD) is a group of inherited disorders with progressive degeneration of symmetrical skeletal muscle groups.

CEREBRAL PALSY (CP)

Overview

- CP is the most common permanent physical disability in children.

- CP may cause abnormal perception and sensation; visual, hearing, and speech impairments; seizures; and cognitive disabilities.

- CP manifests differently in each child. Developmental outcomes vary and are dependent on the severity of the injury. Many children with CP are able to perform most, if not all, developmental tasks, and more than half will be able to work outside the home as adults. Others will require complete care for their entire lives.

Data Collection

- Risk Factors

  - The exact cause of CP is not known. Prenatal, perinatal, and postnatal risk factors known to be associated with CP include:

    - Existing brain anomalies, cerebral infections, head trauma (shaken baby syndrome), and /or anoxia to the brain

    - Premature birth

    - Multiple births

    - Extremely low or very low birth weights in newborns

    - Inability of the placenta to provide the developing fetus with oxygen and nutrients

    - Interruption of oxygen delivery to the fetus during birth

    - Kernicterus as a result of high levels of bilirubin in the neonatal period

- Subjective Data

  - Parents may describe concerns with development.

  - Developmental early warning signs about which parents may be concerned

    - Poor head control or absence of smiling in a 3-month-old infant

    - Difficulty with dressing and diaper changes due to stiff arms or legs during infancy and early childhood. The child may push away or arch his back.

    - A floppy or limp body in infants

    - An inability to sit up without support in an 8-month-old infant

    - Use of only one side of the body to play or move about

    - Feeding difficulties (moving food from side to side with tongue, inability to swallow safely)

  - Painful muscle spasms

- Objective Data

  - Physical Assessment Findings

    - Persistent primitive reflexes (Moro or tonic neck)

    - Motor function showing muscle tightness or spasticity, involuntary movements, and disturbance in gait or mobility

    - Findings associated with specific types of CP

      - Spastic

        - Spastic CP is characterized by hypertonicity (muscle tightness or spasticity); increased deep tendon reflexes; clonus; and poor control of motion, balance, and posture.

        - Spastic CP may cause impairments of fine and gross motor skills.

- Spastic CP may present in all extremities (quadriplegia), similar parts of the body (diplegia), three limbs (triplegia), one limb (monoplegia), or one side of the body (hemiplegia). It often causes affected limbs to be shorter and thinner.

- Associated scoliosis may be present.

- Gait may appear crouched with a scissoring motion of the legs with intoeing and use of primarily the balls of the feet in a tip-toe fashion.

- Spastic CP may present with contractures, especially the heel cord, hips, or knees. Wrists and elbows are in a flexed position with clenching of the hand.

- Flexor, adductor, and internal rotator muscles are more affected than the extensor and external adductor or rotator muscles.

□ Dyskinetic

- Movements increase with stress but are absent with sleep. Normal deep tendon reflexes are present with absence of clonus.

- Speech may be impaired.

□ Athetoid

- Findings include involuntary jerking movements that appear slow, writhing, and wormlike. These movements involve the trunk, neck, face, and tongue.

□ Dystonic

- Slow, twisting movements occur that affect the trunk and extremities.

□ Ataxic

- Evidence of wide-based gait and difficulty with coordination

- Poor ability to do repetitive movements

- Difficulty with quick or precise movements (writing or buttoning a shirt)

- Jerky speech pattern is present

○ Diagnostic Procedures

■ Complete neurological assessment

■ MRI

□ Used to evaluate structures or abnormal areas located near bone (Sedation may be necessary.)

□ Nursing Actions

- Tell the child to remain still during the procedure.

- Assist with sedation of the child if prescribed.

□ Client Education

- Provide emotional support.

Collaborative Care

- Nursing Care

  - Monitor developmental milestones.

  - Evaluate the need for hearing and speech evaluations.

  - Promote independence with self-care activities as much as possible. Assist the child to maintain a positive self-image and a high level of self-esteem.

  - Determine the extent of family coping and support.

  - Determine the family's awareness of available resources.

  - Determine the child's developmental level and approach the child in a way that is appropriate for the child's developmental level, rather than chronological age.

  - Communicate with children directly, but include the parents as needed.

  - Help children to use augmented communication, such as electronic devices for speech and other types of communication tools.

  - Include families in physical care of hospitalized children with cerebral palsy.

    - Ask families about routine care and encourage them to provide it if appropriate.

    - Encourage families to help verify the child's needs if communication is impaired.

  - Maintain an open airway by elevating the head of the child's bed (this is especially important if the child has increased oral secretions).

  - Ensure suction equipment is available if required. Suction oral secretions as needed.

  - Monitor for pain (especially with muscle spasms) using a developmentally appropriate pain tool.

  - Administer medication for pain and/or spasms as prescribed.

  - Ensure adequate nutrition.

    - Check for the possibility of aspiration for children who are severely disabled.

    - Determine the child's ability to take oral nutrition.

    - Ascertain the correct positioning for feeding children. Use head positioning and manual jaw control methods as needed.

    - Provide foods that are similar to foods eaten at home when possible. Administer supplements as prescribed.

    - Administer feedings by gastric tube as prescribed.

    - Maintain weight/height chart.

- ○ Provide skin care.

  - Observe the skin under splints and braces if applicable.

  - Maintain skin integrity by turning the child to keep pressure off bony prominences.

  - Keep skin clean and dry.

  - ○ Provide rest periods as needed.

- Medications

  - ○ Baclofen (Lioresal)

    - Use as a centrally acting skeletal muscle relaxant that decreases muscle spasm and severe spasticity.

    - Nursing Considerations

      - □ Administer orally or assist with intrathecal administration via a specialized, surgically implanted pump.

      - □ Monitor effectiveness of the medication.

      - □ Monitor for muscle weakness, increased fatigue, or less-common side effects (diaphoresis, constipation).

    - Client Education

      - □ Reinforce with families about expected responses to medications.

      - □ Reinforce with families the side effects of medications, such as drowsiness, and when to call the provider.

      - □ Instruct families to bring children to see the provider every 4 to 6 weeks to monitor effectiveness of therapy and to receive refills.

  - ○ Diazepam (Valium)

    - Skeletal muscle relaxant used to decrease muscle spasms and severe spasticity

    - Nursing Considerations

      - □ Use in older children and adolescents.

      - □ Monitor for drowsiness and fatigue.

    - Client Education

      - □ Reinforce with families about expected responses to medications.

      - □ Reinforce with families the side effects of the medication and when to call the provider.

- Interdisciplinary Care

  - ○ Coordinate care with other professionals, such as speech therapists, physical and recreational therapists, education specialists, and/or medical specialists.

  - ○ Request a referral for technical aids that can assist with coordination, speaking, mobility, and an increased level of independence, such as that which may be achieved with the use of a voice activated wheelchair.

- Care After Discharge
  - Client Education
    - Reinforce the therapeutic plan of care.
    - Reinforce the need for rest periods.
    - Reinforce feeding schedule and feeding techniques if changes were made during hospitalization.
    - Reinforce adherence to medication regimen.
    - Encourage regular dental care.
    - Encourage the parents to provide developmental stimulation.
    - Reinforce teaching about wound care if needed.
    - Help families identify resources needed (respite care).
    - Suggest participation in a support group for CP.
- Client Outcomes
  - The child will develop and maintain optimal functioning.
  - The child will maintain adequate nutrition and growth.

Complications

- Aspiration of oral secretions
  - Nursing Actions
    - Keep the child's head elevated.
    - Keep suction available if copious oral secretions are present or the child has difficulty with swallowing foods and/or fluids.
  - Client Education
    - Reinforce to families about feeding techniques to decrease the risk of aspiration.
    - Encourage families to take CPR classes.
- Potential for injury
  - Nursing Actions
    - Make sure the child's bed rails are raised to prevent falls from the bed.
    - Pad side rails and wheelchair arms to prevent injury.
    - Secure children in mobility devices, such as wheelchairs.
    - Encourage children to receive adequate rest to prevent injury at times of fatigue.
    - Encourage the use of helmets, seat belts, and other safety equipment.
  - Client Education
    - Reinforce to children and their families about safety precautions.

SPINA BIFIDA

 Overview

- Neural tube defects (NTDs) are present at birth and affect the CNS and osseous spine.

- The degree of neurologic dysfunction is determined by the level of sac protrusion and tissue involvement.

  o Spina bifida occulta – A defect in the bony spine that is invisible to the eye and has no manifestations or problems

  o Spina bifida cystica

    ▪ Meningocele – A spinal defect and sac-like protrusion are present, only spinal fluid and meninges are present in the sac. After the sac is repaired, no further symptoms are usually seen because spinal nerves are not damaged.

    ▪ Myelomeningocele – The sac includes meninges, spinal fluid, and nerves.

      □ Impairments will present depending on the level of spinal injury, from complete paralysis to a slightly decreased sensation in the lower extremities. Other findings may include joint deformities, bowel and bladder incontinence, developmental delays, hydrocephalus, and a high risk for latex allergy.

View Media Supplement: Spina Bifida (Image)

Data Collection

- Risk Factors

  o Neural tube defects are caused by the failure of the neural tube to close in the first 3 to 5 weeks of gestation.

  o Neural tube defects have been linked to insufficient folic acid in the maternal diet.

  o An elevated alpha-fetoprotein (AFP) may indicate the presence of a neural tube defect.

- Subjective Data

  o Collect prenatal history, especially exposure to and intake of folic acid.

  o Ask about family history for neural tube defects.

- Objective Data

  o Physical Assessment Findings

    ▪ Assist the nurse with inspection of the sac to determine whether it is intact.

    ▪ Assist the nurse with inspection of the lumbosacral area for dimpling. This may indicate spina bifida occulta.

    ▪ Ongoing assessments

- □ Measure head circumference, which may increase rapidly with hydrocephalus until normal cranial growth is reached.

- □ Observe skin integrity for pressure ulcers caused by decreased sensation in the affected trunk and extremities.

- □ Identify allergies. Specifically ask about latex allergy.

- □ Determine cognitive development. This may be permanently delayed in some children.

- □ Determine bladder/bowel functioning. Functioning is permanently affected in all children with spina bifida.

- □ Monitor for manifestations of infection, including elevation of body temperature, nausea, vomiting, and fatigue.

- ○ Laboratory Tests

  - ▪ Laboratory studies may be used to determine causative pathogens for meningitis or UTI.

- ○ Diagnostic Procedures

  - ▪ Maternal serum analysis

    - □ Maternal serum should be tested for serum alpha-fetoprotein levels between 15 and 20 weeks of gestation (it is best to test between 16 and 18 weeks). Elevated levels will require further testing, such as an amniocentesis.

  - ▪ Amniocentesis

    - □ An amniocentesis should be performed to test amniotic fluid for levels of alpha-fetoprotein. Elevated levels may indicate neural tube defects.

  - ▪ MRI, ultrasound, CT, and myelography

    - □ These tests may be used to determine brain and spinal cord involvement.

  - ▪ Radioallergosorbent test (RAST)

    - □ A RAST detects the presence of latex allergy.

Collaborative Care

- ● Nursing Care

  - ○ Observe for infant-parent attachment.

  - ○ Provide care of the sac.

    - ▪ Check the integrity of the sac at least every 2 hr.

    - ▪ Avoid activities that may damage or break the sac.

    - ▪ Assist with the application of moist, nonadherent dressing to cover the sac.

  - ○ Place children in the prone position until the sac is repaired.

    - ▪ Promote skin integrity.

    - ▪ Keep skin clean and dry.

- - Keep pressure off bony prominences.

  - Reposition children hourly.

  - Observe skin under splints or braces.

- Provide range of motion to legs. This may be passive or active, depending on the disability.

- Position the extremities to maintain alignment and prevent contractures or deformities, especially in children who have paralysis.

- Use an appropriate pain assessment tool.

- Check for self-esteem and body image disturbances, which arise due to bowel and bladder incontinence, use of mobility aids, inability to keep up with peers, and other physical and social problems.

- Determine the family's knowledge of available resources.

- Evaluate the family's coping ability and support system.

- Monitor head circumference for signs of increasing intracranial pressure or shunt failure.

- Monitor for elevations in body temperature and other signs and symptoms of infection.

- Use nonlatex gloves, catheters, and other equipment to decrease the risk of latex allergy.

- Work with children and parents on bladder control measures.

  - Show how to perform clean, intermittent self-catheterization (CIC) to the parents and to the child if the child is developmentally capable of performing the skill.

  - Work with families on other strategies for acceptable bladder care (incontinence supplies, condom catheters).

  - Note color, clarity, odor, and amount of urine. Monitor for UTIs. Administer antibiotics as prescribed.

- Monitor bowel function for constipation and incontinence.

  - Avoid taking temperatures rectally to prevent irritation of rectal sphincter.

  - Administer laxatives or enemas as ordered to assist bowel function.

- Provide instruction about principles of nutrition and work with families to prevent obesity.

- Medications

  - Oxybutynin chloride (Ditropan) and tolterodine (Detrol)

    - These are antispasmodics that are used to improve bladder capacity and continence.

- Client Education
  - Reinforce to families about the need for proper and timely administration of medications.
  - Reinforce to families about the need for periodic monitoring of medication levels.

- Interdisciplinary Care
  - Occupational therapy, physical therapy, and social services may all be involved in the care of a child who has spina bifida.

- Therapeutic Procedures
  - The insertion of feeding tubes may be necessary.
    - Nursing Actions
      - Prepare children and parents for the procedure.
    - Client Education
      - Explain the procedure and anticipated postoperative care.

- Surgical Interventions
  - Closure of a myelomeningocele sac is done as soon as possible to prevent complications of injury and infection.
    - Nursing Actions
      - Preoperative
        - Reinforce the information that was provided by the provider.
        - Maintain a sterile, moist (with 0.9% sodium chloride), nonadherent dressing over the exposed sac until surgery.
        - Place the newborn in a prone position until surgery to protect the sac.
    - Client Education
      - Reinforce teaching with the parents about what to expect postoperatively.
      - Reinforce teaching with the parents about proper positioning techniques.
      - Tell the parents to avoid touching the sac.
  - Surgical shunt
    - Will be inserted if hydrocephalus develops
    - Nursing Actions
      - Postoperatively
        - Measure the head circumference and abdominal girth of infants.
        - Observe for signs of increased intracranial pressure (high-pitched cry, bulging fontanels, vomiting, irritability).
        - Avoid positioning children on the shunt site.

- ■ Client Education
  - □ Reinforce teaching with families about the signs and symptoms of shunt malfunction.
  - □ Reinforce the need to seek care with any sign of shunt malfunction.
- o Bladder surgery
  - ■ May be performed to manage bladder dysfunction (either spasms or flaccidity)
  - ■ Nursing Actions
    - □ Monitor for signs of bladder dysfunction.
    - □ Monitor for signs of bladder infection.
    - □ Monitor for bleeding.
    - □ Reinforce teaching with children and families about care of stoma (vesicostomy) if applicable.
- o Orthopedic surgeries
  - ■ Corrections of associated potential problems, such as clubfoot, scoliosis, and other malformations of the feet and legs
  - ■ Nursing Actions
    - □ Monitor for signs of infection.
    - □ Administer pain medications.
    - □ Provide cast care if cast is present.
    - □ Monitor for neurosensory deficits.
  - ■ Client Education
    - □ Reinforce to families about signs and symptoms of infection.
    - □ Reinforce to families about cast and splint care if indicated.
- • Client Outcomes
  - o The child will reach and maintain optimal levels of functioning.
  - o The child will be free from injury.

Complications

- • Skin ulceration
  - o Caused by prolonged pressure in one area
  - o Nursing Actions
    - ■ Monitor skin for breakdown.
    - ■ Reposition frequently to prevent pressure on bony prominences.
    - ■ Monitor skin under splints and braces.

- ○ Client Education
    - Reinforce teaching with children and parents about how to monitor skin integrity.

- Latex allergy

    - ○ These children have a high risk of allergy to latex. Allergy responses range from urticaria to wheezing, which may progress to anaphylaxis. There may also be an allergy to certain foods (bananas, avocados, kiwi, chestnuts).

    - ○ Nursing Actions
        - Recommend testing for allergies.
        - Reduce exposure to known allergens.

    - ○ Client Education
        - Reinforce to the parents to avoid exposing children to latex.
        - Provide families with a list of household items that may contain latex (disposable diapers, cleaning or kitchen gloves, elastic found in clothing).
        - Reinforce to families about how to identify signs and symptoms of allergic reaction and report them to the provider.
        - Provide instruction in the use of epinephrine (EpiPen).

- Increased intracranial pressure

    - ○ Signs and symptoms
        - Infants – High-pitched cry, lethargy, vomiting, bulging fontanels, and/or widening cranial suture lines
        - Children – Headache, lethargy, nausea, vomiting, double vision, decreased school performance of learned tasks, decreased level of consciousness, and seizures

    - ○ Caused by shunt malfunction

    - ○ Nursing Actions
        - Use gentle movements when performing range-of-motion exercises.
        - Minimize environmental stressors (noise, frequent visitors).
        - Check pain level and manage it.

    - ○ Client Education
        - Reinforce teaching about the signs and symptoms of shunt malfunction and instruct children and family to report any signs and symptoms to the provider immediately.

DOWN SYNDROME

 Overview

- Clinical manifestations of Down syndrome

    o Hypotonicity, congenital heart defects, thyroid dysfunction, congenital hypothyroidism, dysfunctional immune system, and high risk for leukemia

    o The presence of cognitive defects with an IQ that will vary in range with an average of 50

Data Collection

- Risk Factors

    o The exact etiology of Down syndrome is probably multifactorial. There is a higher incidence in infants born to mothers who are older than 35 years of age.

- Objective Data

    o Physical Assessment Findings

        ■ Small head

        ■ Flattened forehead

        ■ Low-set ears

        ■ Upward slant to eyes

        ■ Protruding tongue and narrow, high-arched palate

        ■ Underdeveloped nasal bone (results in a flattened appearance to the nasal bridge)

        ■ Hypotonia (decreased muscle tone)

        ■ Transverse palmar crease

        ■ Plantar space and wide space between the great toe and second toe

        ■ Congenital heart defects (may be present)

    o Diagnostic Procedures

        ■ Prenatal testing for alpha-fetoprotein in maternal serum – Low in the presence of Down syndrome

        ■ Chromosome analysis

            □ Prenatal testing, such as an amniocentesis, should be conducted for chromosome analysis to confirm the genetic abnormality.

Collaborative Care

- Nursing Care

    o Swaddle infants to maintain warmth and security.

- ○ Support the parents and child at the time of diagnosis.

- ○ Reinforce physical care of children.

  - ▪ Feeding

  - ▪ Management of secretions and prevention of upper respiratory infections

  - ▪ Skin care

  - ▪ Positioning

- ○ Emphasize the child's strengths while being aware of limitations to ensure safety.

- • Interdisciplinary Care

  - ○ Encourage families and children to begin early interventions with speech, physical, and occupational therapy.

  - ○ Identify and recommend children and parents to a support group.

- • Surgical Interventions

  - ○ Interventions for surgical repair will depend on the associated congenital anomalies. These may include cardiac defects or strabismus.

    - ▪ Nursing Actions

      - □ Listen to concerns of the parents and discuss ethical dilemmas regarding treatment for physical defects.

      - □ Provide standard postoperative care with emphasis on wound care, respiratory care, and pain management.

    - ▪ Client Education

      - □ Reinforce teaching about postoperative and home care management.

      - □ Reinforce the therapeutic plan of care.

- • Care After Discharge

  - ○ Client Education

    - ▪ Reinforce with the parents that children need holding and cuddling but may not be able to cling or hold the parent due to associated hypotonia, not a lack of attachment.

    - ▪ Show parents how to position children to prevent injury or complications due to hypotonicity and laxity of joints.

    - ▪ Encourage parents to change infants' positions frequently to help promote aeration of the lungs and prevent pooling of secretions.

    - ▪ Reinforce the follow-up of associated physical conditions.

      - □ Hearing and vision

      - □ Thyroid function

      - □ Ear, nose, and throat (highly prone to otitis)

- When it is age appropriate, a radiological exam should be used to rule out atlantoaxial instability before the children are allowed to participate in certain sports.

- Reinforce teaching with the parents about the importance of providing food and fluids to maintain adequate nutrition and prevent issues with constipation.

- Emphasize the need to provide a well-balanced diet for adequate nutrition. Poor eating habits may result in obesity later in life.

- Reinforce feeding techniques with parents.

- Plot the child's height and weight on Down syndrome growth charts.

- Reinforce care of the skin. Use mild soaps to prevent drying and apply moisturizing creams daily or as needed (highly prone to dry and cracking skin and lips).

- Instruct the parents about how to prevent physical complications.

  □ Avoid infection by engaging in proper hand hygiene.

  □ Increase fiber in diet to avoid constipation.

  □ Encourage physical activity.

  o Follow-up

- Encourage parents to seek regular checkups for their children.

Complications

- Respiratory infections

  o Respiratory infections are common due to decreased muscle tone and poor drainage of mucus because of hypotonicity and associated under-developed nasal bone.

  o Nursing Actions

- Rinse the child's mouth with water after feeding and at other times of the day when it is dry. Mucous membranes are dry due to constant mouth breathing, which also increases the risk for respiratory infection.

- Provide cool mist humidification and clearing of the nasal passages with a bulb syringe as needed.

- Encourage exercise in older children.

  o Client Education

- Instruct the parents and child about proper hand hygiene. Encourage frequent repositioning of children to promote respiratory function.

- Instruct the parents how to perform postural drainage and percussion if needed.

- Reinforce the need for routine immunizations.

- Tell parents to seek health care at the earliest sign of infection.

- Reinforce the need to follow the antibiotic schedule if prescribed.

JUVENILE IDIOPATHIC ARTHRITIS (JIA)

Overview

- Classifications of JIA include systemic arthritis, oligoarthritis, and polyarthritis with or without rheumatoid factor.

- No definitive diagnosis is available, but the onset of the disorder starts prior to 16 years of age, and symptoms occur in one or more joints and last for 6 weeks or longer with no other cause identified.

- Peak incidence is between 1 and 3 years of age.

- JIA is rarely life-threatening, and it may subside over time, but it can result in residual joint deformities and altered joint function.

Data Collection

- Risk Factors

    o Susceptible individuals who have an autoimmune response to internal or external triggers

- Subjective and Objective Data

    o Joint swelling, stiffness, redness, and warmth

    o Mobility limitations

    o Fever

    o Rash

    o Nodules under the skin

    o Delayed growth and development

    o Enlarged lymph nodes

    o Visual changes and uveitis (inflammation in the anterior chamber of the eye)

    o Laboratory Tests

        ▪ Erythrocyte sedimentation rate (ESR) – May or may not be elevated

        ▪ CBC with differential may demonstrate elevated WBCs, especially during exacerbations.

        ▪ Antinuclear antibodies (ANA) indicate an increased risk for uveitis.

        ▪ Rheumatoid factor may or may not be present.

o Diagnostic Procedures

- Radiographic studies

  □ Radiographic studies may be used for baseline comparison. X-rays may demonstrate increased synovial fluid in the joint, which causes soft tissue swelling or widening of the joint. Later findings may include osteoporosis and narrowed joint spaces.

  □ Nursing Actions

  ▸ Assist with positioning.

  ▸ Ensure that adolescent females are not pregnant.

Collaborative Care

- Nursing Care

  o Care of children who have JIA is primarily outpatient.

  o Include the family in the child's care so they are prepared for home care.

  o Regularly evaluate the child's pain and response to prescribed analgesics.

  o Encourage children to participate in a physical therapy program to increase mobility and prevent deformities.

  o Encourage activity as tolerated.

  o Instruct parents to apply splints for nighttime sleep. Splints should be applied to knees, wrists, and hands to decrease pain and prevent flexion deformities.

  o Encourage proper positioning with sleep. Encourage the use of electric blankets or sleeping bags for extra warmth.

  o Provide firm mattress and discourage use of pillows under knees. Use no pillow or flat pillow for head.

  o Encourage full range-of-motion exercises when pain and inflammation have subsided.

  o Apply heat or warm moist packs to the child's affected joints prior to exercise.

  o Encourage warm baths.

  o Identify alternate ways for children to meet developmental needs, especially during periods of exacerbation.

  o Encourage self-care by allowing adequate time for completion.

  o Encourage a well-balanced diet that is high in fiber and contains adequate fluids to prevent constipation from immobility.

  o Encourage participation in school and contact with peers.

  o Collaborate with the school nurse and teachers to arrange for care during the school day (medication administration, rest periods, extra time to get to classes, extra sets of books, split days).

- Medications

  - NSAIDs – Naproxen (Naprelan), ibuprofen (Motrin), and tolmetin sodium (Tolectin)

    - NSAIDs control pain and inflammation.

    - Nursing Considerations

      - Instruct children and families to administer NSAIDs as prescribed.

      - Instruct children and families that NSAIDs should be taken with food to minimize gastric irritation.

    - Client Education

      - Instruct children and families to report changes in stool and GI discomfort or increase in bruising immediately.

  - Methotrexate (Rheumatrex)

    - A cytotoxic disease modifying antirheumatic drug (DMARD) that slows joint degeneration and progression of rheumatoid arthritis when NSAIDs do not work alone

    - Nursing Considerations

      - Monitor liver function tests and CBC regularly.

    - Client Education

      - Tell adolescents to avoid alcohol.

      - Discuss the use of effective birth control to avoid birth defects while taking this medication.

  - Corticosteroids

    - Glucocorticoids provide symptomatic relief of inflammation and pain. They are reserved for life-threatening complications, severe arthritis, and uveitis.

    - Nursing Considerations

      - Administer as ophthalmic drops, orally, or assist with intravenous administration.

      - Administer at the lowest effective dose for short-term therapy and then discontinue by tapering the dose. An injection into the intraarticular space may provide effective pain relief.

    - Client Education

      - Advise children and families that weight gain, especially in the face, is a common side effect.

      - Monitor height and weight.

      - Advise families that an alteration in growth is a possible long-term complication of corticosteroids.

      - Advise children to avoid exposure to potentially infectious agents.

      - Advise children and families to practice healthy eating habits.

- ○ Etanercept (Enbrel)
    - ■ Etanercept is a tumor necrosis factor alpha-receptor blocker, another DMARD, that is used when methotrexate is not effective for immunosuppressive action.
    - ■ Nursing Considerations
        - ☐ Administer etanercept once or twice each week by subcutaneous injection.
    - ■ Client Education
        - ☐ Reinforce to children and families about the potential for allergic reactions.
        - ☐ Instruct children and families to avoid exposure to infectious agents.
- ● Interdisciplinary Care
    - ○ Occupational therapy, and physical therapy may be involved when caring for children who have JIA.
- ● Care After Discharge
    - ○ Client Education
        - ■ Assist parents in obtaining accommodations in school.
        - ■ Reinforce exercises prescribed by physical and occupational therapy. These may include exercise in a warm water pool.
        - ■ Caution parents against using aspirin during viral illnesses due to the risk of Reye syndrome.
        - ■ Instruct children and parents about nonpharmacological pain management techniques (distraction, relaxation).
        - ■ Encourage regular eye exams.
- ● Client Outcomes
    - ○ The child will remain free from deformities and impaired joint mobility.
    - ○ The child will reach and maintain optimal levels of functioning.

Complications

- ● Joint deformity and functional disability
    - ○ Nursing Actions
        - ■ Reinforce the individualized therapeutic plan of care.
        - ■ Advocate for children when treatments are not producing expected results.
    - ○ Client Education
        - ■ Encourage children and families to adhere to the treatment regimen.
        - ■ Encourage self-care and active participation in an exercise program.

MUSCULAR DYSTROPHY (MD)

Overview

- Muscular dystrophy (MD) is the largest group of diseases that affects muscle function in children.

- Loss of muscular strength is insidious.

- Developmental milestones are likely to be met until the onset of the disease.

- Onset of disease, rate of progression, and muscle group affected depend on the type of MD.

- Duchenne (pseudohypertrophic) muscular dystrophy (DMD) is the most common form of MD. Inherited as an X-linked recessive trait, DMD has an onset between 3 and 7 years of age. Life expectancy with current technology for DMD reaches into early adulthood.

- Management of DMD is symptomatic to assist with maintaining the highest level of mobility and preventing complications as the disease progresses.

Data Collection

- Risk Factors

  o DMD – Family history of MD

- Subjective Data

  o Family reports of delay in walking; changes in gait; and difficulties with running, climbing stairs, and riding a bike

- Objective Data

  o Physical Assessment Findings

    ▪ Muscular weakness in lower extremities

    ▪ Muscular hypertrophy, especially in calves

    ▪ Mild delay in motor skill development

    ▪ Mobility with general muscle strength declining over time

    ▪ Unsteady, wide-based or waddling gait and loss of walking ability (usually by age 12)

    ▪ Difficulty riding a tricycle, running, and rising from a seated position

    ▪ Mild cognitive delay with learning disabilities

    ▪ Cardiovascular complications (associated with the progression of DMD) – Weight loss, increased fatigue during usual ADLs, and orthopnea

  o Laboratory Tests

    ▪ DNA analysis using peripheral blood, serum polymerase chain reaction (PCR) for the dystrophin gene mutation, or muscle tissue biopsy

- Serum creatine kinase (CK) – Elevated
- Electromyography (EMG) may also be used

Collaborative Care

- Nursing Care
  - Collect baseline data and monitor:
    - The child's ability to perform ADLs
    - The child's respiratory function, including depth, rhythm, and rate of respirations during sleep and daytime hours
    - The child's cardiac function
    - The child and parent's understanding of long-term effects
    - The child and parent's coping and support
  - Maintain optimal physical function for as long possible.
    - Encourage children to be independent for as long as possible and to perform ADLs.
    - Perform range of motion exercises and provide appropriate physical activity. Include stretching exercises, strength and muscle training, and breathing exercises.
    - Maintain proper body alignment and encourage children to reposition self frequently to avoid skin breakdown.
    - Apply splints and braces as prescribed.
  - Maintain respiratory functioning.
    - Encourage the use of incentive spirometry.
    - Position children to enhance expansion of lungs.
    - Provide oxygen as prescribed.
    - Provide noninvasive ventilation as prescribed.
  - Encourage adequate fluid intake.
  - Monitor and encourage adequate nutritional intake.
- Medications
  - Prednisone (Deltasone)
    - Prednisone is a corticosteroid that increases muscle strength.
    - Nursing Considerations
      - Monitor for infection.
    - Client Education
      - Instruct children and parents to avoid potentially infectious agents.
      - Encourage children and family to practice healthy eating habits.

- Interdisciplinary Care

  ○ Encourage the parents to consider assistance with care as disease progresses (respite care, long-term care, home health care).

  ○ Discuss support groups for MD with children and parents.

- Surgical Interventions

  ○ Surgery may be indicated for release or repair of contractures or for insertion of a gastrostomy tube or tracheostomy.

  ○ Surgical release of contractures

    ■ Nursing Actions

      □ Provide standard postoperative care with emphasis on monitoring respiratory status, cast care (if applicable), skin and wound care, and elimination.

    ■ Client Education

      □ Provide preoperative teaching for children and parents.

      □ Reinforce to families about signs and symptoms of infection.

- Care After Discharge

  ○ Client Education

    ■ Provide information regarding social supports and programs available to children and parents.

    ■ Provide information regarding respite care and home care services available to children and parents.

    ■ Encourage routine physical exams and immunizations.

    ■ Facilitate discussion of end-of-life decisions when appropriate, including the use of mechanical ventilation and feeding tubes.

    ■ Encourage and provide for genetic counseling for parents.

- Client Outcomes

  ○ The child will maintain optimal levels of functioning.

Complications

- Respiratory compromise

  ○ Respiratory muscles impair the child's ability to maintain adequate respirations.

  ○ Nursing Actions

    ■ Help children turn hourly or more frequently.

    ■ Have children use deep breathing and coughing.

    ■ Suction as needed.

- Administer oxygen as prescribed.

- Use intermittent positive pressure ventilation and mechanically-assisted cough devices if indicated.

- Administer antibiotics as prescribed.

○ Client Education

- Direct children and parents to the provider for questions about mechanical ventilation options.

(A) APPLICATION EXERCISES

1. A nurse is caring for a child who has cerebral palsy. Which of the following medications should the nurse expect to administer to treat painful muscle spasms? (Select all that apply.)

    _____ Baclofen (Lioresal)

    _____ Diazepam (Valium)

    _____ Oxybutynin chloride (Ditropan)

    _____ Methotrexate (Rheumatrex)

    _____ Prednisone (Deltasone)

2. A nurse is caring for a school-age child who has juvenile idiopathic arthritis. Which of the following are appropriate home care instructions? (Select all that apply.)

    ___✓___ Sleep on a firm mattress.

    _____ Use cold compresses for joint pain.

    _____ Take ibuprofen (Motrin) on an empty stomach.

    ___✓___ Plan rest periods during the day.

    ___✓___ Perform range-of-motion exercises when inflammation has subsided.

3. A nurse in the newborn nursery is assigned to care for a newborn with Down syndrome, and is reviewing teaching with the mother. Which of the following statements by the mother indicates a need for further teaching?

    A. "I'm glad he will be assigned a physical therapist."

    B. "I know he will not sit or crawl at the same time as babies his same age."

    C. "He will look better as he starts to grow and his tongue stops protruding."

    D. "He has an appointment with the cardiologist in two weeks."

4. Match the following types of cerebral palsy with their associated physical assessment findings.

    _____ Spastic   1. Involuntary jerky movements, can be worm-like

    _____ Dyskinetic   2. Scissoring motion of legs, appear to be on tip-toe

    _____ Athetoid   3. Wide-based gait which is uncoordinated

    _____ Dystonic   4. Movements absent in sleep, worse with stress

    _____ Ataxic   5. Slow, twisting movements affecting trunk and extremities

5. A nurse is caring for an antenatal client who is to undergo an amniocentesis. Which of the following laboratory tests of amniotic fluid may be used to identify a fetus with a neural tube defect?

    A. Lecithin/sphingomyelin (L/S) ratio

    B. Erythrocyte sedimentation rate (ESR)

    C. Antinuclear antibodies (ANA)

    D. Alpha-fetoprotein (AFP)

6. A nurse is assisting with the admission of a 7-year old child with suspected Duchenne muscular dystrophy (DMD) to the pediatric unit. Which of the following data should the nurse expect to collect about this child? (Select all that apply.)

    _____ Mother describes child meeting infant developmental milestones sooner than children of same age.

    _✓__ Mother describes child having difficulty feeding himself.

    _✓__ Mother describes child as not having gained weight and being smaller than children of same age.

    _✓__ Child describes being tired often and needing rest periods.

    _✓__ Gait is unsteady and wide-based.

7. List risk factors for the development of cerebral palsy to include one prenatal factor, one perinatal factor and one postnatal factor.

    A. Prenatal factor: _____

    B. Perinatal factor: _____

    C. Postnatal factor: _____

(A) **APPLICATION EXERCISES ANSWER KEY**

1. A nurse is caring for a child who has cerebral palsy. Which of the following medications should the nurse expect to administer to treat painful muscle spasms? (Select all that apply.)

   __X__ **Baclofen (Lioresal)**

   __X__ **Diazepam (Valium)**

   _____ Oxybutynin chloride (Ditropan)

   _____ Methotrexate (Rheumatrex)

   _____ Prednisone (Deltasone)

   Baclofen and diazepam are muscle relaxants used to treat painful muscle spasms. Oxybutynin chloride is an anti-spasmodic, anticholinergic medication used to decrease bladder spasms. Methotrexate is a cytotoxic disease modifying anti-rheumatic drug (DMARD) that slows joint degeneration and progression of rheumatoid arthritis and is used for children with juvenile idiopathic arthritis. Prednisone is a corticosteroid that increases muscle strength for children who have muscular dystrophy.

(N) **NCLEX® Connection: Pharmacological Therapies, Expected Actions/Outcomes**

2. A nurse is caring for a school-age child who has juvenile idiopathic arthritis. Which of the following are appropriate home care instructions? (Select all that apply.)

   __X__ **Sleep on a firm mattress.**

   _____ Use cold compresses for joint pain.

   _____ Take ibuprofen (Motrin) on an empty stomach.

   __X__ **Plan rest periods during the day.**

   __X__ **Perform range-of-motion exercises when inflammation has subsided.**

   The child with juvenile idiopathic arthritis should sleep on a firm mattress to prevent joint deformities and maintain body alignment, rest periodically throughout the day to conserve energy, and perform range-of-motion exercises when inflammation has subsided to minimize pain. Heat (warm, moist packs), rather than cold compresses, provides comfort and relieves stiffness. Ibuprofen should be taken with food to prevent gastrointestinal upset.

(N) **NCLEX® Connection: Basic Care and Comfort, Mobility/Immobility**

3. A nurse in the newborn nursery is assigned to care for a newborn with Down syndrome, and is reviewing teaching with the mother. Which of the following statements by the mother indicates a need for further teaching?

   A. "I'm glad he will be assigned a physical therapist."

   B. "I know he will not sit or crawl at the same time as babies his same age."

   C. "He will look better as he starts to grow and his tongue stops protruding."

   D. "He has an appointment with the cardiologist in two weeks."

   Infants with Down syndrome have characteristics that are permanent such as a large protruding tongue, low-set ears, and upward slant of the eyes. These characteristics may become less prominent as the child grows, but do not disappear. Physical therapists work with children who have Down syndrome to promote meeting developmental milestones which can be delayed due to hypotonicity. A cardiology consult is important because congenital heart defects are often associated with Down syndrome.

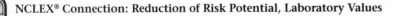 NCLEX® Connection: Reduction of Risk Potential, Potential for Alterations in Body Systems

4. Match the following types of cerebral palsy with their associated physical assessment findings.

__2__	Spastic	1. Involuntary jerky movements, can be worm-like
__4__	Dyskinetic	2. Scissoring motion of legs, appear to be on tip-toe
__1__	Athetoid	3. Wide-based gait which is uncoordinated
__5__	Dystonic	4. Movements absent in sleep, worse with stress
__3__	Ataxic	5. Slow, twisting movements affecting trunk and extremities

   NCLEX® Connection: Reduction of Risk Potential, Potential for Alterations in Body Systems

5. A nurse is caring for an antenatal client who is to undergo an amniocentesis. Which of the following laboratory tests of amniotic fluid may be used to identify a fetus with a neural tube defect?

   A. Lecithin/sphingomyelin (L/S) ratio

   B. Erythrocyte sedimentation rate (ESR)

   C. Antinuclear antibodies (ANA)

   D. Alpha-fetoprotein (AFP)

   An alpha-fetoprotein (AFP) test is used to identify the presence of a neural tube defect. The L/S ratio is used to evaluate fetal lung maturity as part of the analysis of amniotic fluid. An ESR is a blood test used to identify the presence of inflammation and is used in cases of juvenile idiopathic arthritis (JIA). The ANA test is another diagnostic blood test used in cases of JIA.

   NCLEX® Connection: Reduction of Risk Potential, Laboratory Values

6. A nurse is assisting with the admission of a 7-year old child with suspected Duchenne muscular dystrophy (DMD) to the pediatric unit. Which of the following data should the nurse expect to collect about this child? (Select all that apply.)

_____ Mother describes child meeting infant developmental milestones sooner than children of same age.

_____ Mother describes child having difficulty feeding himself.

___X___ **Mother describes child as not having gained weight and being smaller than children of same age.**

___X___ **Child describes being tired often and needing rest periods.**

___X___ **Gait is unsteady and wide-based.**

Expected findings in a child with DMD include weight loss and increased fatigue which can indicate cardiovascular complications. The child's gait is increasingly unsteady, wide-based and waddling with loss of walking ability usually by age 12. Children with DMD are delayed in motor skill and cognitive development. Muscular weakness is present in lower extremities.

Ⓝ NCLEX® Connection: Basic Care and Comfort, Mobility/Immobility

7. List risk factors for the development of cerebral palsy to include one prenatal factor, one perinatal factor and one postnatal factor.

A. Prenatal factor: _____

A. Prenatal factors include: premature birth, multiple births, extremely low or low newborn birth weight, placental insufficiency

B. Perinatal factor: _____

B. Perinatal factor: interruption of oxygen to the fetus during birth

C. Postnatal factor: _____

C. Postnatal factor: kernicterus resulting from high bilirubin levels in the neonatal period

Ⓝ NCLEX® Connection: Physiological Adaptations, Basic Pathophysiology

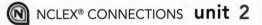

UNIT 2: NURSING CARE OF CHILDREN WITH SYSTEM DISORDERS

Section: Integumentary Disorders

- Skin Infections and Infestations

- Dermatitis and Acne

- Burns

NCLEX® CONNECTIONS

When reviewing the chapters in this section, keep in mind the relevant sections of the NCLEX® outline, in particular:

CLIENT NEEDS: BASIC CARE AND COMFORT	CLIENT NEEDS: REDUCTION OF RISK POTENTIAL	CLIENT NEEDS: PHYSIOLOGICAL ADAPTATION
Relevant topics/tasks include:	Relevant topics/tasks include:	Relevant topics/tasks include:
• Non-Pharmacological Comfort Interventions	• Changes/Abnormalities in Vital Signs	• Alterations in Body Systems
○ Assist in planning comfort interventions for client with impaired comfort.	○ Reinforce client teaching about normal and abnormal vital signs.	○ Provide care to correct client alteration in body system.
• Nutrition and Oral Hydration	• Diagnostic Tests	• Fluid and Electrolyte Imbalances
○ Reinforce client teaching on special diets based on client diagnosis/nutritional needs and cultural considerations.	○ Reinforce client teaching about diagnostic test.	○ Apply knowledge of pathophysiology to monitoring client for alterations in body systems.
• Rest and Sleep	• Potential for Complications of Diagnostic Tests/ Treatments/Procedures	
○ Identify client usual rest and sleep patterns.	○ Suggest change in interventions based on client response to diagnostic tests/ treatments/procedures.	

UNIT 2	NURSING CARE OF CHILDREN WITH SYSTEM DISORDERS
Section:	Integumentary Disorders
Chapter 29	**Skin Infections and Infestations**

◎ Overview

- More than 50% of skin disorders in children are a form of dermatitis. The inflammatory response appears similar, but the causative agent and course of the dermatitis have wide variations.

- Most changes caused by dermatitis are reversible, unless complicated by ulceration, infection, and/or scratching.

- Viruses cause epidermal inflammation and formation of vesicles or warts.

- Dermatophytoses cause fungal infections, which affect the stratum corneum, hair, and nails. The lesions are superficial and not in the skin.

- Pediculosis (head lice) is a contagious parasitic infestation.

  - Pediculosis is transmitted through the sharing of personal items (hair brushes, combs, hats) or when personal items are kept close together.

  - Female lice lays eggs (nits) that attach to the hair follicles and hatch within 7 to 10 days.

  - Lice can live up to 1 month on the host, but only 48 hr without the host.

  - Movement and saliva of the lice cause pruritus.

- Scabies is a contagious skin infestation caused by a microscopic mite.

- Lyme disease is caused by a spirochete, which is contained within the saliva and feces of ticks (mainly deer ticks). The spirochete is transferred to an individual's bloodstream when the tick attaches to the person's skin.

Data Collection

- Risk Factors

  - Causes of skin lesions in children include genetic factors and systemic illnesses (rheumatic fever, cancer).

  - Causative agents include bacteria, viruses, fungi, mites, and infected insects.

- o Risks for developing bacterial skin infections include:

    - Immunodeficiency disorders (AIDS, leukemia, solid tumors [lymphoma])

    - Long-term immunosuppressive therapy (corticosteroids)

  - o Lice infestation can occur during periods of time when children are in close contact (day care, school, summer camp) and sharing personal care items (comb/hair brush, hats).

  - o Scabies spreads quickly under crowded conditions. Infestation may also occur with the sharing of infested clothing, towels, and bedding. Individuals with weakened immune systems are at the greatest risk for infestation.

- Subjective Data

  - o Nursing history information should include:

    - Recent exposure to a causative agent, such as a virus, food, medication, animal, or plant.

    - Reports of itching and/or pain in areas such as the head, genitals, joints, and back.

- Objective Data

  - o Physical Assessment Findings

INFECTION/CAUSATIVE AGENTS	MANIFESTATIONS
Impetigo contagiosa bacteria • Staphylococcus	• Appears as a red macule that becomes a vesicle and ruptures • Has thick, crusted, amber-colored exudate (honey-colored crust) • Spreads easily
Verruca (warts) • Human papillomavirus	• Appears as a well-circumscribed grey or brown papule with rough papillomatous texture
Cold sores and fever blisters • Herpes simplex virus type1 Genital herpes • Herpes simplex virus type 2	• Appears as a group of vesicles on inflamed skin, usually around the lips or genitalia • Is accompanied by a painful burning sensation • Dries, exfoliates, and heals within 8 to 10 days
Tinea capitis (ringworm) – Fungus on the head • *Trichophyton tonsurans* • *Microsporum canis*	• Appears as circular, scaly patches on scalp with or without areas of alopecia • Begins in the scalp and possibly progresses to the neck or hairline

INFECTION/CAUSATIVE AGENTS	MANIFESTATIONS
Tinea corporis (ringworm) – Fungus on the body • *Trichophyton rubrum* • *Trichophyton mentagrophytes* • *Microsporum canis*	• Appears as circular, scaly, red patches • Has a clear center that spreads peripherally to the edges of the lesion
Candidiasis (thrush) – Fungus • *Candida albicans*	• Appears as inflamed areas with white exudate that peel and bleed easily
Pediculosis (lice) – Parasite • *Pediculus humanus capitis* (head lice) • *Pediculus corporis* (body lice) • *Pediculus pubis* (pubic lice)	• Begins with generalized itching on head or genital area • Progresses to visible lesions from scratching, which can become infected with bacteria or fungi • Involves nits in hair that are visible, behind ears, at base of scalp, and occasionally in eyelashes and brows (With heavy infestations, live lice may also be seen.)
Scabies mite • *Sarcoptes scabiei*	• Appears as grayish-brown, threadlike burrows with a black dot at the end (mite) • Involves eczematous eruption in infants • Is accompanied by intense itching that can cause sores to become infected • Appears as lesions in interdigital, antecubital, popliteal, and inguinal areas

Lyme disease
• *Borrelia burgdorferi*
	• Has symptoms of viral-like illness
	• Has three stages
	  ○ Stage 1 – Rash of red ring about 3 to 31 days after possible tick bite
	  ○ Stage 2 – Neurologic, cardiac, and musculoskeletal involvement
	  ○ Stage 3 – Musculoskeletal pain in joints and supporting structures, as well as neurological problems

(M) View Media Supplement:

• Impetigo (Image)   • Lice (Image)

- ○ Laboratory Tests
    - ▪ Wound culture (for bacterial infections)
    - ▪ Serologic testing (for Lyme disease)
- ○ Diagnostic Procedures
    - ▪ Identify the parasite.
        - ▫ *Pediculus humanus capitis* (head lice) are small (but visible), wingless, free-moving, and grayish tan in color.
        - ▫ Nits (small, white oval eggs) attach to hair follicles about 6 mm (0.25 in) from the scalp and are difficult to remove from hair shafts. They may resemble dandruff.
        - ▫ Translucent (empty) nits may be found farther down the hair shaft.
        - ▫ Nursing Actions
            - ▸ Conduct a microscopic exam of tissue or lesions.
        - ▫ Client Education
            - ▸ Instruct the child and parents how to eliminate the infestation. Treatment will depend on which parasite is identified.
            - ▸ Reinforce the need to follow the therapeutic plan to prevent reinfestation and spread.

Collaborative Care

- Nursing Care
    - ○ Evaluate the general condition of the skin, hair, and nails, including color (redness, pallor, cyanosis), cleanliness, warmth, swelling, and bleeding of mucous membranes.
    - ○ Observe for presence, pattern, and location of vesicles, warts, rash, hives, or open wounds.
    - ○ Evaluate for signs of a wound infection.
        - ▪ Swelling
        - ▪ Purulent drainage
        - ▪ Pain
        - ▪ Increased temperature
        - ▪ Redness extending beyond the wound margin
    - ○ Gently clean affected areas.
    - ○ Apply topical antibiotics or antifungal creams as prescribed.
    - ○ Trim and clean the child's fingernails.
    - ○ Encourage the child to wear gloves at night to prevent scratching.

- Care After Discharge

  - Client Education

    - Instruct families how to avoid the spread of infections.

      - Use proper hand hygiene.

      - Avoid sharing clothing, hats, combs, brushes, and/or towels.

      - Keep the child from touching the affected area by using distraction.

      - Do not squeeze vesicles.

      - Apply topical medications as prescribed.

      - Administer oral medications as prescribed.

        - Remind parents to bring children taking griseofulvin for periodic laboratory tests to monitor renal and liver function.

      - Clean surfaces that might be harboring causative agents, including bed linens, clothing, and furniture.

    - Discourage the use of home remedies for lice.

    - Instruct the family how to prevent arthropod bites.

      - Avoid tick-infested areas. If bitten, carefully remove ticks and observe skin for development of any reactions.

      - Wear light-colored clothing when going into areas that may have ticks so that ticks can be identified and removed.

      - Apply insect repellants cautiously to avoid neurologic complications.

- Client Outcomes

  - The child will be free of infection.

Complications

- Secondary infection (staphylococcus, streptococcus, *Haemophilus influenzae*)

  - Clinical manifestations may include:

    - Red inflammation of skin with swelling

    - Lymphangitis (red streaking)

    - Enlargement of lymph nodes

    - Development of abscess

    - Fever and malaise

  - Nursing Actions

    - Administer antibiotics, antipyretics, and antipruritics as prescribed.

    - Monitor effects of prescribed medications.

- Keep lesions clean and dry.
- Apply dressings as prescribed.

o Client Education

- Reinforce the therapeutic management plan with emphasis on maintaining health and hygiene.
- Reinforce hand hygiene as a good way to prevent infections.
- Encourage children and the parents to trim nails short and discourage scratching.

Ⓐ APPLICATION EXERCISES

1. Which of the following is a manifestation of scabies? (Select all that apply.)

    _____ Nits present

    _____ Thread-like rash between fingers and other moist areas

    _____ Circular rash on extremities

    _____ Pruritus

    _____ Eczematous eruptions in infants

2. Match the following infections with the appropriate medication used in treatment.

    _____ Ringworm   1. Pediculicide

    _____ Thrush   2. Amoxicillin (Amoxil)

    _____ Head lice   3. Griseofulvin (Grifulvin)

    _____ Lyme disease   4. Nystatin (Mycostatin)

3. A nurse is reinforcing teaching to a parent about the cause of Lyme disease. Which of the following statements by the parent indicates the teaching was effective?

    A. "I'll spray the yard to get rid of the mosquitoes."

    B. "Washing the sheets in hot water will get rid of the fungus."

    C. "I'll check his skin for any ticks after he's been hiking."

    D. "Using a special shampoo on the dog will get rid of the fleas."

4. A nursing is caring for a 6-month-old infant with impetigo. Which of the following discharge instructions should be reviewed with the infant's mother? (Select all that apply.)

    _____ Clean nipples and pacifiers frequently in hot, soapy water and air dry.

    _____ Apply topical antibacterial ointment to the infected areas.

    _____ Leave the antibacterial ointment on for 6 to 8 hrs, then wash it off.

    _____ Use clean towels when bathing the infant.

    _____ Check the infant's hair often for the presence of nits.

APPLICATION EXERCISES ANSWER KEY

1. Which of the following is a manifestation of scabies? (Select all that apply.)

_____ Nits present

__X__ **Thread-like rash between fingers and other moist areas**

_____ Circular rash on extremities

__X__ **Pruritus**

__X__ **Eczematous eruptions in infants**

Scabies is caused by the scabies mite, which burrows into the skin. The mite is often found between the fingers or in other moist areas, such as antecubital, popliteal, or inguinal areas. The burrows seen on the skin often appear grayish-brown and thread-like with a black dot at the end (the mite). Skin lesions are pruritic in nature. In infants, skin lesions may look like eczema. The presence of nits indicates pediculosis, not scabies; and a circular rash on extremities may indicate Lyme disease or ringworm.

N NCLEX® Connection: Safety and Infection Control, Standard/Transmission-Based/Other Precautions/Surgical Asepsis

2. Match the following infections with the appropriate medication used in treatment.

__3__ Ringworm   1. Pediculicide

__4__ Thrush   2. Amoxicillin (Amoxil)

__1__ Head lice   3. Griseofulvin (Grifulvin)

__2__ Lyme disease   4. Nystatin (Mycostatin)

N NCLEX® Connection: Pharmacological Therapies, Expected Actions/Outcomes

3. A nurse is reinforcing teaching to a parent about the cause of Lyme disease. Which of the following statements by the parent indicates the teaching was effective?

A. "I'll spray the yard to get rid of the mosquitoes."

B. "Washing the sheets in hot water will get rid of the fungus."

C. "I'll check his skin for any ticks after he's been hiking."

D. "Using a special shampoo on the dog will get rid of the fleas."

Lyme disease is caused by a spirochete contained in the saliva and feces of ticks (mainly deer ticks). When the tick attaches to the person's skin, blood containing the spirochete is transferred to the individual. Lyme disease is not caused by mosquitoes, fungus, or fleas.

N NCLEX® Connection: Safety and Infection Control, Standard/Transmission-Based/Other Precautions/Surgical Asepsis

4. A nursing is caring for a 6-month-old infant with impetigo. Which of the following discharge instructions should be reviewed with the infant's mother? (Select all that apply.)

   X   **Clean nipples and pacifiers frequently in hot, soapy water and air dry.**

   X   **Apply topical antibacterial ointment to the infected areas.**

       Leave the antibacterial ointment on for 6 to 8 hrs, then wash it off.

   X   **Use clean towels when bathing the infant.**

       Check the infant's hair often for the presence of nits.

Impetigo is caused by staphylococcus and is easily spread. It often occurs around the nose and mouth, so keeping pacifiers clean will reduce the risk of recontamination. Apply a topical antibacterial ointment to the infected areas according to the prescription and do not remove after application. Using clean towels when bathing the infant will reduce the spread of infection to other family members. Nits are found with head lice, not impetigo.

NCLEX® Connection: Physiological Adaptations, Alterations in Body Systems

UNIT 2   NURSING CARE OF CHILDREN WITH SYSTEM DISORDERS

Section: Integumentary Disorders

Chapter 30   Dermatitis and Acne

Overview

- Common skin conditions of the pediatric population include:

    o   Contact dermatitis

    o   Atopic dermatitis

    o   Acne

CONTACT DERMATITIS

Overview

- Contact dermatitis is an inflammatory reaction of the skin. It is caused when the skin comes into contact with chemicals or other irritants (feces, urine, soaps, poison ivy, animals, metals, dyes, medications).

    o   Diaper dermatitis may be caused by detergents, soaps, and/or chemicals that come in contact with the genital area. It may also be a result of *Candida albicans*.

    o   Contact dermatitis is a result of exposure to urushiol, an oil found in poisonous plants.

    o   Seborrheic dermatitis (cradle cap) has an unknown etiology but is most common in infancy and then again at puberty.

Data Collection

- Risk Factors

    o   Use of diapers

    o   Exposure to wild plants

- Subjective Data

    o   Constant pruritus

- Objective Data

  - Physical Assessment Findings

    - Diaper dermatitis

      - Red, inflamed skin on areas in most contact with urine, feces, and/or chemical irritants. Note whether the irritation is within or across the inguinal folds.

      - Lesions manifested are varied in type and pattern. Satellite lesions are characteristic of *Candida albicans*.

      - Involved areas usually include folds of the buttocks, inner thighs, and scrotum.

    - Contact dermatitis

      - The area of reaction will vary depending on exposure. The reaction may be mild to severe and include redness, swelling, blisters, and pruritus.

    - Medication reactions

      - Reactions may occur immediately after administration of the medication, if previously taken, or they may be delayed. It may take up to 7 days for a child who has never been exposed to a particular medication to have an adverse response.

      - Reactions may range from a simple rash to a full body response, and they may be mild to severe. These reactions may look similar to other skin disorders.

      - A sudden onset of a generalized inflammatory response with itching and gastrointestinal (GI) discomfort may occur. However, this response can progress to anemia and kidney and/or liver dysfunction.

    - Seborrheic dermatitis

      - Thick, yellowish, scaly adhesions occur on the scalp, eyelids, and external ear canals.

Collaborative Care

- Nursing Care

  - Diaper dermatitis

    - Promptly remove the wet diaper.

    - Clean urine off the perineal area with a nonirritating cleanser. Cleanse the perineal area of feces with warm water and mild soap.

    - Wash skin folds and the genital area frequently with water.

    - Expose the affected area to air.

    - Use superabsorbent disposable diapers to reduce skin exposure.

- Apply a skin barrier, such as zinc oxide. Do not wash it off with each diaper change.

- Use cornstarch to reduce friction between the diaper and the skin. Instruct the parents to shake the cornstarch into their hand and then apply to the infant's skin.

o Contact dermatitis

- Rinse areas that have been exposed to poisonous plants with cold running water.

View Media Supplement: Poison Ivy Rash and Poison Ivy Plant (Image)

- Remove all clothing that has come into contact with the plant and wash with alcohol followed by water.

- Use calamine lotion or compresses of ammonium acetate in water (Burow's solution) on affected skin.

- Encourage baths with commercial colloidal oatmeal.

- Apply a topical corticosteroid gel.

- Encourage the child not to scratch skin to prevent a secondary infection from developing.

o Medication reactions

- Discontinue the medication.

- Initiate emergency response for anaphylaxis.

o Seborrheic dermatitis

- Treat by gently scrubbing the scalp with mild pressure and shampoo daily with mild soap or antiseborrheic shampoo.

- Medications

o Antihistamines – Hydroxyzine (Atarax) or diphenhydramine (Benadryl)

- Administer in cases of allergic/medication reactions.

- Nursing Considerations

□ Administer the medication as prescribed.

- Client Education

□ Reinforce to families the importance of the medication and administering on schedule.

□ Reinforce the sedating effect of some antihistamines and the need for parents to monitor the child and provide for safety during use.

- o Antibiotics
  - ▪ Use to treat secondary infections.
  - ▪ Nursing Considerations
    - ▫ Administer medications as prescribed.
  - ▪ Client Education
    - ▫ Reinforce to families about the importance of continuing the medication as prescribed.
- Care After Discharge
  - o Client Education
    - ▪ Encourage frequent diaper changes.
    - ▪ Advise parents that their child should avoid bubble baths and harsh soaps.
    - ▪ Encourage children to wear long sleeves and pants.
    - ▪ Educate parents to remove an offending agent as soon as exposure takes place.
- Client Outcomes
  - o The child's skin will heal without complications and will remain intact.
  - o The child will be free of infections.

Complications

- Infection
  - o Caused by breaks in the skin from scratching
  - o Nursing Actions
    - ▪ Monitor the area for signs of infection.
    - ▪ Keep fingernails trimmed short.
    - ▪ Cleanse the area with mild soap and water.
    - ▪ Administer antipruritics as prescribed.
  - o Client Education
    - ▪ Educate the family and child about avoiding offending agents.

ATOPIC DERMATITIS (AD)

Overview

- Atopic dermatitis (AD) is a type of eczema (eczema describes a category of integumentary disorders, not a specific disorder with a determined etiology) that is characterized by pruritus and associated with a history of allergies that are of an inherited tendency (atopy).

- New lesions develop with continued scratching and increase the risk of secondary infection.

- Classifications of atopic dermatitis are based on the child's age, how the lesions are distributed, and the appearance of the lesions.

- AD cannot be cured but can be well controlled.

Data Collection

- Risk Factors

  ○ Presence of allergic condition and family history of atopy

  ○ Previous skin disorder and exacerbation of present skin disorder

  ○ Exposure to irritating and/or causative agents

- Subjective Data

  ○ Recent exposure to any irritant (medication, food, soap, contact with animals)

  ○ Intense pruritus

- Objective Data

  ○ Physical Assessment Findings

CLASSIFICATION	DISTRIBUTION	LESIONS
Infants – Onset at 2 to 6 months of age with spontaneous remission by 3 years of age	• Generalized distribution of lesions on cheeks, scalp, trunk, hands and feet, as well as extensor surfaces of extremities	• Usually symmetric • Weeping and oozing or crusty and scaly • Erythematous vesicles and papules
Children 1 to 12 years of age – Progression of infant form or starts at 2 years of age with full symptoms evident by 5 years of age	• Redness or irritation in the flexor spaces (the antecubital and popliteal fossae, on wrists, ankles, and feet)	• Red or tan-colored patches or clusters of papules • Hyperpigmented • Dry • Thickened skin • Keratosis pilaris
Adolescents – Onset at 12 years of age and may continue into adulthood	• Similar distribution to children	• Same as for children • Papules that appear blended together • Larger, dry, thickened patches

- Unaffected skin may appear dry and rough.

- Hypopigmentation of skin may occur in small, diffuse areas.

- Pallor surrounds the nose, mouth, and ears.
- A bluish discoloration is present underneath the eyes.
- Numerous infections of the nails are present.
- Lymphadenopathy occurs, especially around affected areas.
- Signs of a wound infection are present (swelling, purulent drainage, pain, increased temperature, redness extending beyond the wound margin).

Collaborative Care

- Nursing Care
  - Keep skin hydrated with tepid baths (with/without soap or emulsifying oil), then apply an emollient within 3 min of bathing. Two or three baths may be given daily with one prior to bedtime.
  - Dress children in cotton clothing. Avoid wools or synthetic fabrics.
  - Avoid excessive heat and perspiration, which increases itching.
  - Avoid irritants (bubble baths, soaps, perfumes, fabric softeners).
  - Provide support to the child and family.
  - Wash skin folds and genital area frequently with water.
    - Assist in identifying causative agent.
- Medications
  - Antihistamines – Hydroxyzine (Atarax) or diphenhydramine (Benadryl)
    - Administer in cases of medication reactions.
    - Client Education
      - Reinforce the sedating effect of some antihistamines and the need for parents to monitor the child during use.
      - Reinforce safety of children when using sedating antihistamines.
  - Antihistamines – Loratadine (Claritin) or fexofenadine (Allegra)
    - Oral antihistamine for antipruritic effect
    - Nursing Considerations
      - Administer the medication as prescribed.
    - Client Education
      - Inform the parents that it is preferred for use during the daytime.
  - Antibiotics
    - Antibiotics should be used to treat secondary infections.

- o Topical corticosteroids
  - ■ Use topical corticosteroids intermittently to reduce or control flare-ups. They may be low, moderate, or high potency, and are prescribed based on the degree of skin involvement (extremity versus eyelids), age of the child, and consequences from side effects.
- o Nonsteroidal agents
  - ■ Used to decrease inflammation during flare-ups
  - ■ Nursing Considerations
    - □ Use for children older than 2 years of age.
    - □ Use at the start of an exacerbation of AD when skin turns red and starts to itch.
- o Client Education
  - ■ Reinforce the signs of infection.
  - ■ Instruct families to:
    - □ Change diapers when wet or soiled.
    - □ Keep nails short and trimmed.
    - □ Place gloves or cotton socks over hands for sleeping.
    - □ Dress young children in soft, cotton, one-piece, long-sleeve, long-pant outfits.
    - □ Remove items that may promote itching (woolen blankets, scratchy fabrics). Use cotton whenever possible.
    - □ Use mild detergents to wash clothing and linens. The wash cycle may be repeated without soap.
    - □ Avoid latex products, second-hand smoke, furry pets, dust, and molds.
    - □ Encourage tepid baths without the use of soap. Avoid oils and powders.
    - □ Follow specific directions regarding topical medications, soaks, and baths. Emphasize the importance of understanding the sequence of treatments to maximize the benefit of therapy and prevent complications.
    - □ Avoid overheating the bedroom during winter months. Use a room humidifier.
    - □ Maintain treatment to prevent flare-up.
    - □ Follow up with the provider as directed.
    - □ Participate in support groups.
- • Client Outcomes
  - o The child will be free from exacerbations.
  - o The child will remain free from itching.

- o   The child's skin will remain intact.

- o   The child will remain free from infection.

- o   The child will maintain a positive self-image.

Complications

- Infection

    - Caused by breaks in the skin from scratching

- o   Nursing Actions

    - Keep nails trimmed.

    - Administer antipruritics as prescribed.

    - Monitor the area for signs of infection.

    - Cleanse the area with mild soap and water.

- o   Client Education

    - Educate children and families to avoid offending agents.

ACNE

Overview

- Acne is the most common skin condition during adolescence.

- Acne is self-limiting and non life-threatening. However, it poses a threat to self-image for adolescents.

- Acne involves the pilosebaceous follicles (hair follicle and sebaceous gland complex) of the face, neck, chest, and upper back.

- *Propionibacterium acnes* (*P. acnes*) is the bacteria associated with inflammation in acne.

Data Collection

- Risk Factors

    - o   Acne may be genetic.

    - o   Acne is more common in males than in females.

    - o   Hormonal fluctuations may result in acne flares in females.

    - o   The use of cosmetic products containing ingredients such as petrolatum and lanolin may increase acne outbreaks.

    - o   Although there is no dietary intake link with acne, adolescents working at fast food restaurants may have an increased incidence of acne due to exposure to cooking grease.

- Subjective and Objective Data

  o Report of exacerbations and remissions

  o Physical Assessment Findings

    ■ Lesions (comedones) are either open (blackheads) or closed (whiteheads). Both are most often found on the face, neck, back, and chest.

    ■ *P. acnes* may lead to inflammation manifesting as papules, pustules, nodules, or cysts.

Collaborative Care

- Nursing Care

  o Discuss the process of acne with adolescents and their families.

  o Discuss the importance of adherence with the prescribed plan of care.

  o Provide written instructions to accompany verbal instructions.

  o Instruct adolescents to gently wash the face and other affected areas, avoiding scrubbing and abrasive cleaners.

  o Inform adolescents and their families about the medications prescribed, especially side effects.

  o Monitor for signs of mood changes or suicidal ideation in adolescents who are taking isotretinoin 13-cis-retinoic acid (Accutane)

  o Provide support and encouragement to adolescents and their families.

MEDICATION	ACTION	NURSING INTERVENTIONS/CLIENT EDUCATION

Tretinoin (Retin-A)	• Interrupts abnormal keratinization that causes microcomedones	• Inform adolescents that tretinoin may irritate the skin. Instruct the child to apply within 20 to 30 min after washing the face.
		• Tell adolescents to:
		  o Use a pea-size amount of medication and apply at night.
		  o Avoid sun exposure.
		  o Use sunscreen (SPF 15 or greater) to avoid sunburn.

Benzoyl peroxide	• Antibacterial agent • Inhibits growth of *P. acnes*	• Inform adolescents that benzoyl peroxide may bleach bed linens, towels, and clothing, but not skin.

MEDICATION	ACTION	NURSING INTERVENTIONS/CLIENT EDUCATION
Topical antibacterial agents	• Inhibits growth of *P. acnes*	• Inform adolescents that various topical or oral antibacterial agents are available. However, be alert to allergic reactions. • Tell adolescents to avoid overexposure to the sun. • Use sunscreen with an SPF of 15 or greater when exposure to sun is unavoidable.
Isotretinoin 13-cis-retinoic acid (Accutane)	• Affects factors involved in the development of acne	• Isotretinoin 13-cis-retinoic acid is only prescribed by dermatologists. • Side effects include dry skin and mucous membranes, dry eyes, decreased night vision, headaches, photosensitivity, elevated cholesterol and triglycerides, depression, suicidal ideation, and/or violent behaviors. • Monitor for behavioral changes. • Isotretinoin 13-cis-retinoic acid is teratogenic. Therefore, it is contraindicated in women of childbearing age who are not taking oral contraceptives.

- Care After Discharge
  - Client Education
    - Reinforce that adherence to the therapeutic plan is essential to preventing acne flares.
    - Encourage adolescents to eat a balanced, healthy diet.
    - Encourage sleep, rest, and daily exercise.
    - Tell adolescents to wash the affected area gently with a mild cleanser once or twice daily, and not to pick or squeeze comedones.
    - Encourage frequent shampooing.
    - Encourage family members to assist adolescents in coping with body-image changes.
    - Instruct adolescents to wear protective clothing and sunscreen when outside.
    - Tell adolescents to avoid the use of tanning beds.

- Reinforce the need for follow-up and monitoring of cholesterol and triglycerides, especially in adolescents who are taking isotretinoin 13-cis-retinoic acid.

- Reinforce with adolescent females about the importance of using oral contraceptives while taking isotretinoin 13-cis-retinoic acid.

- Client Outcomes

  o The adolescent's skin will heal without complications.

  o The adolescent will experience relief from pruritus.

  o The adolescent will maintain a positive self-image.

  o The adolescent will remain free from infection.

Complications

- Infection and cellulitis

  o Caused by lesions of dermatitis, acne, or breaks in the skin from scratching

  o Nursing Actions

    - Monitor the area for signs of infection.

    - Cleanse the area with mild soap and water.

    - Check for signs of redness, swelling, and pain, which may indicate cellulitis.

    - Check for fever.

  o Client Education

    - Reinforce with adolescents and their families about avoidance of offending agents.

    - Instruct adolescents and their families to keep fingernails trimmed and short.

    - Use antipruritics as prescribed.

    - Reinforce teaching with adolescents and their families about signs and symptoms of cellulitis and to notify the provider if they occur.

Ⓐ APPLICATION EXERCISES

1. An infant is brought to the public health clinic by his mother. The mother shows the nurse the infant's scalp, which is half-covered by crusty, yellow patches. The mother asks, "Is this something he caught from other children at day care?" Which of the following responses by the nurse is appropriate?

   A. "These patches occur when the infant's head is not washed regularly."

   B. "Let's first review how this problem started."

   C. "The patches are due to a scalp infection."

   D. "Yes, he probably came in contact with another child with this at day care."

2. A nurse is talking with a group of adolescents when a question is asked about the cause of acne. Which of the following is the appropriate response by the nurse? (Select all that apply.)

   _____ "One explanation is that acne may be genetic."

   _____ "Products containing lanolin may cause acne outbreaks."

   _____ "Eating too much chocolate is one reason why acne occurs."

   _____ "Acne is due to the presence of a virus on the skin surface."

   _____ "The inflammation of hair follicles by bacteria is one cause of acne."

3. A nurse is reviewing discharge instructions with the mother of a child with contact dermatitis. Which of the following statements by the mother indicates a need for further teaching?

   A. "Calamine lotion reduces the associated itching."

   B. "I can use corticosteroid cream on the skin."

   C. "I should gently scrub the area to remove the crusty areas."

   D. "I need to wash the clothes he wore when the problem occurred with alcohol."

4. A nurse is reviewing ways to prevent diaper dermatitis with a group of new mothers. Which of the following methods should be included in the discussion? (Select all that apply.)

   _____ Use superabsorbent disposable diapers.

   _____ Change diapers when wet and as soon as possible.

   _____ Use perfumed diaper wipes to cleanse the skin.

   _____ Apply a barrier ointment such as zinc oxide in between diaper changes.

   _____ Keep a diaper in place at all times.

5. The oil in plants that is the cause of contact dermatitis is called _____.

6. A common name used for seborrheic dermatitis is _____.

7. A term used to describe allergies of an inherited tendency is _____.

APPLICATION EXERCISES ANSWER KEY

1. An infant is brought to the public health clinic by his mother. The mother shows the nurse the infant's scalp, which is half-covered by crusty, yellow patches. The mother asks, "Is this something he caught from other children at day care?" Which of the following responses by the nurse is appropriate?

   A. "These patches occur when the infant's head is not washed regularly."

   B. "Let's first review how this problem started."

   C. "The patches are due to a scalp infection."

   D. "Yes, he probably came in contact with another child with this at day care."

   An appropriate response by the nurse is to ask the mother how the problem started. The responses about the patches caused by a lack of washing the scalp, an infection, or the infant acquiring it from another child are not appropriate until data has been collected about the mother's concern.

   NCLEX® Connection: Reduction of Risk Potential, Alterations in Body Systems

2. A nurse is talking with a group of adolescents when a question is asked about the cause of acne. Which of the following is the appropriate response by the nurse? (Select all that apply.)

       X   **"One explanation is that acne may be genetic."**

       X   **"Products containing lanolin may cause acne outbreaks."**

       _____ "Eating too much chocolate is one reason why acne occurs."

       _____ "Acne is due to the presence of a virus on the skin surface."

       X   **"The inflammation of hair follicles by bacteria is one cause of acne."**

   Acne is the most common skin condition in adolescence and may be genetic. The use of cosmetics containing ingredients such as lanolin and petroleum may increase acne outbreaks. Inflammation of hair follicles is due to the *P. acnes* bacteria. There is no dietary link with acne but exposure to cooking grease when working in fast food restaurants may be a possible cause. Acne is not due to a virus on the skin surface.

   NCLEX® Connection: Reduction of Risk Potential, Potential for Alterations in Body Systems

3. A nurse is reviewing discharge instructions with the mother of a child with contact dermatitis. Which of the following statements by the mother indicates a need for further teaching?

    A. "Calamine lotion reduces the associated itching."

    B. "I can use corticosteroid cream on the skin."

    C. "I should gently scrub the area to remove the crusty areas."

    D. "I need to wash the clothes he wore when the problem occurred with alcohol."

Calamine lotion and the use of a corticosteroid gel are appropriate in cases of contact dermatitis. Clothing that came in contact with the irritant should be washed in alcohol followed by water. The exposed skin should be rinsed and bathed in a solution of commercial colloid oatmeal. Avoid scrubbing the area.

(N) NCLEX® Connection: Physiological Adaptations, Alterations in Body Systems

4. A nurse is reviewing ways to prevent diaper dermatitis with a group of new mothers. Which of the following methods should be included in the discussion? (Select all that apply.)

    __X__   **Use superabsorbent disposable diapers.**

    __X__   **Change diapers when wet and as soon as possible.**

    _____   Use perfumed diaper wipes to cleanse the skin.

    __X__   **Apply a barrier ointment such as zinc oxide in between diaper changes.**

    _____   Keep a diaper in place at all times.

Prevent diaper dermatitis by using highly absorbent diapers, removing the diaper as soon as possible after urination or a bowel movement, and applying a barrier ointment to the skin in between diaper changes. Use a mild soap and water for cleansing the skin. Avoid the use of bubble bath and perfumed wipes, soaps, or powders. Exposing the diaper area to air can also prevent diaper rash.

(N) NCLEX® Connection: Physiological Adaptations, Alterations in Body Systems

5. The oil in plants that is the cause of contact dermatitis is called **urushiol**.

6. A common name used for seborrheic dermatitis is **cradle cap**.

7. A term used to describe allergies of an inherited tendency is **atopy**.

(N) NCLEX® Connection: Physiological Adaptations, Basic Pathophysiology

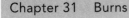

UNIT 2	NURSING CARE OF CHILDREN WITH SYSTEM DISORDERS
Section:	Integumentary Disorders

Chapter 31	Burns

Overview

- Thermal, chemical, electrical, and radioactive agents can cause burns that result in cellular destruction of the skin layers and underlying tissue. The type of burn and the severity of the burn impact the treatment plan.

  o Thermal burns occur when there is exposure to flames, steam, or hot liquids.

  o Chemical burns occur when there is exposure to a caustic agent. Cleaning agents used in the home (drain cleaner, bleach) and agents used in the industrial setting (caustic soda, sulfuric acid) cause chemical burns.

  o Electrical burns occur when an electrical current passes through the body. This type of burn may result in severe damage, including loss of organ function, tissue destruction with the subsequent need for amputation of a limb, and cardiac and/or respiratory arrest.

  o Radiation burns most frequently occur as a result of therapeutic treatment for cancer or from sunburn.

- In addition to destruction of body tissue, a burn injury results in loss of:

  o Temperature regulation

  o Sweat and sebaceous gland function

  o Sensory function

- Metabolism increases to maintain body heat.

- Burns are initially considered clean due to a lack of pathogens. However, they may become contaminated by dirt or unclean water.

 View Media Supplement: Percentage of Burns (Image)

- The severity of the burn is based on the percentage of total body surface area (TBSA). Standardized charts for age groups are used to identify the extent of the injury.

  o Depth of the burn

  o Body location of the burn

- Age of the child
- Causative agent
- Presence of other injuries
- Involvement of the respiratory system
- Overall health of the child

- Burn management occurs in three phases.

  - Emergent (resuscitative phase)
    - Occurs the first 24 to 48 hr after the burn occurs
  - Acute
    - Begins when resuscitation is finished
    - Ends when the wound is covered by tissue
  - Rehabilitative
    - Begins when most of the burn area is healed
    - Ends when reconstructive and corrective procedures are complete (may last for years)

Data Collection

- Risk Factors

  - Lack of supervision
  - Developmental level of children

- Subjective Data

  - To evaluate the extent of damage when observing burns, it is important to know:
    - The type of burning agent (dry heat, moist heat, chemical, electrical, ionizing radiation)
    - The duration of contact
    - The area of the body in which the burn occurred

- Objective Data

  - Physical Assessment Findings

DEPTH	APPEARANCE	SENSATION/HEALING	EXAMPLE
Superficial • Damage to epidermis	• Pink to red in color with no blisters, mild edema, and no eschar	• Painful • It heals within 5 to 10 days • No scarring	• Sunburn

DEPTH	APPEARANCE	SENSATION/HEALING	EXAMPLE
Superficial partial thickness • Damage to the entire epidermis and some parts of the dermis	• Pink to red in color with blisters, mild to moderate edema, and no eschar	• Pain is present. • It heals within 14 days. • No scarring is present.	• Flame or burn scalds
Deep partial thickness • Damage to the entire epidermis and some parts of the dermis	• Red to white in color with no blisters, moderate edema, and soft and dry eschar	• Pain is present and the burn is sensitive to touch. • It heals within 14 to 36 days. • Scarring is likely. • Possible grafting is involved.	• Flame and burn scalds • Grease, tar, or chemical burns • Exposure to hot objects for prolonged time
Full thickness • Damage to the entire epidermis and dermis, and possible damage to the subcutaneous tissue • Nerve damage	• Red to tan, black, brown, or white in color with no blisters, severe edema, and hard and inelastic eschar	• As burn heals, painful sensations return and severity of pain increases. • It heals within weeks to months. • Scarring is present. • Grafting is required.	• Burn scalds • Grease, tar, chemical, or electrical burns
Deep full thickness • Damage to all layers of the skin that extends to muscle, tendons, and bones	• Black in color with no edema and hard and inelastic eschar	• No pain is present. • It heals within weeks to months. • Scarring is present.	• Flame, electrical, grease, tar, and chemical burns

 View Media Supplement: Stages of Burns (Image)

- Inhalation damage findings may include burn injury on the lips and face, singed eyebrows/eyelashes and nasal hairs, soot around the mouth and nose, and edema of the larynx. Clinical manifestations may not be evident for 24 to 48 hr, and are seen as wheezing, hoarseness, and increased respiratory secretions.

- Carbon monoxide inhalation (suspected if the injury took place in an enclosed area) findings include erythema and edema, followed by sloughing of the respiratory tract mucosa.

- Altered level of consciousness, spiking fever, and hypoactive bowel signs may be signs of impending sepsis.

- Irritability, crying, and restlessness

- Hypotension, tachycardia, and decreased cardiac output may occur indicating hypovolemia or shock.

  o Laboratory tests

- Evaluate – CBC, serum electrolytes, BUN, ABGs, fasting blood glucose, random blood glucose, liver enzymes, urinalysis, and clotting studies.

  ▸ WBC – Initially increased and then decreased with left shift

  ▸ Blood glucose – Elevated due to stress response

  ▸ ABGs – Slight hypoxemia, metabolic acidosis

  ▸ Total protein and albumin – Low due to fluid loss

Collaborative Care

- Nursing Care

  o Minor burns

- Stop the burning process.

  □ Remove clothing or jewelry that may conduct heat.

  □ Apply cool water soaks or run cool water over the injury; do not use ice.

  □ Flush chemical burns with large amounts of water.

  □ Cover the burn with a clean cloth to prevent contamination and hypothermia.

  □ Provide warmth.

  □ If necessary, bring the child to a health care facility for medical care.

  □ Provide analgesia.

  □ Cleanse with mild soap and tepid water (Avoid excess friction.).

  □ Use antimicrobial ointment.

  □ Apply dressing (nonadherent, hydrocolloid) if the burn area is irritated by clothing.

  □ Educate families to avoid using greasy lotions or butter on burns.

- ☐ Educate families to monitor for signs of infection.
- ☐ Check immunization status for tetanus and determine the need for immunization.

- ○ Moderate and major burns
  - Maintain airway and ventilation.
  - Provide humidified supplemental oxygen as prescribed.
  - Monitor vital signs.
  - Maintain cardiac output.
    - ☐ Monitor fluid replacement.
      - ▸ Rapid fluid replacement is needed during the emergent phase to maintain tissue perfusion and prevent hypovolemic (burn) shock.
      - ▸ Fluid resuscitation is based on individual child needs (evaluation of urine output, cardiac output, blood pressure, status of electrolytes).
      - ▸ Isotonic crystalloid solutions, such as 0.9% sodium chloride or lactated Ringer's solution, are used during the early stage of burn recovery.
      - ▸ Colloid solutions, such as albumin or synthetic plasma expanders (Hespan), may be used after the first 24 hr of burn recovery.
      - ▸ Maintain urine output of 1 to 2 mL/kg/hr if the child weighs less than 30 kg (66 lb).
      - ▸ Maintain urine output of 30 mL/hr if the child weighs more than 30 kg (66 lb).
      - ▸ Monitor children receiving blood products.
    - ☐ Monitor for manifestations of septic shock.
      - ▸ Alterations in sensorium (confusion)
      - ▸ Increased capillary refill time
      - ▸ Spiking fever
      - ▸ Decreased bowel sounds
      - ▸ Decreased urine output
    - ☐ Notify the provider of findings.
  - Pain management
    - ☐ Establish ongoing monitoring of pain and effectiveness of pain treatment.
  - Monitor children receiving intermittent IV bolus pain medications or IV patient controlled analgesia.
    - ☐ Avoid IM or subcutaneous injections.
    - ☐ Monitor for respiratory depression when using opioid analgesics.

- □ Administer pain medications prior to dressing changes or procedures.

- □ Use nonpharmacologic methods for pain control (guided imagery, music therapy, therapeutic touch) to enhance the effects of analgesic medications and lead to more effective pain management.

- ■ Infection prevention

  - □ Follow standard precautions when performing wound care.

  - □ Restrict plants and flowers due to the risk of contact with pseudomonas.

  - □ Restrict consumption of fresh fruits and vegetables.

  - □ Limit visitors.

  - □ Use reverse isolation if prescribed.

  - □ Monitor for signs and symptoms of infection and report them to the provider.

  - □ Use client-designated equipment, such as blood pressure cuffs and thermometers.

  - □ Administer tetanus toxoid if indicated.

  - □ Administer antibiotics if infection is present.

- ■ Nutritional support

  - □ Encourage increased caloric intake to meet increased metabolic demands and prevent hypoglycemia.

  - □ Encourage increased protein intake to prevent tissue breakdown and promote healing.

  - □ Provide enteral therapy if necessary due to decreased gastrointestinal motility and increased caloric needs.

  - □ Monitor children who are receiving total parenteral nutrition (TPN).

- ■ Restoration of mobility

  - □ Maintain correct body alignment, splint extremities, and facilitate position changes to prevent contractures.

  - □ Maintain active and passive range of motion.

  - □ Assist with ambulation as soon as children are stable.

  - □ Apply pressure dressings to prevent contractures and scarring.

  - □ Closely monitor areas at high risk for pressure sores (heels, sacrum, back of head).

- ■ Psychological support

  - □ Provide developmentally appropriate support for children.

  - □ Assist with coping.

- Medications

  o Topical agents

ANTIMICROBIAL CREM	USES AND ADVANTAGES	DISADVANTAGES
Silver nitrate 0.5%	• Use on wounds that are exposed to air or with modified or occlusive dressings • May affect joint movement • Reduces fluid evaporation • Bacteriostatic against pseudomonas and staphylococcus • Inexpensive	• Does not penetrate eschar • Stains clothing and linen • Discolors the wound, making assessment difficult • Painful upon application
Silver sulfadiazine 1% (Silvadene)	• Use with occlusive dressings • Maintains joint mobility • Effective against gram-negative and gram-positive bacteria	• May cause transient neutropenia • Does not penetrate eschar • Painful to remove from the wound • Decreases granulocyte formation • Contraindicated for children who have allergies to sulfa
Mafenide acetate (Sulfamylon)	• Use on wounds that are exposed to air • Use as a solution for occlusive dressings to keep the dressing moist • Penetrates eschar and goes into underlying tissues • Effective with electrical and infected wounds • Biostatic against gram-positive and gram-negative organisms	• Painful to apply and remove (cream) • May cause metabolic acidosis or hypercapnia • Inhibits wound healing • May cause hypersensitivity
Bacitracin	• Use on wounds that are exposed to air or with modified dressings • Maintains joint mobility • Bacteriostatic against gram-positive organisms • Painless and easy to apply	• Limited effectiveness on gram-negative organisms

- o Morphine sulfate
  - Analgesia
  - Nursing Considerations
    - □ Monitor for respiratory depression.
    - □ Monitor pain relief.
  - Client Education
    - □ Educate children and families on the safety precautions needed with opioid administration.
- o Midazolam (Versed), fentanyl (Sublimaze), propofol (Diprivan), and nitrous oxide
  - Sedation and analgesia
  - Nursing Considerations
    - □ Identify the need for sedation.
    - □ Monitor pain relief.
  - Client Education
    - □ Educate children and families about the safety precautions needed with opioid administration.

- Interdisciplinary Care
  - o Involvement of a dietician, social worker, home health nursing care, psychological counselor, or occupational/physical therapist if indicated.
  - o Respiratory therapy may be necessary to improve pulmonary status.
- Therapeutic Procedures
  - o Wound care
    - Nursing Actions
      - □ Monitor pain and discomfort level.
      - □ Ensure children are premedicated with analgesic and antipruritic agents as prescribed prior to all wound care.
      - □ Remove all previous dressings.
      - □ Observe for odors, drainage, and discharge.
      - □ Cleanse the wound as prescribed, removing all previous ointments (It is important to cleanse the wound thoroughly.).
      - □ Assist with debridement.

- ▸ Mechanical – Use of scissors and forceps to cut away the dead tissue during the hydrotherapy treatment.
- ▸ Hydrotherapy (children placed in a warm tub of water or use of warm running water, as if to shower) to cleanse the wound.
  - ▹ Assist with hydrotherapy by using mild soap or detergent to gently wash burns and then rinsing with room-temperature water. Usually performed once or twice a day for up to 20 min.
    - ◆ Encourage children to exercise their joints during the hydrotherapy treatment.
    - ◆ Ensure that children do not become hypothermic during the treatment.
- ▸ Enzymatic
  - ▹ Apply a topical enzyme to break down and remove dead tissue.
  - ▹ Apply a thin layer of topical antibiotic ointment as prescribed and cover with a dressing using surgical aseptic technique.
- ○ Skin coverings
  - ■ Biologic skin coverings may be used to promote healing of large burns.
    - ☐ Allograft (homograft) – Skin donated by human cadavers that is used for partial and full thickness burn wounds
    - ☐ Xenograft – Obtained from animals, such as pigs, for partial thickness burn wounds
    - ☐ Synthetic skin coverings – Used for partial thickness burn wounds
  - ■ Permanent skin coverings may be the treatment of choice for burns covering large areas of the body.
    - ☐ Autografts
      - ▸ Sheet graft – Sheet of skin used to cover the wound
      - ▸ Mesh graft – Sheet of skin placed in a mesher so skin graft has small slits in it; allows graft to cover larger areas of burn wound
      - ▸ Artificial skin – Synthetic product that is used for partial and full-thickness burn wounds (healing is faster)
      - ▸ Cultured epithelium – Epithelial cells cultured for use when grafting sites are limited
  - ■ Nursing Actions
    - ☐ Maintain immobilization of the graft site.
    - ☐ Elevate the extremity.
    - ☐ Provide wound care to the donor site.

  ☐ Administer pain medication.

  ☐ Monitor for signs of infection before and after skin coverings or grafts are applied.

  ▸ Discoloration of unburned skin surrounding burn wound

  ▸ Green color to subcutaneous fat

  ▸ Degeneration of granulation tissue

  ▸ Development of subeschar hemorrhage

  ▸ Hyperventilation indicating systemic involvement of infection

  ▸ Unstable body temperature

- Client Education

  ☐ Instruct children to keep the extremity elevated.

  ☐ Instruct families to report signs and symptoms of infection.

● Care After Discharge

  ○ Client Education

  - Instruct children to continue to perform range-of-motion exercises and to work with a physical therapist to prevent contractures.

  - Provide instructions about how to observe the wound for infection and how to perform wound care.

  - Reinforce age-appropriate safety measure for the home (covering electrical outlets, supervising children in the bath, keeping irons out of reach of children, teaching the dangers of playing with matches).

  - Instruct families to store matches and lighters out of reach and sight of children.

  - Reinforce to families to avoid sun exposure between 10 a.m. and 4 p.m., wear protective clothing, and apply sunscreen to prevent sunburn.

  - Instruct families to have adequate number and placement of fire extinguishers and smoke alarms in the home and that they should be operable.

  - Instruct families to keep emergency numbers near the phone.

  - Have families develop an exit and meeting plan for fires.

  - Review with children and families that in the event that clothing or skin is on fire, they should "Stop, drop, and roll" to extinguish the fire.

● Client Outcomes

  ○ The child will remain free of complications.

  ○ The child will be able to perform ADLs.

  ○ The family will demonstrate wound care.

Complications

- Airway Injury

    o Thermal injuries to the airway may result from steam or chemical inhalation, aspiration of scalding liquid, and explosion while breathing. If the injury took place in an enclosed space, carbon monoxide poisoning should be suspected.

    o Clinical manifestations may be delayed for 24 to 48 hr.

    o Signs and symptoms include progressive hoarseness, brassy cough, difficulty swallowing, drooling, increased secretions, adventitious breath sounds, and expiratory sounds that include audible wheezes, crowing, and stridor.

    o Nursing Actions

        ■ Maintain airway and ventilation, and provide oxygen as prescribed.

    o Client Education

        ■ Educate children and families about airway management (deep breathing, coughing, elevating the head of the bed).

- Wound Infections

    o Nursing Actions

        ■ Observe for discoloration, edema, odor, and drainage.

        ■ Check for fluctuations in temperature and heart rate.

        ■ Obtain a wound culture.

        ■ Administer antibiotics as prescribed.

        ■ Monitor laboratory results, observing for anemia and infection.

        ■ Maintain surgical aseptic technique with dressing changes.

    o Client Education

        ■ Educate children and families about the importance of infection control.

Ⓐ APPLICATION EXERCISES

Scenario: A nurse is preparing for the admission of two children burned in an accident. The first child is a 10 year old with burns to the lower arms and anterior thorax. The second child is a 13 year old with burns to the anterior and posterior legs.

1. What data should the nurse collect that could indicate the children also experienced inhalation injuries?

2. The children are prescribed a colloid solution to be given as a continuous IV infusion for fluid management. Which of the following solutions should the nurse administer?

    A. Lactated Ringer's

    B. 0.9% sodium chloride

    C. Albumin

    D. 0.45% sodium chloride with 20 mEq potassium chloride

3. Which of the following interventions should the nurse contribute to the plan of care for a child being treated with skin grafts? (Select all that apply.)

    _____ Elevate the involved extremity.

    _____ Apply topical enzymes.

    _____ Provide wound care to the donor site.

    _____ Exercise the joints of the involved extremity.

    _____ Assess for color changes to tissues around the graft site.

4. A nurse is reinforcing teaching to a parent with a child who has a sunburn. The nurse should instruct the parent to apply

    A. butter or margarine.

    B. cool, wet compresses.

    C. an ice pack.

    D. a petroleum-based ointment.

(A) APPLICATION EXERCISES ANSWER KEY

Scenario: A nurse is preparing for the admission of two children burned in an accident. The first child is a 10 year old with burns to the lower arms and anterior thorax. The second child is a 13 year old with burns to the anterior and posterior legs.

1. What data should the nurse collect that could indicate the children also experienced inhalation injuries?

   The nurse should observe for burn injuries to the lips and face, singed nasal hair, soot around the nose and mouth, singed or absent eyebrows and eyelashes, and difficulty speaking. Wheezing, increased respiratory secretions, and hoarseness may not be apparent for 24 to 48 hr post-inhalation injury.

    NCLEX® Connection: Physiological Adaptations, Medical Emergencies

2. The children are prescribed a colloid solution to be given as a continuous IV infusion for fluid management. Which of the following solutions should the nurse administer?

   A. Lactated Ringer's

   B. 0.9% sodium chloride

   C. Albumin

   D. 0.45% sodium chloride with 20 mEq potassium chloride

   A colloid solution, such as albumin, should be used after the first 24 hr of burn recovery. Lactated Ringer's and sodium chloride solutions are isotonic crystalloids. Potassium chloride is a medication added to IV solution.

    NCLEX® Connection: Physiological Adaptations, Fluid and Electrolyte Imbalances

3. Which of the following interventions should the nurse contribute to the plan of care for a child being treated with skin grafts? (Select all that apply.)

__X__	**Elevate the involved extremity.**
_____	Apply topical enzymes.
__X__	**Provide wound care to the donor site.**
_____	Exercise the joints of the involved extremity.
__X__	**Assess for color changes to tissues around the graft site.**

   Elevate the burned extremity to decrease the risk of edema. Treat the donor site now as an open wound. Monitor graft site for signs of infection including color changes to the unburned tissue around the graft site, which may indicate interrupted circulation. Use topical enzymes for debridement of a burn and not on grafts. Immobilize the involved extremity to promote adherence of the grafts.

    NCLEX® Connection: Reduction of Risk Potential, Therapeutic Procedures

4. A nurse is reinforcing teaching to a parent with a child who has a sunburn. The nurse should instruct the parent to apply

    A. butter or margarine.

    B. cool, wet compresses.

    C. an ice pack.

    D. a petroleum-based ointment.

The child has sustained a superficial burn that involves damage only to the epidermis. Cool, wet compresses are appropriate to hydrate the skin. Ice to the injured area reduces circulation. Avoid the application of butter, margarine, or a petroleum-based ointment as they cause heat to be retained and prolong the burn process.

Ⓝ NCLEX® Connection: Reduction of Risk Potential, Therapeutic Procedures

UNIT 2: NURSING CARE OF CHILDREN WITH SYSTEM DISORDERS

Section: Endocrine Disorders

- Diabetes Mellitus

- Growth Hormone Deficiency

NCLEX® CONNECTIONS

When reviewing the chapters in this section, keep in mind the relevant sections of the NCLEX® outline, in particular:

CLIENT NEEDS: PHARMACOLOGICAL THERAPIES

Relevant topics/tasks include:
- Adverse Effects/ Contraindications/Side Effects/Interactions
  - Implement procedures to counteract adverse effects of medications.
- Expected Actions/ Outcomes
  - Reinforce education to client regarding medications.
- Medication Administration
  - Administer a subcutaneous (SQ), intradermal, or intramuscular (IM) medication.

CLIENT NEEDS: REDUCTION OF RISK POTENTIAL

Relevant topics/tasks include:
- Diagnostic Tests
  - Perform diagnostic testing.
- Potential for Complications of Diagnostic Tests/ Treatments/Procedures
  - Suggest change in interventions based on client response to diagnostic tests/ treatments/procedures.
- Therapeutic Procedures
  - Reinforce client teaching on treatments and procedures.

CLIENT NEEDS: PHYSIOLOGICAL ADAPTATION

Relevant topics/tasks include:
- Alterations in Body Systems
  - Identify/intervene to control signs of hypoglycemia or hyperglycemia.
- Basic Pathophysiology
  - Identify signs and symptoms related to acute or chronic illness.
- Fluid and Electrolyte Imbalances
  - Provide interventions to restore client fluid and/or electrolyte balance.

UNIT 2   NURSING CARE OF CHILDREN WITH SYSTEM DISORDERS

Section: Endocrine Disorders

Chapter 32   Diabetes Mellitus

Overview

- Diabetes mellitus is characterized by chronic hyperglycemia due to problems with insulin secretion and/or the effectiveness of endogenous insulin (insulin resistance).

- Diabetes mellitus is a contributing factor for the development of cardiovascular disease, hypertension, renal failure, blindness, and stroke as individuals age.

Data Collection

- Risk Factors

  ○ Genetics can predispose a person to the occurrence of type 1 and type 2 diabetes mellitus.

  ○ Toxins and viruses can predispose an individual to diabetes by destroying the beta cells of the islets of Langerhans in the pancreas, leading to type 1 diabetes mellitus.

  ○ Obesity, physical inactivity, high triglycerides (greater than 250 mg/dL), and hypertension may lead to the development of insulin resistance and type 2 diabetes mellitus.

- Subjective and Objective Data

  ○ Blood glucose alterations

    ▪ Hypoglycemia – Blood glucose level less than 70 mg/dL, rapid onset

AUTONOMIC NERVOUS SYSTEM RESPONSES RAPID ONSET	IMPAIRED CEREBRAL FUNCTION GRADUAL ONSET
• Hunger, lightheadedness, and shakiness • Drowsiness • Anxiety, nervousness, and irritability • Pale, cool skin • Diaphoresis • Normal or shallow respirations • Tachycardia and palpitations	• Strange or unusual feelings • Decreasing level of consciousness • Difficulty in thinking and inability to concentrate • Change in emotional behavior • Slurred speech • Headache and blurred vision • Seizures leading to coma

- ■ Hyperglycemia – Blood glucose levels usually greater than 250 mg/dL, gradual onset
  - ☐ Mental status varies from alertness to stupor
  - ☐ Thirst
  - ☐ Frequent urination
  - ☐ Nausea and vomiting
  - ☐ Skin that is warm, dry, and flushed with poor turgor
  - ☐ Dry mucous membranes
  - ☐ Soft eyeballs
  - ☐ Weakness
  - ☐ Rapid, weak pulse; hypotension
  - ☐ Rapid, deep respirations with acetone/fruity odor due to ketones (Kussmaul respirations)
- ○ Laboratory Tests
  - ■ Diagnostic criteria for diabetes include two of the following findings (on separate days):
    - ☐ Symptoms of diabetes plus a random plasma glucose concentration of greater than 200 mg/dL (without regard to time since last meal)
    - ☐ A fasting blood glucose greater than 126 mg/dL
    - ☐ A 2-hr glucose of greater than 200 mg/dL with an oral glucose tolerance test
  - ■ Fasting blood glucose
    - ☐ Nursing Actions
      - ▸ Postpone administration of antidiabetic medication until after the level is drawn.
    - ☐ Client Education
      - ▸ Ensure that children have fasted (no food or drink other than water) for 8 hr prior to the blood draw. Antidiabetic medications should be postponed until after the level is drawn.
  - ■ Oral glucose tolerance test
    - ☐ Obtain a blood sample to determine a fasting blood glucose level at the start of the test.
    - ☐ Instruct children to consume a specified amount of glucose.
    - ☐ Obtain a blood sample for blood glucose levels every 30 min for 2 hr.

- □ Monitor children for hypoglycemia throughout the procedure.

- □ Client Education

    ▸ Instruct children to consume a balanced diet for the 3 days prior to the test. Then instruct children to fast for the 8 to 10 hr prior to the test.

- ■ Glycosylated hemoglobin (HbA1c)

    - □ The expected reference range is 4% to 6%, but an acceptable target for children who have diabetes may be 6.5% to 8%, with a total target goal of less than 7%.

- ○ Diagnostic Procedures

    - ■ Self-monitored blood glucose (SMBG)

        - □ Nursing Actions

        - □ Follow or ensure that children and families follow the proper procedure for blood sample collection and use of a glucose meter. Supplemental short-acting insulin may be prescribed for elevated pre-meal glucose levels.

        - □ Client Education

            ▸ Instruct children and families to check the accuracy of the strips with the control solution provided.

            ▸ Advise children and families to keep a record of the SMBG that includes time, date, serum glucose level, insulin dose, food intake, and other events that may alter glucose metabolism, such as activity level or illness.

Collaborative Care

- • Nursing Care

    - ○ Monitor the following:

        - ■ Blood glucose levels and factors affecting levels (other medications)

        - ■ I&O and weight

        - ■ Skin integrity and healing status of any wounds, paying close attention to the feet and folds of the skin

        - ■ Sensory alterations (tingling, numbness)

        - ■ Visual alterations

        - ■ Presence of recurrent infections

        - ■ Dietary practices

        - ■ Exercise patterns

        - ■ The child's proficiency at self-monitoring blood glucose

        - ■ The child's proficiency at self-administering medication

- ○ Follow agency policy for nail care. Some protocols allow for trimming toenails straight across with clippers and filing edges with a nail file. If clippers or scissors are contraindicated, children should file the nails straight across.

- ○ Reinforce proper foot care.

  - ■ Inspect feet daily, using a mirror to check the bottom of the feet as needed.

  - ■ Wash feet daily with mild soap and warm water.

  - ■ Pat feet dry gently, especially between the toes.

  - ■ Use mild foot powder (powder with cornstarch) on sweaty feet.

  - ■ Do not use commercial remedies for the removal of calluses or corns.

  - ■ Perform nail care after a bath/shower if possible.

  - ■ Separate overlapping toes with cotton or lambs' wool.

  - ■ Avoid open-toe, open-heel shoes. Leather shoes are preferred to plastic ones. Wear slippers with soles. Do not go barefoot. Shake out shoes before putting them on.

  - ■ Wear clean, absorbent socks or stockings that are made of cotton or wool and have not been mended.

  - ■ Do not use hot water bottles or heating pads to warm feet. Wear socks for warmth.

  - ■ Avoid prolonged sitting, standing, and crossing of legs.

- ○ Instruct children and families to cleanse cuts with warm water and mild soap, gently dry, and apply a dry dressing. Instruct the child and parents to monitor healing and to seek intervention promptly.

- ○ Provide nutritional guidelines.

  - ■ Plan meals to achieve appropriate timing of food intake, activity, onset, and peak of insulin. Calories and food composition should be similar each day.

  - ■ Eat at regular intervals and do not skip meals.

  - ■ Count grams of carbohydrates consumed.

  - ■ Recognize that 15 g of carbohydrates are equal to 1 carbohydrate exchange.

  - ■ Restrict calories and increase physical activity as appropriate to facilitate weight loss (for children who are obese or to prevent obesity).

  - ■ Include fiber in the diet to increase carbohydrate metabolism and to help control cholesterol levels.

  - ■ Avoid concentrated sweets.

  - ■ Use artificial sweeteners.

  - ■ Keep fat content below 30% of the total caloric intake.

○ Instruct children and families in appropriate techniques for SBGM, including obtaining blood samples, recording and responding to results, and correctly handling supplies and equipment.

○ Instruct children and their families in guidelines to follow when sick.

- Monitor blood glucose levels every 3 to 4 hr.

- Continue to take insulin or oral antidiabetic agents.

- Consume 4 oz of sugar-free, non-caffeinated liquid every 0.5 hr to prevent dehydration.

- Meet carbohydrate needs by eating soft foods if possible. If not, consume liquids that are equal to the usual carbohydrate content.

- Test urine for ketones and report if abnormal (should be negative to small).

- Rest.

- Call the provider if:

  □ Blood glucose is higher than 240 mg/dL.

  □ Fever higher than 38.9° C (102° F), fever does not respond to acetaminophen (Tylenol), or fever lasts more than 12 hr.

  □ Disorientation or confusion occurs.

  □ Rapid breathing is experienced.

  □ Vomiting occurs more than once.

  □ Diarrhea occurs more than five times or for longer than 24 hr.

  □ Liquids cannot be tolerated.

  □ Illness lasts longer than 2 days.

○ Instruct children and their families what to do if they experience signs and symptoms of hypoglycemia (shakiness, diaphoresis, anxiety, nervousness, irritability, pallor, palpitations, drowsiness, headache, dizziness, confusion).

- Check blood glucose levels.

- Follow guidelines outlined by the provider/diabetes educator. Guidelines may include:

  □ Treat with 15 to 20 g carbohydrates.

  □ Recheck blood glucose in 15 min.

  □ If still low (less than 70 mg/dL), give 15 to 20 g more of carbohydrates.

    ▸ Examples – 4 oz orange juice, 2 oz grape juice, 8 oz milk, glucose tablets per manufacturer's suggestion to equal 15 g

□ Recheck blood glucose in 15 min.

□ If blood glucose is within normal limits, take 7 g protein (if the next meal is more than an hour away).

▸ Examples – 1 oz of cheese (1 string cheese), 2 tablespoons of peanut butter, or 8 oz of milk

■ Instruct family members to administer glucagon SC or IM if the child is unconscious or unable to swallow and to notify the provider. Administer liquid with glucose as soon as tolerated. Watch for vomiting and take precaution against aspiration.

o Instruct children and their families regarding signs and symptoms of hyperglycemia (hot, dry skin, fruity breath) and measures to take in response to hyperglycemia.

■ Encourage oral fluid intake.

■ Administer insulin as prescribed.

■ Restrict exercise when blood glucose levels are greater than 240 mg/dL or until blood glucose is controlled.

■ Test urine for ketones and report if findings are abnormal.

■ Consult the provider if symptoms progress.

o Encourage children to wear a medical identification wristband.

• Medications

o Most children are on an insulin regimen that frequently consists of more than one type of insulin (rapid, short, intermediate, long acting). Insulin given in this manner is administered one or more times per day and is based on a child's blood glucose level.

o Some children are given an insulin pump, which is a small pump that is worn externally, contains insulin, and delivers insulin as programmed via a needle inserted into the subcutaneous tissue. The catheter should be changed at least every 3 days.

o The rate of onset, peak, and duration of action varies for each different type of insulin.

TYPE	TRADE NAME	ONSET	PEAK	DURATION
Rapid acting	Insulin lispro (Humalog)	Less than 15 min	0.5 to 1 hr	3 to 4 hr
Short acting	Regular insulin (Humulin R)	0.5 to 1 hr	2 to 3 hr	5 to 7 hr
Intermediate acting	NPH insulin (Humulin N)	1 to 2 hr	4 to 12 hr	18 to 24 hr
Long acting	Insulin glargine (Lantus)	1 hr	none	10.4 to 24 hr

■ Nursing Considerations

□ Observe children performing self-administration of insulin and offer additional instruction as indicated.

- Client Education
  - Provide information regarding self-administration of insulin.
    - ‣ Rotate injection sites (prevent lipohypertrophy) within one anatomic site (prevent day-to-day changes in absorption rates).
    - ‣ Inject at a 90° angle (45° angle if thin). Aspiration for blood is not necessary.
    - ‣ When mixing a rapid- or short-acting insulin with a longer-acting insulin, draw up the shorter-acting insulin into the syringe first and then the longer-acting insulin (this reduces the risk of introducing the longer-acting insulin into the vial of the shorter-acting insulin).
    - ‣ Do not mix insulin glargine (Lantus) with other insulins due to incompatibility.

- Interdisciplinary Care
  - Diabetes educator should be involved to provide comprehensive education in diabetes management.

- Client Outcomes
  - The child will have blood glucose levels within an acceptable range.
  - The child will be able to self-administer insulin.
  - The child will be able to monitor for complications and intervene as necessary.
  - The child will maintain adequate dietary intake to support growth and development.

Complications

- Diabetic ketoacidosis (DKA)
  - DKA is an acute, life-threatening condition characterized by hyperglycemia (greater than 300 mg/dL), resulting in the breakdown of body fat for energy and an accumulation of ketones in the blood and urine. The onset is rapid, and the mortality rate is high.
  - Causes of DKA include insufficient insulin (usually failure to take the appropriate dose), acute stress (as from trauma or surgery), and poor management of acute illness.
  - Nursing Actions
    - Collect subjective and objective data for a blood glucose level greater than 300 mg/dL.
      - Reports of nausea, vomiting, and/or abdominal pain (DKA/metabolic acidosis)
      - Reports of frequent urination, thirst, and hunger
      - Reports of confusion
      - Change in mental status

           □ Signs of dehydration (dry mucous membranes, weight loss, sunken eyeballs resulting from fluid loss such as polyuria)

           □ Kussmaul respiration pattern, rapid and deep respirations, fruity scent to the breath (DKA/metabolic acidosis)

      ■ Assist with the emergency management

           □ Children should receive rapid isotonic fluid (0.9% sodium chloride) replacement to maintain perfusion to vital organs. Often large quantities are required to replace losses and should be done cautiously. Monitor children for evidence of fluid volume excess.

           □ Children should then receive a hypotonic fluid (0.45% sodium chloride) to continue replacing losses to total body fluid.

           □ When serum glucose levels approach 250 mg/dL, add glucose to IV fluids to minimize the risk of cerebral edema associated with drastic changes in serum osmolality.

           □ Children should receive regular insulin 0.1 unit/kg as an IV bolus dose and then start on a continuous intravenous infusion of regular insulin at 0.1 unit/kg/hr.

      ■ Monitor glucose levels hourly.

      ■ Monitor serum potassium levels. Potassium levels will initially be elevated. With insulin therapy, potassium will shift into cells and children should be monitored for hypokalemia. Provide potassium replacement therapy in all replacement IV fluids as indicated by lab values. Make sure urinary output is adequate before administering potassium.

   ○ Client Education

      ■ Reinforce instructions to manage blood glucose levels.

- Hypoglycemia

   ○ Decreased level of consciousness

   ○ Nursing Actions

      ■ Follow facility protocol for hypoglycemia.

      ■ Administer glucagon as prescribed.

      ■ Monitor unresponsive children.

      ■ Follow with a planned meal or snack when child is awake or add a snack of 10% of daily calories as tolerated.

      ■ Monitor blood glucose levels every hour.

Ⓐ APPLICATION EXERCISES

1. A nurse is reinforcing teaching about foot care with a group of mothers and school-age children who have diabetes. Which of the following points should the nurse include in the teaching? (Select all that apply.)

   _____ Wear shoes with open heels.

   _____ Remove sand or other debris from shoes before putting them on.

   _____ Wear thin, white, polyester socks.

   _____ Wear leather footwear.

   _____ Apply a cornstarch-based powder to sweaty feet.

2. Glycosylated hemoglobin is also known as _____.

3. The target range for glycosylated hemoglobin for children who have diabetes is _____ with a total target goal of less than _____.

4. Which of the following should the nurse include when identifying causes of a hypoglycemic reaction? (Select all that apply.)

   _____ Urinary tract infection

   _____ Skipping breakfast

   _____ Exercising strenuously

   _____ Taking an extra dose of insulin

   _____ Stress

5. Which of the following should the nurse include when instructing adolescents who have diabetes about signs and symptoms related to hyperglycemia? (Select all that apply.)

   _____ Palpitations

   _____ Elevated blood pressure

   _____ Hunger

   _____ Kussmaul respirations

   _____ Warm, dry skin

6. Describe the diagnostic criteria for diabetes.

APPLICATION EXERCISES ANSWER KEY

1. A nurse is reinforcing teaching about foot care with a group of mothers and school-age children who have diabetes. Which of the following points should the nurse include in the teaching? (Select all that apply.)

            Wear shoes with open heels.

     X   **Remove sand or other debris from shoes before putting them on.**

            Wear thin, white, polyester socks.

     X   **Wear leather footwear.**

     X   **Apply a cornstarch-based powder to sweaty feet.**

   Proper foot care includes removing any debris from shoes before putting them on, wearing leather rather than plastic shoes, using a cornstarch-based powder on sweaty feet, avoiding open-toe and open-heel shoes, and wearing clean, absorbent cotton or wool socks or stockings that have not been mended. Avoid polyester socks.

 NCLEX® Connection: Physiological Adaptations, Alterations in Body Systems

2. Glycosylated hemoglobin is also known as **HbA1c.**

3. The target range for glycosylated hemoglobin for children who have diabetes is **6.5% to 8%** with a total target goal of less than **7%.**

 NCLEX® Connection: Reduction of Risk Potential, Laboratory Values

4. Which of the following should the nurse include when identifying causes of a hypoglycemic reaction? (Select all that apply.)

            Urinary tract infection

     X   **Skipping breakfast**

     X   **Exercising strenuously**

     X   **Taking an extra dose of insulin**

            Stress

   Skipping a meal (especially if usual insulin dose is taken), exercising strenuously, and taking an extra dose of insulin may cause hypoglycemia. Infections and stress may cause hyperglycemia.

NCLEX® Connection: Physiological Adaptations, Alterations in Body Systems

5. Which of the following should the nurse include when instructing adolescents who have diabetes about signs and symptoms related to hyperglycemia? (Select all that apply.)

    _____   Palpitations

    _____   Elevated blood pressure

    __X__   **Hunger**

    __X__   **Kussmaul respirations**

    __X__   **Warm, dry skin**

    Signs and symptoms of hyperglycemia include hunger, Kussmaul respirations (rapid and deep with acetone/fruity odor due to ketones), warm, dry skin that is flushed with poor turgor, thirst, frequent urination, soft eyeballs, weakness, malaise, and hypotension. Palpitations are more likely to occur with hypoglycemia.

    (N) **NCLEX® Connection: Physiological Adaptations, Alterations in Body Systems**

6. Describe the diagnostic criteria for diabetes.

    Two of the following findings (on separate days):

    A. Symptoms of diabetes plus a random plasma glucose of greater than 200 mg/dL without regard to time since the last meal.

    B. A fasting blood glucose greater than 126 mg/dL

    C. A 2 hr glucose of greater than 200 mg/dL with an oral glucose tolerance test.

    (N) **NCLEX® Connection: Reduction of Risk Potential, Laboratory Values**

UNIT 2	NURSING CARE OF CHILDREN WITH SYSTEM DISORDERS
Section:	Endocrine Disorders
Chapter 33	**Growth Hormone Deficiency**

 Overview

- Human growth hormone (GH), somatotropin, is a naturally occurring substance that is secreted by the pituitary gland.

- GH is important for normal growth, development, and cellular metabolism.

- A deficiency in GH prevents somatic growth throughout the body.

- Other hormones that work with GH to control metabolic processes include adrenocorticotropic hormone (ACTH), thyroid stimulating hormone (TSH), and the gonadotropins (follicle-stimulating hormone [FSH] and luteinizing hormone [LH]).

- Hypopituitarism is the diminished or deficient secretion of pituitary hormones (primarily GH). Consequences of the condition depend on the degree of the deficiency.

Data Collection

- Risk Factors

  o Structural factors (tumors, trauma, structural defects, surgery)

  o Heredity disorders

  o Other pituitary hormone deficiencies (deficiencies of TSH or ACTH)

  o Most often, GH deficiencies are idiopathic.

- Subjective Data

  o Reports of lack of activity

- Objective Data

  o Physical Assessment Findings

    ▪ Short stature with growth during the first year within expected percentile ranges

      □ A decrease in percentiles usually starts by the second year and may be as low as the fifth percentile.

      □ Height is usually more delayed than weight, which appears appropriate.

- Normal skeletal proportions
- Delayed eruption of permanent teeth
- Underdeveloped jaw resulting in overcrowding of teeth

○ Laboratory Tests

- Plasma insulin-like growth factor-1 (IGF-1) and IGF binding protein-3 (IGFBP-3) levels
  - □ Further evaluation is indicated if the values are 1 standard deviation below the mean for age and gender.
- Blood studies to determine hypothyroidism, hypoadrenalism, and hypoaldosteronism
- Radioimmunoassays to determine GH levels

○ Nursing Actions

- Collect the appropriate amount of blood for the test.
- Explain the laboratory procedure to children and their families.

○ Client Education

- Children should fast the night before the test.

○ Diagnostic Procedures

- GH stimulation
  - □ GH stimulation testing is generally done for children who have a low level of IGF-1 and IGFBP-3 and poor growth.
  - □ GH secretion is stimulated by administering glucose or having the child exercise. Blood samples are then taken at set time intervals to measure the release of GH.
- Radiologic assessments
  - □ Measure the child's skeletal maturity by comparing epiphyseal centers on an x-ray to age-appropriate published standards.
  - □ Perform a general skeletal survey in children under 3 years of age, or survey the hands and wrists in older children. This will provide information about growth as well as epiphyseal function.
  - □ Nursing Actions
    - ▸ Assist in positioning the child.
- CT and MRI scans and skull x-rays
  - □ Use to identify tumors or other structural defects
  - □ Nursing Actions
    - ▸ Monitor children during the procedure.
    - ▸ Assist with sedation of children, if prescribed.

- □ Client Education
  - ‣ Provide emotional support.
- ■ Evaluation of the growth curve
  - □ Nursing Actions
    - ‣ Accurately obtain and plot height and weight measurements.
    - ‣ Determine height velocity or height over time.
    - ‣ Determine height-to-weight relationship.
    - ‣ Project target height in context of genetic potential.

Collaborative Care

- ● Nursing Care
  - ○ Measure the child's height and weight and mark on a growth chart at every visit to the provider.
    - ■ The height of a child is more affected than weight. Bone age usually matches height age.
    - ■ Measure children who are younger than 3 years of age at least every 6 months and children older than 3 years of age every year.
  - ○ Monitor effectiveness of GH replacement. GH is supplied by recombinant DNA technology.
  - ○ Administer other hormone replacements (thyroid hormone) if prescribed.
  - ○ Provide support to children and their families regarding psychosocial concerns (altered body image, depression). Reassure children and their families that there are no cognitive delays or deficits.
  - ○ Stress the importance of maintaining realistic expectations based on the child's age and abilities.
- ● Medications
  - ○ Somatropin
    - ■ Use as a human growth hormone that is a replacement for deficiency in growth hormones
    - ■ Nursing Considerations
      - □ Administer the medication via subcutaneous injections.
      - □ Use cautiously in children who are receiving insulin.
- ● Interdisciplinary Care
  - ○ An endocrinologist coordinates care and treatment.
  - ○ Psychological counseling may be needed to help children and their families cope during this period of time.

- Care After Discharge

  - Nursing Actions

    - Inform children and their families that there should not be any significant side effects when GH replacement therapy is used in appropriate doses for GH deficiency.

    - Inform children and their families that GH will assist with muscle growth and help improve self-esteem.

  - Client Education

    - Instruct children and their families how to administer medication by subcutaneous injection for home use.

    - Instruct children and their families that GH should be administered 6 to 7 days a week.

    - Inform children and their families that GH is usually continued until bone maturation takes place. This may be 16 years of age or older for boys and 14 years of age or older for girls.

    - Encourage children and their families to seek evaluation during early adulthood. Children with GH deficiency in childhood should be evaluated in early adulthood to determine the need for continued replacement therapy.

- Client Outcomes

  - The child will show improvement in growth patterns.

  - The child will show improvement in self-esteem.

Complications

- GH deficiency without hormone replacement may result in disruption of vertical growth, delayed epiphyseal closure, retarded bone age, delayed sexual development, and premature aging later in life.

Ⓐ APPLICATION EXERCISES

1. Match the following diagnostic tests with their findings related to growth disorders.

    _____ X-rays of wrist and hand   1. Determines GH level

    _____ IGF-1   2. Identifies pituitary gland tumor

    _____ MRI   3. Determines bone age

    _____ GH stimulation/suppression test   4. Measures effect of glucose on GH

2. A nurse is reviewing the care plan of a 4-year-old child who has a growth hormone deficiency. Which of the following actions should the nurse plan to take? (Select all that apply.)

    _____ Administer other hormone replacements as prescribed.

    _____ Measure height and weight every 6 months.

    _____ Plot the height and weight at each visit to the provider.

    _____ Encourage parents to be realistic in their expectations.

    _____ Discuss the issue of cognitive delays that may begin to appear.

(A) APPLICATION EXERCISES ANSWER KEY

1. Match the following diagnostic tests with their findings related to growth disorders.

   3   X-rays of wrist and hand   1. Determines GH level

   1   IGF-1   2. Identifies pituitary gland tumor

   2   MRI   3. Determines bone age

   4   GH stimulation/suppression test   4. Measures effect of glucose on GH

(N) NCLEX® Connection: Reduction of Risk Potential, Diagnostic Tests

2. A nurse is reviewing the care plan of a 4-year-old child who has a growth hormone deficiency. Which of the following actions should the nurse plan to take? (Select all that apply.)

   X   **Administer other hormone replacements as prescribed.**

   _____   Measure height and weight every 6 months.

   X   **Plot the height and weight at each visit to the provider.**

   X   **Encourage parents to be realistic in their expectations.**

   _____   Discuss the issue of cognitive delays that may begin to appear.

   Nursing actions to be taken with a 4-year-old child who has growth hormone deficiency include administering hormone replacements (thyroid) as prescribed, plotting height and weight on a growth chart at each visit, and encouraging parents to be realistic. After age 3, measure height and weight on a yearly basis, not every 6 months. Cognitive delays and deficits are not related to growth hormone deficiency.

(N) NCLEX® Connection: Physiological Adaptations, Alterations in Body Systems

UNIT 2: NURSING CARE OF CHILDREN WITH SYSTEM DISORDERS

Section: Immune and Infectious Disorders

- Immunizations

- Communicable Diseases

- Acute Otitis Media

- HIV/AIDS

NCLEX® CONNECTIONS

When reviewing the chapters in this section, keep in mind the relevant sections of the NCLEX® outline, in particular:

CLIENT NEEDS: SAFETY AND INFECTION CONTROL	**CLIENT NEEDS: HEALTH PROMOTION & MAINTENANCE**	**CLIENT NEEDS: PHYSIOLOGICAL ADAPTATION**
Relevant topics/tasks include:	Relevant topics/tasks include:	Relevant topics/tasks include:
• Standard Precautions/ Transmission-Based Precautions/Surgical Asepsis ○ Use standard/universal precautions.	• Aging Process ○ Provide care that meets the special needs of adolescents aged 13 to 18 years. * • Developmental Stages and Transitions ○ Modify approaches to care in accordance with client development stage. • Health Promotion/Disease Prevention ○ Identify precautions and contraindications to immunizations.	• Alterations in Body Systems ○ Intervene to improve client respiratory status. • Pathophysiology ○ Apply knowledge of pathophysiology to monitoring client for alterations in body systems. • Unexpected Response to Therapies ○ Document client unexpected response to therapy.

UNIT 2	NURSING CARE OF CHILDREN WITH SYSTEM DISORDERS
Section:	Immune and Infectious Disorders
Chapter 34	Immunizations

Overview

- Administration of a vaccine causes production of antibodies that prevents illness from a specific microbe.

- Active immunity is long-term and occurs over time as the body produces antibodies in response to an infection or to an immunization and becomes immune as a result of the primary immune response.

- Passive natural immunity occurs when antibodies are passed from the mother to the newborn/infant through the placenta and breastfeeding. Passive artificial immunity is temporary, and occurs after antibodies, in the form of immune globulins, are administered to an individual who requires immediate protection against a disease after exposure has occurred.

- Most immunizations consist of killed or live viruses that are attenuated or weakened.

MEDICATION CLASSIFICATION: VACCINATIONS

- 2011 Centers for Disease Control and Prevention (CDC) immunization recommendations for healthy children (To see a listing of vaccinations by age and updates, go to the Web site of the Centers for Disease Control and Prevention [http://www.cdc.gov] for updates).

  - Diphtheria and tetanus toxoids and acellular pertussis vaccine (DTaP) – Doses at 2, 4, 6, and 15 to 18 months and again at 4 to 6 years of age

  - Tetanus and diphtheria toxoids and pertussis vaccine (DTaP) – One dose at 11 to 12 years of age

  - Tetanus and diphtheria (Td) booster – One dose every 10 years following DTaP

  - *Haemophilus influenza* type b (Hib) – Doses at 2, 4, 6, and at 12 to 15 months

  - Rotavirus (RV) oral vaccine – Available in two formulations

    - RotaTeq requires three doses beginning at 6 weeks of age, with subsequent doses 4 to 10 weeks apart. RotaTeq vaccination should be completed before 32 weeks of age. Vaccination should not be initiated for infants 15 weeks of age or older.

    - Rotarix requires 2 doses beginning at 6 weeks of age with the next dose 4 weeks later. All doses should be completed by 8 months of age.

- Inactivated poliovirus vaccine (IPV) – Doses at 2, 4, and 6 to 18 months and again at 4 to 6 years

- Measles, mumps, and rubella vaccine (MMR) – Doses at 12 to 15 months and at 4 to 6 years

- Varicella vaccine – One dose at 12 to 15 months and again at 4 to 6 years or 2 doses administered 4 weeks apart if administered after age 13

- Pneumococcal conjugate vaccine (PCV) – Doses at 2, 4, 6, and 12 to 15 months

- Hepatitis A (Hep A) – Two doses 6 months apart after 12 months of age

- Hepatitis B (Hep B) – Within 12 hr after birth with additional doses at 1 to 2 months and 6 to 18 months of age

- Seasonal influenza vaccine – Annually beginning at 6 months, the trivalent inactivated influenza vaccine (TIV) should be given. Starting at 2 years of age, the live attenuated influenza vaccine (LAIV) (nasal spray) should be used. October through November is the ideal time, but December is acceptable.

- Meningococcal vaccine (MCV4) – One dose at 11 to 12 years of age (earlier if specific risk factors are present)

- Human Papilloma Virus (HPV2, HPV4) – Three doses should be given over a 6-month interval for females at 11 to 12 years of age (minimum age is 9 years). The second dose should be administered 2 months after the first dose, and the third dose should be administered 6 months after the first dose. HPV4 may be given to males starting at age 9 years of age.

Purpose

- Expected Pharmacological Action

  - Immunizations produce antibodies that provide active immunity. Immunizations may take months to have an effect, but they provide long-lasting protection against infectious diseases.

- Therapeutic Uses

  - Eradication of infectious diseases (polio, smallpox)

  - Prevention of childhood and adult infectious diseases and their complications (measles, diphtheria, mumps, rubella, tetanus, *H. influenza*)

Ⓢ Complications/Contraindications/Precautions

- An anaphylactic reaction to a vaccine is a contraindication for receiving further doses of that vaccine.

- An anaphylactic reaction to a vaccine is a contraindication for using other vaccines containing that substance.

- Contraindications to all immunizations include severe allergies to any component of a vaccine.

- Moderate or severe illnesses with or without fever are contraindications to receiving immunizations. With acute febrile illness, vaccination is deferred until symptoms resolve. The common cold and other minor illnesses are not contraindications.

- Contraindications to vaccinations require health care providers to analyze data and weigh the risks that come with vaccinating or not vaccinating.

- Immunocompromised individuals are defined by the Centers for Disease Control and Prevention (CDC) as those with hematologic or solid tumors, congenital immunodeficiency, or long-term immunosuppressive therapy, including corticosteroids.

IMMUNIZATION	SIDE EFFECTS	CONTRAINDICATIONS/PRECAUTIONS
DTaP	• Local reaction at the injection site • Fever and irritability • Crying that cannot be consoled and lasts up to 3 hr • Seizures • Rare – Acute encephalopathy	• An occurrence of encephalopathy 7 days after the administration of the immunization • An occurrence of seizures within 3 days of the immunization • A history of uncontrollable, inconsolable crying lasting more than 3 hr or temperature of 40.5° C (105° F) or higher occurring within 48 hr of vaccination
Hib	• Mild local reactions and a low grade fever • Rare – Fever (temperature greater than 38.5° C [101.3° F]), vomiting, and crying	• Children less than 6 weeks of age
RV	• Diarrhea, vomiting, and possibly ear infection	• Diarrhea and vomiting (in infants) • Use caution with infants who are immunocompromised (with HIV infection or from medication administration).
IPV	• Local reaction at injection site • Possible allergic reaction in children allergic to streptomycin, neomycin, or bacitracin (These medications are contained in the vaccine in small amounts.) • Rare – Vaccine-associated paralytic poliomyelitis	• Allergy to neomycin, streptomycin, and polymyxin B • Pregnancy

IMMUNIZATION	SIDE EFFECTS	CONTRAINDICATIONS/PRECAUTIONS
MMR	• Local reactions (rash; fever; swollen glands in cheeks, in the neck, and under the jaw) • Possibility of joint pain lasting for days to weeks • Risk for anaphylaxis and thrombocytopenia	• Pregnancy • Allergy to gelatin and neomycin • History of thrombocytopenia or thrombocytopenic purpura • Immunosuppression (with HIV infection or from medication administration) • Recent transfusion with blood products or immunoglobulins
Varicella vaccine	• Varicella-like rash that is local or generalized (vesicles on the body)	• Pregnancy • Cancers of blood and lymphatic system • Allergy to gelatin and neomycin • Immunosuppression (with HIV or from medication administration) • Children receiving corticosteroids
PCV	• Mild local reactions, fever, and no serious adverse effects	• Pregnancy

Hep A and Hep B	• Local reaction at the injection site and mild fever
	• Anaphylaxis
		• Hep A
		  o Pregnancy (may be a contraindication)
		• Hep B
		  o Allergy to baker's yeast

Seasonal influenza vaccine	• TIV – Mild local reaction and fever
	• LAIV – Headache, cough, and fever
	• Rare – Risk for Guillain-Barré syndrome (ascending paralysis, weakness of lower extremities, difficulty breathing)
		• Hypersensitivity to eggs
		• LAIV
		  o Fewer than 2 years
		  o Immunosuppression
		  o Chronic disease

Meningococcal conjugate vaccine (MCV4)	• Mild local reaction • Rare – Risk for allergic response	• History of Guillain-Barré syndrome
HPV2 and HPV4	• Mild local reaction and fever • Fainting (shortly after receiving the vaccination) • Rare – Risk for Guillain-Barré syndrome	• Pregnancy • Hypersensitivity to yeast

Nursing Administration

- Infants and Children

  - Obtain parental consent for children.

  - Note the date, route, and site of vaccination on the child's immunization record at the time of immunization.

  - Give intramuscular vaccinations in the vastus lateralis or ventrogluteal muscle in infants and young children, and into the deltoid muscle for older children and adolescents.

  - Give subcutaneous injections in the outer aspect of the upper arm or anterolateral thigh.

  - Use an appropriately sized needle for the route, site, age, and amount of medication.

  - Use strategies to minimize discomfort.

  - Provide for distraction.

  - Do not allow children to delay the procedure.

  - Encourage the parents to use comforting measures during the procedure (cuddling, pacifiers) and after the procedure (application of cool compresses to injection site, gentle movement of the involved extremity).

  - Provide praise afterward.

  - Apply a colorful bandage, if appropriate.

  - Have emergency medications and equipment on standby in case the child experiences an allergic response, such as anaphylaxis (rare).

  - Follow storage and reconstitution directions. If reconstituted, use within 30 min.

  - Provide written vaccine information sheets and review the content with parents or clients.

  - Instruct the parents and child to observe for complications and to notify the provider if side effects occur.

  - Encourage the parents to maintain up-to-date immunizations for the child.

  - Document the administration of the vaccine, including the date, route, and site of vaccination; type, manufacturer, lot number, and expiration date of the vaccine; and name, address, and signature of the child and/or parent.

  - Instruct the parents to avoid administering aspirin to the child to treat fever or local reaction, due to the risk of the development of Reye syndrome

  - Instruct the parents to premedicate infants and children with nonopioid analgesics/antipyretics prior to immunizations and for the following 24 hr. Use acetaminophen for infants 2 to 6 months of age. Ibuprofen may be administered starting at 6 months of age.

  - Instruct the parents to apply a topical anesthetic prior to the injection.

Nursing Evaluation of Medication Effectiveness

- Depending on therapeutic intent, effectiveness may be evidenced by:

  o Improvement of local reaction to vaccination with absence of pain, fever, and swelling at the site of injection

  o Development of immunity

Ⓐ APPLICATION EXERCISES

Scenario: The parents of a 4-year-old have arrived at the clinic for their daughter's pre-kindergarten physical exam and immunizations. The family recently moved to the area and has a copy of the child's immunization record from the previous health care provider.

1. Prior to giving an immunization, what data should the nurse collect about the child?

2. The child is to receive an intramuscular injection. Which of the following injection sites should the nurse select?

   A. Deltoid region

   B. Outer aspect of the upper arm

   C. Ventrogluteal site

   D. Anterolateral thigh

3. Which of the following actions should the nurse take to administer the immunization? (Select all that apply.)

   _____ Obtain parental consent for the immunization.

   _____ Document the date, route, and site of the injection on the child's immunization record.

   _____ Use a reconstituted vial of vaccine that was prepared 6 hr ago.

   _____ Apply a warm compress to the injection site immediately after the immunization.

   _____ Remind parents to give acetaminophen or ibuprofen as needed for the next 24 hr.

4. A nurse is providing information to a group of parents regarding immunizations. Which of the following actions should the nurse suggest parents take prior to bringing their children to the clinic for the next immunization? (Select all that apply.)

   _____ Premedicate the child with ibuprofen or acetaminophen.

   _____ Withhold food for 4 hr prior to the vaccination.

   _____ Bring comfort items, such as pacifiers, favorite toys, or blankets.

   _____ Apply a topical anesthetic to the injection site.

   _____ Avoid giving fluids for 2 hr prior to the vaccination.

(A) APPLICATION EXERCISES ANSWER KEY

Scenario: The parents of a 4-year-old have arrived at the clinic for their daughter's pre-kindergarten physical exam and immunizations. The family recently moved to the area and has a copy of the child's immunization record from the previous health care provider.

1. Prior to giving an immunization, what data should the nurse collect about the child?

   The parents should be asked if the child has allergies and if so, these need to be reviewed. The nurse should also ask if the child had any previous reactions to vaccines, and if the child has any current illness or fever. The temperature of the child should be taken if the parents indicate the presence of a fever.

   (N) NCLEX® Connection: Health Promotion and Maintenance, Health Promotion/Disease Prevention

2. The child is to receive an intramuscular injection. Which of the following injection sites should the nurse select?

   A. Deltoid region

   B. Outer aspect of the upper arm

   C. Ventrogluteal site

   D. Anterolateral thigh

   The ventrogluteal muscle is the preferred intramuscular injection site for children ages 1 and up through adolescents. The deltoid muscle is an appropriate injection site for older children and adolescents. Use the outer aspect of the upper arm or anterolateral thigh for subcutaneous injections.

   (N) NCLEX® Connection: Pharmacological Therapies, Medication Administration

3. Which of the following actions should the nurse take to administer the immunization? (Select all that apply.)

   X   **Obtain parental consent for the immunization.**

   X   **Document the date, route, and site of the injection on the child's immunization record.**

          Use a reconstituted vial of vaccine that was prepared 6 hr ago.

          Apply a warm compress to the injection site immediately after the immunization.

   X   **Remind parents to give acetaminophen or ibuprofen as needed for the next 24 hr.**

Obtain parental consent prior to giving the immunization. Complete documentation after the immunization and include the date, route, site of injection, type of immunization, manufacturer, lot number, and expiration date. Remind parents to give acetaminophen or ibuprofen if needed for 24 hr after the immunization to treat mild fever or a localized reaction. Use a reconstituted vaccine within 30 min of reconstitution. Follow the manufacturer's reconstitution and storage guidelines. Apply cool compresses after the injection to minimize localized reactions.

Ⓝ NCLEX® Connection: Reduction of Risk Potential, Therapeutic Procedures

---

4. A nurse is providing information to a group of parents regarding immunizations. Which of the following actions should the nurse suggest parents take prior to bringing their children to the clinic for the next immunization? (Select all that apply.)

   X   **Premedicate the child with ibuprofen or acetaminophen.**

          Withhold food for 4 hr prior to the vaccination.

   X   **Bring comfort items, such as pacifiers, favorite toys, or blankets.**

   X   **Apply a topical anesthetic to the injection site.**

          Avoid giving fluids for 2 hr prior to the vaccination.

Parents can premedicate the child with ibuprofen or acetaminophen prior to the next scheduled immunization to decrease any possible reactions. Comfort items used during the procedure offer support to the child. Applying a topical anesthetic to reduce discomfort is appropriate. Withholding food or fluids prior to the vaccination is not necessary and can stress the child.

Ⓝ NCLEX® Connection: Reduction of Risk Potential, Therapeutic Procedures

---

UNIT 2	NURSING CARE OF CHILDREN WITH SYSTEM DISORDERS
Section:	Immune and Infectious Disorders
Chapter 35	Communicable Diseases

Overview

- Communicable diseases are easily spread through airborne, droplet, or direct contact transmission.

- Most communicable diseases can be prevented with immunizations.

DISEASE/VIRUS	SPREAD	INCUBATION	COMMUNICABILITY
Varicella (chickenpox)/ varicella-zoster virus	• Direct contact • Droplet • Contaminated objects	14 to 21 days	1 day before to 6 days after first lesions appear
Rubella (German measles)/rubella virus	• Direct contact • Droplet	14 to 21 days	7 days before to 5 days after rash
Rubeola (measles)/ rubeola virus	• Direct contact • Droplet	10 to 20 days	4 days before to 5 days after rash
Pertussis (whooping cough)/*Bordetella pertussis*	• Droplet	6 to 20 days	Catarrhal stage before paroxysms
Erythema infectiosum (fifth disease)	• Respiratory secretions and blood	4 to 21 days	Unknown
Mumps/paramyxovirus	• Direct contact • Droplet	14 to 21 days	Immediately before and after swelling
Epstein-Barr virus (EBV), also known as infectious mononucleosis)	• Direct contact	4 to 6 weeks	Unknown

---

View Media Supplement:

- Chickenpox Vesicles (Image)   • Rubella (Image)   • Mumps (Image)

Data Collection

- Risk Factors

    o Immunocompromised status

    o Crowded living conditions

    o Poor sanitation

    o Poor nutrition

    o Poor oxygenation and impaired circulation

    o Chronic illness

    o Recent exposure to a known case of a communicable disease

- Subjective and Objective Data

    o Varicella (chickenpox)

    - Headache and irritability

    - Abdominal discomfort

    - Intense pruritus

    - Malaise

    - Decrease in oral intake

    - Fever

    - Lesions beginning as macules, rapidly progressing to papules, and then changing to clear, fluid-filled lesions (vesicles) before crusting over. All stages may be present at one time.

    o Rubella (German measles)

    - Low-grade fever and mild rash lasting 2 to 3 days

    - Headache and malaise

    - Rash usually beginning on face, spreading down the trunk, and fading in a few days

    o Measles (rubeola)

    - High fever, malaise

    - Sore throat, cough, and runny nose

    - Enlarged lymph nodes and conjunctivitis

    - Koplik spots on buccal mucosa (small, bright red spots with a blue-white center that usually appear 2 days before rash)

    - Rash of red maculopapular lesions that begins at hairline and usually spreads down the body, eventually turning brown

    - Worsening symptoms that decrease about 2 days after the appearance of the rash

- o Pertussis (whooping cough)
  - Reports of nighttime cough
  - Thick mucus plug that may dislodge with coughing
  - Paroxysmal coughing with eyes bulging and tongue protruding
- o Mumps
  - Fever, headache, and malaise
  - Anorexia for 24 hr
  - Earache that increases with chewing
  - Swollen, tender, and painful parotid glands
- o Infectious mononucleosis
  - Headache, malaise, and fatigue
  - Loss of appetite
  - Fever, sore throat
  - Puffy eyes
  - Cervical adenopathy
  - Splenomegaly (tender upper abdomen), which may persist for months
  - Palatine petechiae
  - Pharyngitis/tonsillitis exudate
  - Elevated WBC and atypical lymphocytes detected
  - Possible liver enzymes elevation (AST, ALT) with possible jaundice
- o Conjunctivitis
  - Pain and tearing (foreign body)
  - Purulent drainage and crusted eyelids (bacterial)
  - Watery drainage (viral or allergic)
- o Laboratory Tests
  - CBC
  - Electrolyte panels
  - Mono spot blood test for infectious mononucleosis

Collaborative Care

- Nursing Care

    - Symptomatic treatment

        - Follow airborne, droplet, and contact precautions for children who are hospitalized.

        - Administer an antipyretic for fever. Do not administer aspirin, due to the risk of Reye syndrome.

        - Administer analgesics for pain.

        - Provide fluids and nutritious foods the child prefers.

        - Skin care

            - Provide calamine lotion for topical relief.

            - Keep the child's skin clean and dry to prevent secondary infection.

            - Keep the child cool, but prevent chilling.

            - Dress the child in lightweight, loose clothing.

            - Give baths in tepid water, possibly with oatmeal.

            - Keep the child's fingernails clean and short.

            - Apply mittens if the child scratches.

            - Teach good oral hygiene. Children may gargle with warm water for a sore throat.

            - Change linens daily.

        - Provide quiet diversional activities.

        - Promote adequate rest with naps if necessary.

        - Keep lights dim if children develop photophobia.

        - Keep children out of the sun.

        - Notify the child's school or day care center of the child's infection. Obtain a plan from the school so that the child can continue working on school work at home.

        - Notify the health department of infection if necessary (pertussis, mumps, and measles).

- Medications

    - Antihistamines – Diphenhydramine hydrochloride (Benadryl) and hydroxyzine (Atarax)

        - Used to controls pruritus

        - Nursing Considerations

            - Monitor the child's reaction to the medication, because some children may become hyperalert with the administration of a medication from this group.

□ Monitor children for drowsiness.

■ Client Education

□ Educate families about safety precautions.

○ Acetaminophen (Tylenol)

■ Decreases fever

■ Nursing Considerations

□ Be alert for allergies.

■ Client Education

□ Instruct the parents about appropriate dosage for acetaminophen.

- Care After Discharge

  ○ Client Education

  ■ Encourage adherence with antibiotic or antiviral therapy.

  ■ Instruct the parents to teach the child to cover her nose and mouth with tissue when coughing or sneezing.

  ■ Instruct the parents to wash the child's bed linens daily in mild detergent.

  ■ Instruct the parents of children who are immunocompromised to seek prompt medical care if symptoms develop.

  ■ Encourage adolescents to participate in decision making.

- Client Outcomes

  ○ The child will experience relief from pruritus.

  ○ The child will be free from injury.

  ○ The spread of the disease will be prevented by practicing measures to reduce transmission.

Complications

- Reye syndrome

  ○ Reye syndrome most commonly occurs after an episode of viral illness (influenza, varicella).

  ○ Reye syndrome may be associated with the use of aspirin during a viral illness.

  ○ The best prognosis for Reye syndrome is achieved with prompt diagnosis and aggressive treatment.

  ○ Nursing Actions

  ■ Nursing care is provided in the ICU and includes maintaining vital functions, assisting with lumbar puncture, obtaining blood samples, administering IV fluids, performing nasogastric intubation, and inserting an indwelling urinary catheter.

- ○ Client Education

    - ■ Instruct parents to eliminate the use of aspirin or aspirin-containing products with children.

- Other Complications

    - ○ Varicella – Secondary bacterial infections (pneumonia, sepsis encephalitis, scarring, chronic or transient thrombocytopenia)

    - ○ Rubella – Few complications, but there is a teratogenic effect on the fetus of exposed pregnant women

    - ○ Rubeola (measles) – Otitis media, pneumonia, bronchiolitis, laryngitis and laryngotracheitis, and encephalitis

    - ○ Pertussis (whooping cough) – Pneumonia, otitis media, seizures, hemorrhage (caused by forceful coughing), hernia, prolapsed rectum, weight loss, and dehydration

    - ○ Mumps – Epididymo-orchitis in males, hearing loss, encephalitis, meningitis, myocarditis, arthritis, hepatitis, and pancreatitis

    - ○ Infectious mononucleosis – Few complications, but ruptured spleen may result from blow to upper abdomen if splenomegaly is present

        - ■ Participation in contact sports is discouraged.

Ⓐ APPLICATION EXERCISES

1. Which of the following communicable diseases may lead to pneumonia? (Select all that apply.)

    _____ Rubella (German measles)

    _____ Rubeola (measles)

    _____ Pertussis (whooping cough)

    _____ Varicella (chickenpox)

    _____ Paramyxovirus (mumps)

Scenario: The parents of a 7-year-old child with the mumps call the clinic to ask what they can do for their child.

2. Which of the following actions should the nurse review with the parents? (Select all that apply.)

    _____ Monitor temperature for pyrexia.

    _____ Give analgesic for discomfort.

    _____ Avoid contact with others until swelling has disappeared.

    _____ Observe for small, bright red spots with a bluish center on the oral mucosa.

    _____ Encourage cool and noncitrus fluids and easy-to-chew foods.

3. What possible complication of the mumps should the nurse advise the parents to be alert for?

_____

4. Infectious mononucleosis is caused by_____.

5. The lesions of chickenpox begin as_____, then progress to_____, and change to_____.

Ⓝ **APPLICATION EXERCISES ANSWER KEY**

1. Which of the following communicable diseases may lead to pneumonia? (Select all that apply.)

    _____ Rubella (German measles)

    __X__ **Rubeola (measles)**

    __X__ **Pertussis (whooping cough)**

    __X__ **Varicella (chickenpox)**

    _____ Paramyxovirus (mumps)

    Rubeola, pertussis, and varicella can cause pneumonia. The other communicable diseases do not result in pneumonia.

Ⓝ NCLEX® Connection: Safety and Infection Control, Standard/Transmission-Based/Other Precautions/Surgical Asepsis

Scenario: The parents of a 7-year-old child with the mumps call the clinic to ask what they can do for their child.

2. Which of the following actions should the nurse review with the parents? (Select all that apply.)

    __X__ **Monitor temperature for pyrexia.**

    __X__ **Give analgesic for discomfort.**

    __X__ **Avoid contact with others until swelling has disappeared.**

    _____ Observe for small, bright red spots with a bluish center on the oral mucosa.

    __X__ **Encourage cool and noncitrus fluids and easy-to-chew foods.**

    Tell parents to monitor the child for a high fever and malaise and to give antipyretics/ analgesics. Children with mumps are communicable immediately prior to and after the swelling appears. Offer the child cool, noncitrus fluids and easy-to-chew foods due to the swelling and earache that occurs. Bright red spots with a bluish center on the oral mucosa are found in cases of measles.

Ⓝ NCLEX® Connection: Reduction of Risk Potential, Potential for Alterations in Body Systems

3. What possible complication of the mumps should the nurse advise the parents to be alert for?

    In males, pain, swelling, and tenderness of the scrotal sac can occur which indicates epididymo-orchitis. Other complications include hearing loss, encephalitis, meningitis, myocarditis, arthritis, and hepatitis.

Ⓝ NCLEX® Connection: Physiological Adaptations, Basic Pathophysiology

4. Infectious mononucleosis is caused by **the Epstein-Barr (EBV) virus.**

Ⓝ NCLEX® Connection: Physiological Adaptations, Alterations in Body Systems

5. The lesions of chickenpox begin as **macules**, then progress to **papules**, and change to **vesicles**.

Ⓝ NCLEX® Connection: Physiological Adaptations, Basic Pathophysiology

UNIT 2   NURSING CARE OF CHILDREN WITH SYSTEM DISORDERS
Section: Immune and Infectious Disorders
Chapter 36   Acute Otitis Media

Overview

- Acute otitis media (AOM) is an infection of the structures in the middle ear.

- Otitis media with effusion (OME) is present when there is a collection of fluid in the middle ear but no infection.

- Repeated infections can cause impaired hearing and speech delays.

- Many infections clear spontaneously in a few days.

Data Collection

- Risk Factors

  - The eustachian tubes in children are shorter and more horizontal than those of adults. Therefore, children have an increased risk for developing otitis media.

  - Otitis media is most common in the first 24 months of life and again when children enter school (ages 5 to 6). Otitis media infrequently occurs after age 7.

  - Otitis media is usually triggered by a bacterial infection (*Streptococcus pneumoniae, Haemophilus influenzae, Moraxella catarrhalis*), a viral infection (respiratory syncytial virus or influenza), allergies, or enlarged tonsils.

  - There is a lower incidence of otitis media in infants who are breastfed (possibly due to the presence of immunoglobulin A [IgA] in breast milk, which protects against infection). Also, reflux of milk into the Eustachian tube is less likely, as the infant is held in a semi-vertical position for breastfeeding.

  - Incidence is higher:

    - In the winter months

    - With exposure to large numbers of children (day care)

    - With exposure to secondhand smoke

    - When a cleft lip and/or cleft palate is present

    - With Down syndrome

- Subjective Data

  ○ Recent history of upper respiratory infection; acute onset of changes in behavior; frequent crying, irritability, and fussiness; inconsolability; tugging at ear; and reports of ear pain, anorexia, nausea, and vomiting.

- Objective Data

  ○ Physical Assessment Findings

    ■ AOM

      □ Rubbing or pulling on ear

      □ Crying

      □ Lethargy

      □ Bulging opacified, yellow or red tympanic membrane

       View Media Supplement: Acute Otitis Media (Image)

      □ Purulent material in middle ear or drainage from external canal

      □ Decreased or no tympanic movement with pneumatic otoscopy

      □ Lymphadenopathy of the neck and head

      □ Temperature (may be as high as 40° C [104° F])

      □ Hearing difficulties and speech delays if otitis media becomes a chronic condition

    ■ OME

      □ Feeling of fullness in the ear

      □ Orange discoloration of the tympanic membrane with decreased movement

      □ Vague findings including rhinitis, cough, and diarrhea

      □ Transient hearing loss and balance disturbances can occur

  ○ Diagnostic Procedures

    ■ Pneumatic otoscopy

      □ A pneumatic otoscope is used to visualize the tympanic membrane and middle ear structures. The otoscope also assesses tympanic membrane movement.

      □ Nursing Actions

        ▸ Gently pull the pinna down and back to visualize the tympanic membrane of a child younger than 3 years old. For a child older than 3 years, gently pull the pinna up and back.

Collaborative Care

- Nursing Care

  - Provide comfort measures.

    - Position an ice compress over the affected ear.

    - Provide diversional activities.

- Medications

  - Acetaminophen (Tylenol) or ibuprofen (Advil)

    - Used to provide analgesia and reduce fever

    - Nursing Considerations

      - Obtain a liquid preparation.

      - Use age-appropriate techniques to administer medication.

  - Amoxicillin (Amoxil) is the first-line antibiotic. Amoxicillin-clavulanate (Augmentin), azithromycin (Zithromax), and cefuroxime (Zinacef) are second-line antibiotics.

  - Antibiotics

    - Nursing Considerations

      - Administer amoxicillin in high doses, usually 80 to 90 mg/kg/day in two divided doses.

      - The usual course of treatment is 10 to 14 days in children younger than 6 years of age. The course may be shorter for older children.

    - Client Education

      - Instruct families that children should complete the total course of treatment.

      - Observe for signs of allergy to the antibiotic, such as rash or difficulty breathing.

  - Benzocaine (Americaine-Otic)

    - Ear drops for topical pain relief

    - Client Education

      - Instruct families how to properly administer ear drops.

      - Discourage the use of decongestants or antihistamines.

- Therapeutic Procedures

  - Myringotomy and placement of tympanoplasty tubes may be indicated for children with multiple episodes of otitis media. This procedure may now be performed by laser treatment.

    - This procedure is performed in an outpatient setting with the administration of general anesthesia. It is usually completed in 15 min.

    - A small incision is made in the tympanic membrane, and tiny pressure-equalizer tubes are placed into the eardrum to equalize pressure and minimize effusion.

    - Recovery takes place in a PACU, and discharge usually occurs within 1 hr.

    - Postoperative pain is not common and, if present, will be mild.

    - Antibiotic ear drops may be prescribed for a few days.

    - The tubes come out by themselves (usually in 6 to 12 months).

    - Client Education

      □ Limit the child's activities for a few days following surgery.

      □ Instruct parents to notify the provider when the tubes come out. This usually does not require replacement of the tubes.

- Surgical Interventions

  - Instruct families to avoid getting water into the child's ears while the tubes are in place. The effectiveness of earplugs is not conclusive. Advise the parents to follow the provider's instructions.

- Care After Discharge

  - Client Education

    - Inform the client/parents about comfort measures.

    - Encourage the parents to feed children in an upright position when bottle or breastfeeding.

    - If drainage is present, clean the external ear with sterile cotton swabs. Apply antibiotic ointment.

    - If possible, instruct the parents to avoid risk factors (secondhand smoke, exposure to individuals with viral/bacterial respiratory infections).

    - Stress the importance of seeking medical care at initial signs and symptoms of infections (change in child's behavior, tugging on ear).

    - Eliminate exposure to secondhand smoke.

    - Encourage the parents to keep the child's immunizations up to date.

- Client Outcomes

  - The child will be free of infection.

Complications

- Hearing loss and/or speech delays
  - ○ Nursing Actions
    - ■ Monitor for deficits.
    - ■ Three months after an acute episode of AOM, children should have audiology testing or language evaluation if OME persists for 3 months or more, or there is evidence of language or learning delays.
  - ○ Client Education
    - ■ Inform families of the need for hearing testing, language evaluation, or speech therapy.

APPLICATION EXERCISES

1. An infant who has signs and symptoms of acute otitis media (AOM) is brought to the outpatient facility by his parent. The nurse should recognize that which of the following factors, if present, places the infant at risk for otitis media? (Select all that apply.)

  _____ Breastfeeding

  _____ Attends day care

  _____ Immunizations are current

  _____ Cleft palate present at birth

  _____ Infant's father smokes cigarettes

2. A nurse is reviewing discharge instructions with the parent of a 2 year old who is recovering from a myringotomy and placement of tympanostomy tubes. Which of the following statements by the parent indicates the need to reinforce teaching?

  A. "The tubes will probably fall out on their own in 6 to 12 months and I know to call my doctor when this happens."

  B. "My child should hardly have any pain when we get home."

  C. "I'll put in the lubricated cotton balls like my doctor showed me to use so my child won't get any water in his ears."

  D. "My son has so much energy so I'm glad he can go to his gymnastics class tomorrow."

3. Which of the following is a long-term complication which can occur after multiple episodes of otitis media? (Select all that apply.)

  _____ Pneumonia

  _____ Speech delay

  _____ Hearing impairment

  _____ Vertigo

  _____ Allergy to antibiotics

(A) **APPLICATION EXERCISES ANSWER KEY**

1. An infant who has signs and symptoms of acute otitis media (AOM) is brought to the outpatient facility by his parent. The nurse should recognize that which of the following factors, if present, places the infant at risk for otitis media? (Select all that apply.)

    _____ Breastfeeding

    __X__ **Attends day care**

    _____ Immunizations are current

    __X__ **Cleft palate present at birth**

    __X__ **Infant's father smokes cigarettes**

    Infants who attend day care have an increased risk of exposure. Infants born with cleft lip and/or palate are more prone to AOM because micro-organisms can more readily move up the eustachian tubes due to reflux of milk. Exposure to second-hand smoke is also a risk factor for AOM. Breastfeeding helps to protect against AOM because breast milk contains secretory IgA. Being up to date with immunizations can help prevent AOM since it is a complication of some communicable diseases, such as measles.

(N) NCLEX® Connection: Reduction of Risk Potential, Potential for Complications From Surgical Procedures and Health Alterations

2. A nurse is reviewing discharge instructions with the parent of a 2 year old who is recovering from a myringotomy and placement of tympanostomy tubes. Which of the following statements by the parent indicates the need to reinforce teaching?

    A. "The tubes will probably fall out on their own in 6 to 12 months and I know to call my doctor when this happens."

    B. "My child should hardly have any pain when we get home."

    C. "I'll put in the lubricated cotton balls like my doctor showed me to use so my child won't get any water in his ears."

    D. "My son has so much energy so I'm glad he can go to his gymnastics class tomorrow."

    Discharge instructions focus on parents knowing that the tubes will probably fall out in 6 to 12 months and parents should notify their provider when this happens. Postoperative pain is not common and should be mild. The child should not get water in his ears and if the provider has instructed the parents on how to prevent this, the information should be reviewed. Tympanostomy tubes allow water to pass into the middle ear which could promote infection. The child's activity should be limited for a few days following surgery so a gymnastics class is not appropriate.

(N) NCLEX® Connection: Reduction of Risk Potential, Potential for Complications from Surgical Procedures and Health Alterations

3. Which of the following is a long-term complication which can occur after multiple episodes of otitis media? (Select all that apply.)

   _____   Pneumonia

   __X__   **Speech delay**

   __X__   **Hearing impairment**

   _____   Vertigo

   _____   Allergy to antibiotics

Long-term complications of otitis media are delayed speech and hearing impairment. These problems result in learning disabilities and affect psychosocial development. Pneumonia is not a long-term complication. Vertigo can occur but is a symptom of otitis media. Allergy to antibiotics is not a complication but the child should be observed for symptoms such as rash or difficulty breathing.

(N) NCLEX® Connection: Physiological Adaptations, Alterations in Body Systems

Overview

- HIV infection is a viral infection in which the virus infects the T-lymphocytes, causing immune dysfunction. This leads to organ dysfunction and a variety of opportunistic infections in a weakened host. In addition, HIV infections that progress to AIDS place children at risk for developing a variety of malignancies (Kaposi's sarcoma, cranial or Burkitt's lymphoma).

- Children who are born to mothers who are HIV positive or are exposed to HIV from other means usually convert to HIV positive status and develop clinical signs more rapidly than adults.

Data Collection

- Risk Factors

  ○ Having a mother with HIV/AIDs can result in vertical transmission of the HIV virus to the fetus. A woman can also vertically transmit the virus when breastfeeding her infant.

  ○ Casual contact (visiting the home of a child with HIV, being in the same classroom as a child with HIV) is not a proven mode of transmission.

- Subjective Data

  ○ Chills

  ○ Anorexia, nausea, weight loss

  ○ Weakness and fatigue

  ○ Headache

  ○ Night sweats

- Objective Data

  ○ Physical Assessment Findings and Laboratory Tests

    ▪ HIV infection – Birth to 12 years

    ▪ HIV infection – 13 to 20 years

      ▫ A confirmed case classification meets the laboratory criteria for a diagnosis of HIV infection and one of the four HIV infection stages (stage 1, stage 2, stage 3, or unknown).

  ○ Exposure – Less than 18 months of age and born to a mother who is HIV-infected

IMMUNOLOGIC CATEGORY	LESS THAN 12 MONTHS		1 TO 5 YEARS		6 TO 12 YEARS	
	CELLS/ MEQ/L*	%**	CELLS/ MEQ/L	%	CELLS/ MEQ/L	%
No suppression	1,500 or more	25 or more	1,000 or more	25 or more	500 or more	25 or more
Moderate suppression	750 to 1,499	15 to 24	500 to 999	15 to 24	200 to 499	15 to 24
Severe suppression	less than 750	less than 15	less than 500	less than 15	less than 200	less than 15

* CD4+ T-lymphocyte count = cells/mEq/L

** CD4+ T-lymphocyte percentage of total lymphocytes = %

NOT SYMPTOMATIC	MILDLY SYMPTOMATIC
No signs or symptoms considered to be the result of HIV infection are present, or the child has only one of the conditions listed in the next column.	Two or more of the conditions listed in this column are present, but the child has none of the conditions listed in the next two columns. • Lymphadenopathy • Hepatomegaly • Splenomegaly • Recurrent upper respiratory infections, sinusitis, or otitis media • Dermatitis • Parotitis

MODERATELY SYMPTOMATIC	SEVERELY SYMPTOMATIC
Children with the following conditions are considered moderately symptomatic. • Anemia • Bacterial meningitis, pneumonia, or sepsis (single episode) • Oropharyngeal candidiasis • Cardiomyopathy • Cytomegalovirus infection, with onset before 1 month of age • Recurrent or chronic diarrhea • Hepatitis • Herpes simplex virus (HSV), stomatitis, bronchitis, pneumonitis, or esophagitis • Herpes zoster • Lymphoid interstitial pneumonitis (LIP) • Nephropathy • Persistent fever (lasting more than1 month) • Toxoplasmosis • Disseminated varicella	Children with the following conditions are considered severely symptomatic. • Multiple or recurrent bacterial infections (meningitis, septicemia, pneumonia) • Esophageal or pulmonary candidiasis, (bronchi, trachea, lungs) • Cytomegalovirus disease • Pneumocystis jiroveci • HIV encephalopathy with developmental delays • HSV stomatitis, bronchitis, pneumonitis, or esophagitis • Kaposi's sarcoma • Brain or Burkitt's lymphoma • Disseminated or extrapulmonary mycobacterium tuberculosis • Pneumocystis carinii pneumonia • Wasting syndrome

STAGE	DEFINING CONDITIONS	CD4+ T-LYMPHOCYTE COUNT	CD4+ T-LYMPHOCYTE PERCENTAGE OF TOTAL LYMPHOCYTES
Stage 1	• None	• 500 cells/mEq/L or more	• 29 or more
Stage 2	• None	• 200 to 499 cells/mEq/L	• 14 to 28
Stage 3 (AIDS)*	• Candidiasis of esophagus, bronchi, trachea, or lungs • Herpes simplex – Chronic ulcers (of more than 1 month's duration) • HIV-related encephalopathy • Disseminated or extrapulmonary histoplasmosis • Kaposi's sarcoma • Burkitt's lymphoma • Mycobacterium tuberculosis of any site • Pneumocystis jiroveci pneumonia • Recurrent pneumonia • Progressive multifocal leukoencephalopathy • Recurrent salmonella septicemia • Wasting syndrome attributed to HIV	• Less than 200 cells/mEq/L	• Less than 14
Stage unknown	• No information available	• No information available	• No information available

* Documentation of an AIDS-defining condition supersedes a CD4+ T-lymphocyte count of 200 cells/mEq/L or more and a CD4+ T-lymphocyte percentage of total lymphocytes of greater than 14.

** Human Immunodeficiency Virus Infection (HIV) (retrieved 3/18/10 from http://www.cdc.gov). To read more about HIV, go to the Web site of the Centers for Disease Control and Prevention (http://www.cdc.gov).

○   Diagnostic Procedures

■   Laboratory criteria for diagnosis

□   Less than 18 months

▸   Positive results on two separate specimens (not including cord blood) from one or more of the following HIV virologic (nonantibody) tests:

▹   HIV nucleic acid (DNA or RNA) detection

▹   HIV p24 antigen test, including neutralization assay (for an infant more than 1 month of age)

▹   HIV isolation (viral culture)

□   18 months to 20 years

▸   Positive result from an HIV antibody screening test (reactive enzyme immunoassay [EIA]) confirmed by a positive result from a supplemental HIV antibody test (Western blot or indirect immunofluorescence assay test)

▸   Positive result or report of a detectable quantity from any of the following HIV virologic (nonantibody) tests:

▹   HIV nucleic acid (DNA or RNA) detection test (polymerase chain reaction [PCR])

▹   HIV p24 antigen test, including neutralization assay

▹   HIV isolation (viral culture)

■   Liver profile, biopsies, and testing of stool for parasites

□   Nursing Actions

▸   Prepare children for the test.

□   Client Education

▸   Inform children about the details of the test, such as length and what to expect.

Collaborative Care

●   Nursing Care

○   Encourage a balanced diet that is high in calories and protein. Obtain the child's preferred food and beverages. Give nutritional supplements. Avoid raw fruits and vegetables.

○   Monitor children receiving total parenteral nutrition (TPN).

○   Provide for good oral care and report abnormalities for treatment.

○   Keep the child's skin clean and dry.

○   Encourage activity alternated with rest periods.

○   Provide nonpharmacological methods of pain relief.

- o Determine the child's pain level and provide adequate pain management. Use of medications may include nonsteroidal anti-inflammatory drugs (NSAIDs), acetaminophen (Tylenol), opioids, muscle relaxants, and/or a eutectic mixture of local anesthetics (EMLA cream) for numerous diagnostic procedures.

- o Protect/prevent infection using standard precautions.

  - Encourage deep breathing and coughing.

  - Maintain good hand hygiene.

  - Monitor for signs of opportunistic infections.

- o Administer medications as prescribed for opportunistic infections (e.g., acyclovir [Zovirax] for herpes simplex virus, amphotericin B [Amphocin] for serious fungal infections).

- Medications

  - o Highly active antiretroviral therapy (HAART) involves using 3 to 4 HIV medications in combination to reduce medication resistance, adverse effects, and dosages.

    - Entry/infusion inhibitors – Enfuvirtide (Fuzeon)

      - This helps to decrease the amount of virus in the body and limit its spread.

    - Nucleoside reverse transcriptase inhibitors (NRTIs) – Zidovudine (Retrovir)

      - These interfere with the virus's ability to convert RNA into DNA.

    - Non-nucleoside reverse transcriptase inhibitors (NNRTIs) – Delavirdine (Rescriptor) and efavirenz (Sustiva)

      - These inhibit viral replication in cells.

    - Protease inhibitors, such as Ritonavir (Norvir), amprenavir (Agenerase), and nelfinavir (Viracept)

      - These inhibit an enzyme needed for the virus to replicate.

    - Nursing considerations

      - Monitor laboratory results (CBC, WBC, liver function tests). Antiretroviral medications may increase serum glutamic oxaloacetic transaminase (SGPT), alanine aminotransferase (ALT), serum glutamic oxaloacetic transaminase (SGOT), aspartate aminotransferase (AST), bilirubin, mean corpuscular volume (MCV), high-density lipoproteins (HDLs), total cholesterol, and triglycerides.

    - Client Education

      - Reinforce to children and families about the side effects of the medications and ways to decrease the severity of the side effects.

      - Reinforce to children and families about the need to take the medication on a regular schedule and to not miss doses.

- o Antibiotics
    - ■ Trimethoprim-sulfamethoxazole (TMP-SMZ)
        - □ Use for prophylaxis treatment of *Pneumocystis jiroveci* pneumonia (PCP) in newborns of mothers who are HIV infected
    - ■ Acyclovir (Zovirax)
        - □ Use for herpes simplex virus
    - ■ Amphotericin B (Amphocin)
        - □ Use for serious fungal infections.
    - ■ Nursing Actions
        - □ Monitor children for side effects.
    - ■ Client Education
        - □ Reinforce to families the importance of ensuring that the full dose of the medication is completed.

- Interdisciplinary Care
    - o Recognize need for social services to help with access to health care and medication acquisition and nutritional support to promote good nutrition.
    - o Support by school may be necessary.

- Care After Discharge
    - o Client Education
        - ■ Reinforce to children and families about the chronicity of the illness and the need for life-long medication administration.
        - ■ Instruct families when to notify the provider. Signs and symptoms requiring medical care include headache, fever, lethargy, warmth, tenderness, redness at joints, and neck stiffness.
        - ■ Remind children and families to avoid individuals who have colds/infections/viruses.
        - ■ Encourage immunizations with killed viruses, to include pneumococcal vaccine (PCV) and yearly seasonal influenza vaccine.
        - ■ Reinforce to children and families about transmission of the virus (high-risk behaviors).
        - ■ Instruct children and families about safe practice when using needles/syringes and administering medications.

- Client Outcomes
    - o The child will be free of infection.
    - o The child will maintain optimal weight.
    - o The child will participate in ADLs.

Complications

- Failure to Thrive

    o Nursing Actions

        ▪ Obtain a baseline height and weight and continue to monitor.

        ▪ Promote optimal nutrition. This may require the administration of TPN.

        ▪ Monitor for growth and development delays.

        ▪ Provide opportunities for normal development (age-appropriate toys, play with children of the same age).

    o Client Education

        ▪ Provide instruction for families about appropriate nutrition and how to meet nutritional needs.

- PCP – the most common opportunistic infection of children infected with HIV; most frequent occurrence is in children 3 to 6 months of age.

    o Nursing Actions

        ▪ Monitor respiratory status, which includes respiratory rate and effort, oxygen saturation, and breath sounds.

        ▪ Administer appropriate antibiotics.

        ▪ Administer an antipyretic and/or analgesics.

        ▪ Provide adequate hydration and maintain fluid and electrolyte balance.

        ▪ Use postural drainage and chest physiotherapy to mobilize and remove fluid from the lungs.

        ▪ Promote adequate rest.

    o Client Education

        ▪ Reinforce to children and families about the infectious process and how to prevent infection.

        ▪ Reinforce to children and families about the importance of medication and the need to maintain the medication regimen.

APPLICATION EXERCISES

1. The parent of a child who is HIV positive is at risk for disease transmission in which of the following situations? (Select all that apply.)

   _____ Sharing the same toothbrush

   _____ Being kissed by the child

   _____ Sharing finger foods with the child from a central plate

   _____ Cleaning up after the child has a nose bleed

   _____ Wiping the child's tears with a handkerchief when crying

2. A nurse is to begin HAART therapy for a child who is HIV positive. These medications are from which of the following classifications of medications?

   A. Antifungals

   B. Antibiotics

   C. Antiretrovirals

   D. Antidiarrheals

3. An adolescent is classified as having AIDS in _____ of the HIV infection.

4. In children less than 12 years of age with HIV infection, the laboratory test used to define the category of immune suppression is _____.

5. A nurse in the prenatal clinic receives a phone call from a client who is positive for HIV infection and asks if breastfeeding can transmit the infection to her newborn after birth. Which of the following is the appropriate response by the nurse?

   A. "It will depend upon the results of your lab tests after delivery."

   B. "No, the HIV virus is not present in breast milk."

   C. "Breastfeeding is one of the modes of transmission of the virus."

   D. "As long as you pump and then give the infant your breast milk, there is no risk to your infant."

APPLICATION EXERCISES ANSWER KEY

1. The parent of a child who is HIV positive is at risk for disease transmission in which of the following situations? (Select all that apply.)

    __X__ Sharing the same toothbrush

    _____ Being kissed by the child

    _____ Sharing finger foods with the child from a central plate

    __X__ Cleaning up after the child has a nose bleed

    _____ Wiping the child's tears with a handkerchief when crying

    The only situations posing any risks are cleaning up after the child has a nose bleed and sharing the same toothbrush. HIV is transmitted by direct contact with blood and body fluids (semen, vaginal secretions). It is important not to share personal hygiene items such as razors or toothbrushes, which could contain blood. None of the other activities should place a person at risk. Even though the virus has been found in small amounts in tears, mucous, and sweat, there is no evidence that transmission has ever occurred unless blood is present.

     NCLEX® Connection: Safety and Infection Control, Standard/Transmission-Based/Other Precautions/Surgical Asepsis

2. A nurse is to begin HAART therapy for a child who is HIV positive. These medications are from which of the following classifications of medications?

    A. Antifungals

    B. Antibiotics

    C. Antiretrovirals

    D. Antidiarrheals

    HAART therapy stands for highly active antiretroviral therapy, which includes using three to four HIV medications in combination to reduce medication resistance, adverse effects, and dosages. Antifungals and antibiotics may be given if the child develops an opportunistic infection, but are not included in the HAART protocol. Antidiarrheals are not included in HAART.

     NCLEX® Connection: Pharmacological Therapies, Expected Actions/Outcomes

3. An adolescent is classified as having AIDS in **stage 3** of the HIV infection.

     NCLEX® Connection: Safety and Infection Control, Standard/Transmission-Based/Other Precautions/Surgical Asepsis

4. In children less than 12 years of age with HIV infection, the laboratory test used to define the category of immune suppression is **the CD4+ T-lymphocyte count.**

     NCLEX® Connection: Reduction of Risk Potential, Laboratory Values

5. A nurse in the prenatal clinic receives a phone call from a client who is positive for HIV infection and asks if breastfeeding can transmit the infection to her newborn after birth. Which of the following is the appropriate response by the nurse?

   A. "It will depend upon the results of your lab tests after delivery."

   B. "No, the HIV virus is not present in breast milk."

   C. "Breastfeeding is one of the modes of transmission of the virus."

   D. "As long as you pump and then give the infant your breast milk, there is no risk to your infant."

A mother who is HIV positive can transmit the virus when breastfeeding her newborn because breast milk is a body secretion. The virus is also transmitted in utero to the fetus through blood. The newborn is exposed to the virus in vaginal secretions at the time of delivery. The decision to breastfeed is not dependent on postpartum laboratory tests. Viral transmission by breast milk is well-documented in medical literature, and pumping breast milk does not alter the presence of the virus in it.

Ⓝ NCLEX® Connection: Safety and Infection Control, Standard/Transmission-Based/Other Precautions/Surgical Asepsis

UNIT 2: NURSING CARE OF CHILDREN WITH SYSTEM DISORDERS

Section: Neoplastic Disorders

- Pediatric Cancers

NCLEX® CONNECTIONS

When reviewing the chapters in this section, keep in mind the relevant sections of the NCLEX® outline, in particular:

CLIENT NEEDS: BASIC CARE AND COMFORT

Relevant topics/tasks include:
- Elimination
  - Identify client at risk for impaired elimination.
- Nonpharmacological Comfort Interventions
  - Monitor client non-verbal signs of pain/discomfort.
- Nutrition and Oral Hydration
  - Monitor and provide for nutritional needs of client.

CLIENT NEEDS: PHARMACOLOGICAL THERAPIES

Relevant topics/tasks include:
- Adverse Effects/Contraindications/Side Effects/Interactions
  - Identify a contraindication to the administration of prescribed over-the-counter medication to the client.
- Expected Actions/Outcomes
  - Apply knowledge of pathophysiology when addressing client pharmacological agents.
- Pharmacological Pain Management
  - Monitor and document client response to pharmacological interventions.

CLIENT NEEDS: REDUCTION OF RISK POTENTIAL

Relevant topics/tasks include:
- Diagnostic Tests
  - Reinforce client teaching about diagnostic test.
- Potential for Complications of Diagnostic Tests/Treatments/Procedures
  - Implement measures to prevent complication of client condition or procedure.
- Therapeutic Procedures
  - Assist with the performance of a diagnostic or invasive procedure.

UNIT 2	NURSING CARE OF CHILDREN WITH SYSTEM DISORDERS
Section:	Neoplastic Disorders
Chapter 38	Pediatric Cancers

Overview

- Wilms' tumor (nephroblastoma) is a malignancy that occurs in the kidneys or abdomen.

    o   It most often occurs during the toddler and preschool years.

    o   Metastasis is rare.

- Neuroblastoma is a malignancy that occurs in the adrenal gland, sympathetic chain of the retroperitoneal area, head, neck, pelvis, or chest.

    o   It occurs before age 10, usually during the toddler years.

    o   Most tumors (70%) have spread by metastasis at the time of diagnosis.

- Cancers that occur in children include leukemia, Wilms' tumor, and neuroblastoma. Presenting signs and symptoms will vary with the type of cancer.

- Leukemia is the term for a group of malignancies that affect the bone marrow and lymphatic system.

- Leukemia is classified by the type of WBCs that becomes neoplastic and is commonly divided into two groups – acute lymphoid leukemia (ALL) and acute myelogenous or nonlymphoid leukemia (AML/ANLL).

- Leukemia causes bone marrow dysfunction that leads to anemia and neutropenia.

- Malignant tumors in bone may originate from all tissues involved in bone growth, including osteoid matrix, blood vessels, and cartilage.

- Soft tissue malignancies arise from undifferentiated cells in any of the soft tissues (muscles, tendons), in connective or fibrous tissue, or in blood or lymph vessels. These malignancies can begin in any area of the body.

- Presenting signs and symptoms will vary with the type of cancer.

WILMS' TUMOR AND NEUROBLASTOMA

Overview

- Treatment for Wilms' tumor and neuroblastoma may be a combination of surgery, chemotherapy, and radiation. The prognosis for children in the low-risk stage include survival rates that range from 88% to 90%. For children in the high-risk stage, survival rates range from 22% to 30%. Generally, the younger the child at diagnosis, the better the survival rate.

Data Collection

- Risk Factors

  ○ There is some evidence of genetic predisposition.

- Subjective and Objective Data

  ○ Wilms' tumor presents as an abdominal swelling or mass that is usually firm, nontender, and unilateral.

  ○ Neuroblastoma presents as an asymmetrical, firm, nontender mass in the abdomen. This mass crosses the midline.

  ○ Wilms' tumor and neuroblastoma can cause urinary symptoms (frequency, urgency) with compression of renal structures.

  ○ Signs and symptoms of metastasis

    ■ Edema (periorbital) with ecchymosis around the eyes

    ■ Lymphadenopathy (predominantly cervical and supraclavicular in neuroblastoma)

    ■ Weight loss, anemia, and fatigue

    ■ Hepatomegaly and splenomegaly

    ■ Possible bone pain

    ■ Respiratory involvement leading to shortness of breath, decreased breath sounds, cough, and respiratory distress

    ■ Paralysis that will have varying degrees (neuroblastoma)

  ○ Laboratory Tests

    ■ Use blood studies to identify anemia and infection.

    ■ Evaluate urine for the presence of breakdown products of catecholamines (vanillylmandelic acid, homovanillic acid, dopamine, norepinephrine) to detect adrenal or sympathetic tumors. Urinary excretion of catecholamines is found in approximately 95% of children with adrenal or sympathetic tumors.

    ■ Obtain liver enzyme studies to assess the quality of liver function.

- ○ Diagnostic Procedures
  - ■ Chest x-ray and CT, MRI, positron emission tomography (PET), and single photon emission computed tomography (SPECT) scans
    - □ Use to visualize tumors and metastasis and determine the stage of the cancer.
    - □ Nursing Actions
      - ▸ Ask about the child's allergies to dye or shellfish.
      - ▸ Assist children to remain still during the procedure.
      - ▸ Instruct children to drink oral contrast if prescribed.
      - ▸ Assist with providing sedation of children if prescribed.
    - □ Client Education
      - ▸ Provide emotional support.
  - ■ Biopsy
    - □ A biopsy may be a local procedure to obtain a sample of tissue for diagnosis. A biopsy can also be obtained during surgery under general anesthesia, possibly in conjunction with excision or resection of the tumor at the same time.
    - □ Nursing Actions
      - ▸ During the procedure, provide emotional support.
      - ▸ Following the biopsy
        - ▹ Observe the site for bleeding.
        - ▹ Prevent infection at the biopsy site.
        - ▹ Provide pain relief.
    - □ Client Education
      - ▸ Instruct the parents to provide emotional support.

Collaborative Care

- Nursing Care
  - ○ Determine the child and family's coping and support.
  - ○ Observe for developmental delays related to illness.
  - ○ Measure physical growth (height and weight).
  - ○ Provide education and support to children and their families regarding diagnostic testing, treatment plan, ongoing therapy, and prognosis.
  - ○ Monitor for signs of infection.
  - ○ Administer antibiotics as prescribed for infection.
  - ○ Keep the child's skin clean, dry, and lubricated.

- ○ Provide oral hygiene and keep the child's lips lubricated.

- ○ Provide age-appropriate diversional activities.

- ○ Provide support to the children and their families.

    - Avoid false reassurance.

    - Listen to the child's concerns.

    - Allow time for children and their families to discuss feelings regarding loss and to grieve.

- Interdisciplinary Care

    - ○ Social services may be of assistance with access to medications and durable medical equipment if needed.

    - ○ A nutritionist may be involved for development of a diet plan.

- Therapeutic Procedures

    - ○ Treatment for Wilms' tumor

        - Preoperative chemotherapy or radiation to decrease the size of the tumor

        - Surgical removal of the tumor and affected organs

        - Chemotherapy treatment that can last from 6 to 15 months

        - Radiation for children who have recurrent diseases, large tumors, and/or metastasis.

    - ○ Treatment for neuroblastoma

        - Staging is performed to establish initial treatment.

        - Surgical removal of the tumor and to obtain biopsies

        - Radiation in an emergency to decrease the size of a tumor that is compressing the spinal cord

        - Radiation to decrease the size of tumors and palliation for metastasis

    - ○ Chemotherapy

        - Chemotherapeutic agents include vincristine (Oncovin), doxorubicin (Adriamycin), cyclophosphamide (Cytoxan), actinomycin D (Dactinomycin) for Wilms' tumor, and cisplatin (Platinol) for neuroblastoma.

        - Medications may be administered orally, intravenously, or locally (such as intrathecally for a CNS tumor).

        - Children may have a long-term central venous access device (VAD) or a peripherally inserted central catheter (PICC) in place.

        - Nursing Actions

            - ☐ Medicate children with an anti-emetic prior to chemotherapy.

            - ☐ Allow children several food choices, and allow them to choose favorite foods.

- □ Observe the mouth for mucosal ulcerations.
- □ Offer cool fluids to prevent dehydration and soothe sore mucous membranes.
  - ■ Client Education
    - □ Educate children and their families about the side effects of chemotherapy (nausea, vomiting, alopecia).
    - □ Educate children and their families about the importance of immunizations (if immune status adequate) and follow-up appointments.
    - □ Educate children and their families about good infection control practices.
  - o Radiation
    - ■ Radiation is dose calculated and usually delivered in divided treatments over several weeks.
    - ■ Radiation affects rapidly growing cells in the body. Therefore, cells that normally have a fast turnover may be affected in addition to cancer cells.
    - ■ Client Education
      - □ Educate children and their families about the targeted areas, procedure, and provide support.
      - □ Instruct children and their families to wash the marked areas with lukewarm water, use hands instead of a washcloth, pat dry, and take care not to remove the markings. Avoid using hot or cold water.
      - □ Instruct children and their families not to wash off marks that outline the targeted areas. They should wash the marked areas with lukewarm water (avoid hot or cold water), use their hands instead of a washcloth, and pat dry.
      - □ Encourage wearing loose cotton clothing.
      - □ Remind children and their families to keep the areas protected from the sun by wearing a hat and long-sleeved shirts.
      - □ Instruct families to seek medical care for blisters, weeping, and red/tender skin.
- Surgical Interventions
  - o Tumor debulking
    - ■ Nursing Actions
      - □ Preoperative
        - ▸ Avoid palpation of Wilms' tumor.
      - □ Postoperative
        - ▸ Monitor gastrointestinal activity (bowel sounds, bowel movements, distention, nausea, vomiting).
        - ▸ Provide pain relief.

        ▸ Monitor vital signs and note any signs and symptoms of infection.

        ▸ Encourage pulmonary hygiene.

- ■ Client Education

  - □ Reinforce preoperative teaching to children and their families that includes length of surgery, where the child will recover, and what equipment will be in place (nasogastric tube, IV line, indwelling urinary catheter).

- Client Outcomes

  - ○ The child will consume adequate nutritional intake to maintain an appropriate weight.

  - ○ The child will experience minimal side effects from treatments.

  - ○ The child will be free from infection.

Complications

- Pancytopenia

  - ○ Bone marrow depression resulting in anemia, neutropenia, and/or thrombocytopenia

  - ○ Nursing Actions

    - ■ Monitor vital signs and report them to the health care provider. Report a temperature greater than 37.8° C (100° F).

    - ■ Monitor for signs of infection (lung congestion; redness, swelling, and pain around IV sites) and lesions in the mouth, and monitor the client's wound site and immunization status.

    - ■ Administer antimicrobial, antiviral, and antifungal medications as prescribed.

    - ■ Protect the child from sources of possible infection.

      - □ Use proper hand hygiene.

      - □ Encourage the child and family to use proper hand hygiene.

    - ■ Encourage children to avoid crowds while undergoing chemotherapy.

    - ■ Instruct children to avoid fresh fruits and vegetables.

    - ■ Avoid invasive procedures (injections, rectal temperatures, catheters). Apply pressure to puncture sites for 5 min.

    - ■ Monitor for signs of bleeding.

    - ■ Avoid aspirin/NSAIDs.

    - ■ Administer filgrastim (Neupogen), a granulocyte colony-stimulating factor that stimulates WBC production, subcutaneously daily.

    - ■ Administer oprelvekin (Interleukin-11, Neumega) subcutaneously daily as prescribed to stimulate platelet formation.

    - ■ Monitor children for headache and mild to moderate bone pain.

- Administer epoetin alfa (Procrit) subcutaneously two to three times per week as prescribed to stimulate RBC formation.
- Encourage the use of a soft toothbrush.
- Use gentle handling and positioning to protect from injury.
- Organize care to provide for rest. Schedule rest periods.

  o Client Education

  - Educate children and their families about infection control procedures at home.
  - Provide support.

- Anorexia, nausea, vomiting

  o These are side effects of chemotherapy and radiation therapy.

  o Nursing Actions

  - Avoid strong odors. Provide a pleasant atmosphere for meals.
  - Suggest and assist in selecting foods/fluids.
  - Provide small, frequent meals.
  - Administer antiemetics as prescribed, usually before meals.

- Alteration in bowel elimination

  o Diarrhea is a result of radiation to the abdominal area. Some chemotherapeutic agents may cause constipation. If mobility and nutrition decrease, the child is more likely to develop constipation.

  o Nursing Actions

  - Provide meticulous skin care.
  - Provide a nutritious diet.
  - Determine if certain foods or drinks (high fiber, lactose rich) worsen the child's condition.
  - Monitor intake and output and daily weight.

- Stomatitis and dry mouth

  o Nursing Actions

  - Provide a soft toothbrush and/or swabs.
  - Lubricate the child's lips.
  - Give soft, nonacidic foods. A puréed or liquid diet may be required.
  - Provide analgesics.

- ○ Client Education
  - ▪ Encourage a dental visit before therapy.
  - ▪ Encourage the use of mouthwashes, such as 1 tsp salt mixed with 1 pint of water or 1 tsp baking soda mixed with 1 quart of water.
- Alopecia
  - ○ Occurs with chemotherapy and radiation of the head and/or neck
  - ○ Nursing Actions
    - ▪ Assess the child's feelings.
    - ▪ Discuss cutting long hair.
    - ▪ Use gentle shampoos. Gently brush the child's hair using a soft brush; avoid using a comb.
    - ▪ Avoid blow dryers and curling irons.
    - ▪ Suggest wearing a cotton hat or scarf.
  - ○ Client Education
    - ▪ Suggest that families purchase a wig.
    - ▪ Instruct children and their families to avoid blow dryers and curling irons.

LEUKEMIA

Overview

- Leukemia causes an increase in the production of immature WBCs, which leads to infiltration of organs and tissues.
  - ○ Bone marrow infiltration causes crowding of cells that would normally produce RBCs, platelets, and mature WBCs.
    - ▪ Deficient RBCs cause anemia.
    - ▪ Deficient mature WBCs (neutropenia) increase the risk for infection.
    - ▪ Deficient platelets (thrombocytopenia) cause bleeding and bruising.
  - ○ Infiltration of the spleen, liver, and lymph nodes leads to tissue fibrosis.
  - ○ Infiltration of the CNS causes increased intracranial pressure.
  - ○ Other tissues may also be infiltrated (testes, prostate, ovaries, gastrointestinal tract).
- Clinical manifestations are related to the area of involvement (bone pain, abdominal pain, neurosensory changes).

Data Collection

- Risk Factors

  o Leukemia is the most common cancer of childhood.

  o ALL is the most common form of leukemia in children. There is an increased incidence in Caucasian boys older than 1 year of age, with peak onset being between 2 and 6 years of age.

  o Children with trisomy 21 (Down syndrome) have a greater risk of developing ALL.

- Subjective Data

  o History and physical assessment findings may reveal vague reports (anorexia, headache, fatigue).

- Objective Data

  o Physical Assessment Findings

    ■ Early manifestations

      □ Low-grade fever

      □ Pallor

      □ Increased bruising and petechiae

 View Media Supplement: Petechiae (Image)

      □ Listlessness

      □ Enlarged liver, lymph nodes, and joints

      □ Abdominal, leg, and joint pain

      □ Constipation

      □ Headache

      □ Vomiting and anorexia

      □ Unsteady gait

    ■ Late manifestations

      □ Pain

      □ Hematuria

      □ Ulcerations in the mouth

      □ Enlarged kidneys and testicles

      □ Signs of increased intracranial pressure

○ Laboratory Tests

- Complete blood counts

  □ Anemia (low blood counts)

  □ Thrombocytopenia (low platelets)

  □ Neutropenia (low neutrophils)

  □ Leukemic blasts (immature WBCs)

○ Diagnostic Procedures

- Bone marrow aspiration or biopsy analysis

  □ Bone marrow aspiration or biopsy is the most definitive diagnostic procedure. If leukemia is present, the specimen will show prolific quantities of immature leukemic blast cells and protein markers indicating a specific type of leukemia. This procedure is performed by an oncologist.

  □ Nursing Actions

    ‣ Assist the provider with the procedure.

    ‣ Topical anesthetic, such as a eutectic mixture of local anesthetics (EMLA), may be applied over the biopsy area 45 min to 1 hr prior to the procedure.

    ‣ Sedation is induced using a general anesthetic, such as propofol (Diprivan).

    ‣ A specimen from the posterior or anterior iliac crest or tibia is obtained by the provider.

    ‣ Postprocedure

      ▷ Apply pressure to the site for 5 to 10 min.

      ▷ Check vital signs frequently.

      ▷ Apply a pressure dressing.

      ▷ Monitor for signs of bleeding and infection for 24 hr.

  □ Client Education

    ‣ Educate children and their families about the procedure and postprocedure care.

- Cerebrospinal fluid (CSF) analysis
  - □ CSF, obtained by lumbar puncture, is used to determine CNS involvement (increased intracranial pressure).
  - □ Nursing Actions
    - ▸ Have children empty their bladder.
    - ▸ Place children in the fetal position and assist in maintaining the position. Distraction may need to be used.
    - ▸ Assist the provider with the procedure.
      - ▷ A topical anesthetic (EMLA cream) may be applied over the biopsy area 45 min to 1 hr prior to the procedure.
    - ▸ Children may be sedated with fentanyl (Sublimaze) and midazolam (Versed).
    - ▸ The provider will clean the skin and inject a local anesthetic.
    - ▸ The provider will take pressure readings and collect three to five test tubes of CSF.
    - ▸ Pressure will be applied after the needle is removed.
    - ▸ Label specimens appropriately and deliver them to the laboratory.
    - ▸ Monitor the site for hematoma or infection.
  - □ Client Education
    - ▸ Instruct children to remain in bed for 4 to 8 hr in a flat position to prevent leakage and a resulting spinal headache. This may not be possible for an infant, toddler, or preschooler.
- Sonograms
  - □ Sonograms are used to detect liver and spleen infiltration, enlargement, and fibrosis.
  - □ Nursing Actions
    - ▸ Assist with positioning children.
  - □ Client Education
    - ▸ Educate children and their families about the procedure.
    - ▸ Provide emotional support.
- Liver and kidney function studies
  - □ These studies are used for baseline functioning before chemotherapy.
  - □ Nursing Actions
    - ▸ Draw the appropriate amount of serum.

        □   Client Education

           ▸   Educate children and their families about the length of time to receive results.

Collaborative Care

- Nursing Care

  - Provide emotional support to the child and parents.

  - Encourage peer contact if appropriate.

  - Use an age-appropriate pain scale to measure pain.

  - Use pharmacological and nonpharmacological interventions to provide around-the-clock pain management.

- Medications

  - Chemotherapy

  - The treatment for leukemia includes chemotherapy. Choice of chemotherapeutic agents is based on the type of leukemia present. Treatment is given in four phases (induction therapy, CNS prophylactic therapy, intensification therapy and maintenance therapy).

    - Nursing Considerations

      - □ Control nausea and vomiting by giving antiemetics prior to treatment.

      - □ Manage side effects of treatment.

SIDE EFFECT	NURSING INTERVENTIONS
Mucosal ulceration	<ul><li>Provide frequent oral care.</li><li>Inspect the child's mouth for ulceration and hemorrhage.</li><li>Use a soft-bristled toothbrush or a soft, disposable toothbrushes for oral care.</li><li>Lubricate lips with lip balm to prevent cracking.</li><li>Offer foods that are soft and bland.</li><li>Assist children to use mouthwashes (such as 1 tsp salt mixed with 1 pint of water or 1 tsp baking soda mixed with 1 qt of water) frequently.</li><li>Apply local anesthetics (hydrocortisone dental paste [Orabase], antiseptic mouth rinse [UlcerEase], aluminum and magnesium hydroxide [Maalox]) to mucosa to minimize pain.</li><li>Use agents (mouthwashes, lozenges) that are effective against fungal and bacterial infections (chlorhexidine gluconate [Peridex]).</li><li>Avoid viscous lidocaine (causes risk of aspiration from depressed gag reflex), hydrogen peroxide (delays healing), milk of magnesia (dries mucous membranes), and lemon glycerin swabs (causes tooth decay and erosion of tissue).</li></ul>

SIDE EFFECT	NURSING INTERVENTIONS
Skin breakdown	• Inspect skin daily. • Check rectal mucosa for fissures. • Avoid rectal temperatures. • Provide sitz baths as needed. • Reposition frequently. • Use a pressure reduction system.

Neuropathy	• Constipation
	  ○ Encourage a diet high in fiber.
	  ○ Administer stool softeners and laxatives as needed.
	  ○ Encourage fluids.
	• Footdrop
	  ○ Use soft splints when in bed.
	• Weakness and numbness of extremities
	  ○ Assist with ambulation.
	• Jaw pain
	  ○ Provide a soft diet.

Loss of appetite	• Monitor fluid intake and hydration status. • Provide small, frequent, well-balanced meals. • Involve children in meal planning. • Administer enteral nutrition if needed. • Weigh children daily. • Monitor electrolyte values. • Administer chemotherapy early in the day.
Hemorrhagic cystitis	• Encourage fluids – at least one and a half times the daily fluid requirement. • Encourage frequent voiding. • Administer chemotherapy early in the morning to promote adequate fluid intake and voiding. • Administer mesna (Mesnex) to provide protection to the bladder.
Alopecia	• Prepare children and their families in advance for hair loss. • Encourage the use of a cotton hat or scarf or a wig if the child is self-conscious about hair loss.

- Client Education
  - Instruct the parents that the use of steroid treatment may cause moon face.
  - Instruct the parents that the child may experience mood changes.
  - Reinforce teaching with the parents about how to recognize signs of infection, skin breakdown, and nutritional deficiency.
  - Encourage children and their families to maintain good hygiene.

- □ Tell children and their families to avoid individuals with infectious diseases.

- □ Instruct children and their families how to administer medications and provide nutritional support at home.

- □ Instruct the parents in the proper use of vascular access devices (VADs).

- □ Instruct children and their families about bleeding precautions and the management of active bleeding.

- **Interdisciplinary Care**

  - ○ Provide information regarding support services for the child and parents.

- **Therapeutic Procedures**

  - ○ Hematopoietic stem cell transplant (HSCT)

    - ■ HSCT may be indicated for children who have AML during the first remission and for children who have ALL after a second remission.

    - ■ Nursing Actions

      - □ Provide emotional support to the child and family who must deal with the effects of high-dose chemotherapy and radiation to destroy tumor cells.

      - □ After the tumor cells are destroyed, the child is given donor bone marrow or other stem cells, such as those cells from cord blood. Implantation of new cells may take 2 to 6 weeks.

      - □ Implement protective isolation.

        - ‣ A private, positive-pressure room

        - ‣ At least 12 air exchanges/hr

        - ‣ HEPA filtration for incoming air

        - ‣ Wearing of respirator mask, gloves, and gowns

        - ‣ No dried or fresh flowers and no potted plants

    - ■ Client Education

      - □ Inform children and their families that there is an increased risk for infection and bleeding until the transfused stem cells grow.

  - ○ Radiation therapy

    - ■ To brain and spinal cord

    - ■ Nursing Actions

      - □ Assist with positioning.

      - □ Provide support to children and their families.

      - □ Manage side effects.

- Client Education
    - Educate children and their families regarding side effects (fatigue, infection).
    - Encourage adequate rest and a healthy diet.
- Client Outcomes
    - The child will be free of infection.
    - The child will consume adequate nutritional intake to maintain an appropriate weight.

Complications

- Infection
    - Infection can be a complication of myelosuppression.
    - Nursing Actions
        - Provide children with a private room. The room should be designed to allow for adequate air flow to reduce airborne pathogens.
        - Restrict visitors and health personnel with active illnesses.
        - Adhere to strict hand hygiene.
        - Assess potential sites of infections (oral ulcer, open cut) and monitor temperature.
        - Administer antibiotics as prescribed.
        - Monitor the child's absolute neutrophil count (ANC).
        - Encourage adequate protein and caloric intake.
    - Client Education
        - Educate about infection control practices.
        - Educate children and their families about signs of infection and when to call the health care provider.
        - Avoid all immunizations while the immune system is depressed.
- Bleeding
    - Bleeding can be a complication of myelosuppression.
    - Nursing Actions
        - Monitor for signs of bleeding (petechiae, ecchymosis, hematuria, bleeding gums, hematemesis, tarry stools).
        - Avoid unnecessary skin punctures and use surgical aseptic technique when performed. Apply pressure for 5 min to stop bleeding.
        - Treat a nosebleed with cold and pressure.
        - Assist with the administration of platelets as ordered.
        - Avoid obtaining temperatures rectally.

- Client Education
  - Encourage/provide meticulous oral care to prevent gingival bleeding. Use a soft toothbrush and avoid astringent mouthwashes.
  - Reinforce teaching with the parents about measures for controlling epistaxis.
  - Tell children and their families to avoid activities that may lead to injury or bleeding.
- Anemia
  - Anemia can be a complication of myelosuppression.
  - Nursing Actions
    - Assist with the administration of blood transfusions as ordered.
    - Allow for frequent rest periods.
    - Administer oxygen therapy.
    - Assist with the administration of IV fluid replacement.
  - Client Education
    - Educate children and their families about foods high in iron.
- Cardiotoxicity
  - Cardiotoxicity is one of the long-term effects of treatment.
  - Nursing Actions
    - Monitor for cardiac dysfunction by checking blood pressure, heart rate, daily weights, capillary refill, and cardiac rhythm disturbances.
  - Client Education
    - Instruct the parents to obtain pulse and blood pressure readings.
    - Educate the parents about the need to obtain daily weights.
    - Educate children and their families about signs to report to the health care provider.
- Delayed growth and development
  - Delayed growth and development is one of the long-term effects of treatment.
  - Nursing Actions
    - Determine the child's developmental status.
    - Recommend occupational and physical therapy.
  - Client Education
    - Suggest occupational therapy and/or physical therapy as needed.
    - Provide support.

BONE AND SOFT TISSUE MALIGNANCIES

Overview

- Types of bone tumors:

  - Osteosarcoma usually occurs in the metaphysis of long bones, most often in the femur. Treatment frequently includes amputation of the affected extremity as well as chemotherapy.

  - Ewing's sarcoma (a primitive neuroectodermal tumor [PNET]) occurs in the shafts of long bones and of trunk bones. Treatment includes surgical biopsy, intensive radiation therapy to tumor site, and chemotherapy, but not amputation.

    - Prognosis depends on how quickly the disease was diagnosed and whether or not metastasis has occurred.

  - Rhabdomyosarcoma is a soft tissue malignancy that originates in skeletal muscle in any part of the body, but it most commonly occurs in the head and neck, with the orbit of the eye frequently affected. Treatment consists of surgical biopsy, local radiation therapy, and chemotherapy, rather than radical surgical procedures.

- Children who undergo irradiation for malignancies in or near the pelvic area may experience sterilization and/or secondary cancers.

Data Collection

- Risk Factors

  - Osteosarcoma occurs most often in males during puberty, when bone growth is most rapid.

  - Ewing's sarcoma occurs most frequently in individuals 4 years of age and older. It is almost completely confined to those under 30 years of age.

  - Rhabdomyosarcoma occurs more frequently in Caucasian children than in African-American children (the ratio is more than 2:1). The highest incidence is in children younger than 5 years of age.

- Subjective and Objective Data

	SUBJECTIVE DATA	OBJECTIVE DATA
Bone cancers	• Nonspecific bone pain that is often mistaken for an injury or growing pains • Temporarily relief of pain when extremity is flexed	• Weakness, swelling, or decreased movement of the extremity • Palpable lymph nodes near the tumor • Anemia, generalized infection, or unexplained weight loss

	SUBJECTIVE DATA	OBJECTIVE DATA

Rhabdomyosarcoma	• May cause pain in local areas related to compression by the tumor (sore throat may occur with tumor of the nasopharynx)
	
	• Possible absence of pain in some parts of the body, such as in the retroperitoneal area, until the tumor begins to obstruct organs
		• Based on affected area
		  ○ Orbit – Strabismus, exophthalmos, generalized swelling, or color change to conjunctiva
		  ○ Nasopharynx – Palpable area of firm swelling, nasal stuffiness, generalized swelling, palpable lymph nodes, and rhinorrhea
		  ○ Retroperitoneal area – Palpable mass and a urinary or intestinal obstruction

- ○ Laboratory Tests
  - ▪ Alkaline phosphatase – may be elevated in bone malignancies
  - ▪ Complete blood count (CBC) and other common tests can help rule out infection, iron deficiency anemia, and other possible causes of findings.
- ○ Diagnostic Procedures
  - ▪ X-rays, CT scans, and magnetic resonance imaging scans
    - □ These tests may be used to:
      - ▸ Diagnose and evaluate tumor characteristic for types of cancer.
      - ▸ Assess soft tissue to tumor boundaries.
      - ▸ Determine involvement of blood or nerve tissue.
      - ▸ Determine the extent of metastasis (lung, liver).
    - □ Bone scan may be performed to evaluate metastasis of bone tumors.
    - □ Bone marrow aspiration may be performed to diagnose lung or bone marrow metastasis.
  - ▪ Bone marrow aspiration
  - ▪ Cerebrospinal fluid (CSF) analysis
    - □ CSF analysis is used for children who have head/neck rhabdomyosarcoma to evaluate for metastasis to the CNS.

Collaborative Care

- Nursing Care

    - Obtain the child's trust by being honest when answering questions and by giving information about the disease and treatment.

    - Allow children time, usually several days, to prepare emotionally for surgery (especially if amputation is involved) and chemotherapy.

    - Avoid overwhelming children with information.

- Medications

    - Chemotherapy

        - Various agents used singly or in combination before or after surgery – High dose methotrexate with citrovorum factor rescue, doxorubicin, bleomycin, actinomycin D, cyclophosphamide, ifosfamide, cisplatin, vincristine, and etoposide

        - Nursing Considerations

            - Control nausea and vomiting with antiemetics prior to treatment.

            - Manage side effects of treatment.

        - Client Education

            - Reinforce teaching with the family about how to recognize signs of infection, skin breakdown, and nutritional deficiency.

            - Encourage children and their families to maintain good hygiene.

            - Direct the family to members of the health care team who can ensure an understanding about the proper use of vascular access devices.

            - Instruct children and their families about bleeding precautions and management of active bleeding.

    - Amitriptyline (Elavil)

        - A tricyclic antidepressant (TCA) for use with neuropathic pain or phantom pain in adolescents who have amputated limbs.

        - Nursing Considerations

            - Monitor the child for drowsiness, orthostatic hypotension, anticholinergic effects, seizures, mania, and cardiac dysfunction.

        - Client Education

            - Instruct children and their families about how to manage side effects.

            - Caution children and their families about taking only the prescribed dosage to prevent toxic reactions.

- Interdisciplinary Care

  ○ Older children and adolescents may benefit from attending a support group for children who have cancer and/or amputations.

  ○ A mental health counselor may be involved to assist the child to resume normal activities.

  ○ Physical and occupational therapy may begin while the child is in the hospital and continue after discharge.

- Therapeutic Procedures

  ○ Localized radiation therapy

    ■ Radiation therapy may be used in combination with chemotherapy and surgery.

    ■ Nursing Actions

      □ Assist the child with positioning.

      □ Monitor for side effects.

    ■ Client Education

      □ Educate children and their families regarding the course of therapy.

- Surgical Interventions

  ○ Surgical biopsy for any of the bone or soft tissue cancers

    ■ The tumor is biopsied under anesthesia to determine presence and/or tissue type of cancer.

    ■ Nursing Actions

      □ Provide routine pre and postoperative care.

      □ Provide for adequate pain relief.

      □ Monitor wound for signs of infection.

      □ Actions vary with extent and area of surgery, but nursing actions should include pre and postprocedure care, including vital signs, medication for pain, and wound care as necessary.

    ■ Client Education

      □ Educate children and their families regarding postoperative care.

  ○ Limb salvage procedure for osteosarcoma

    ■ This procedure is used only for certain children. It involves a preoperative course of chemotherapy to shrink the tumor and then total bone and joint replacement after the tumor and affected bone are removed.

    ■ Nursing Actions

      □ Monitor children who are receiving preoperative chemotherapy.

      □ Assist with managing side effects.

      ☐ Provide routine postoperative care.

      ☐ Provide adequate pain relief.

   ■ Client Education

      ☐ Educate children and their families regarding postoperative care.

      ☐ Reinforce teaching with children and their families about expected effects of preoperative chemotherapy, such as hair loss.

  o Limb amputation for osteosarcoma

   ■ Amputation of the affected limb should occur above the joint or 7.5 cm (3 in) above the proximal edge of the tumor. This may include unilateral removal of the scapula and clavicle for tumors of the upper humerus and removal of portions of the pelvis for tumors of the hip. The child may receive chemotherapy both preoperatively and postoperatively.

   ■ Nursing Actions

      ☐ Provide routine pre and postoperative care.

      ☐ Provide emotional support.

      ☐ Care for the residual limb as prescribed.

      ☐ Ask about phantom limb pain postoperatively and medicate appropriately.

   ■ Client Education

      ☐ Prepare children for fitting of a temporary prosthesis, which may occur immediately after surgery.

      ☐ Encourage cooperation with postoperative physical therapy.

      ☐ Work with children and their families to plan for issues such as appropriate clothing to wear with prosthesis.

      ☐ Role play issues that children will need to deal with after discharge, such as talking to strangers who ask about the prosthesis.

      ☐ Assist the family to recognize that the child's emotions, such as anger, are normal grief reactions after amputation, chemotherapy, and other treatments.

● Care After Discharge

  o Client Education

   ■ Educate children and their families regarding the importance of follow-up care.

  o Community Services

   ■ Discuss appropriate community services to resume normal activities (school attendance, physical activities).

● Client Outcomes

  o The child will be free of postoperative pain, including phantom limb pain for those children who must undergo amputation.

  o The child will learn strategies to manage side effects of radiation and/or chemotherapy.

- o The child will express feelings regarding loss.
- o The child will participate in age-appropriate activities.

Complications

- Skin desquamation (either dry or moist) with permanent hyperpigmentation and possible damage to underlying structures
  - o Nursing Actions
    - Observe the site frequently for signs of infection.
    - Monitor for damage to underlying structures (nerves, blood vessels) by checking circulation and movement.
  - o Client Education
    - Reinforce teaching with the parents about methods to prevent additional irritation to the site (use loose-fitting clothing, prevent exposure to sunlight or extremes of temperature).
    - Reinforce teaching with adolescents about risks of sterilization if indicated.
    - Explain the importance of continuing follow-up examinations.
- Myelosuppression
  - o Elimination of normal blood cells along with cancer cells is a risk with treatment by most chemotherapeutic agents. This may cause infection (reduced leukocytes), hemorrhage (reduced thrombocytes), and anemia (reduced RBCs).
  - o Nursing Actions
    - Evaluate laboratory data and observe for signs of complications.
      - □ Infection – Elevated WBC and fever
      - □ Hemorrhage – Blood in urine or stool, bruising, and petechiae
      - □ Anemia – Fatigue and decreased Hgb/Hct
    - Prevent infection
      - □ Provide a private room when hospitalized.
      - □ Restrict staff/visitors who have infections.
      - □ Promote frequent hand hygiene by staff/visitors.
      - □ Avoid all live-virus vaccines during periods of immunosuppression.
      - □ Ensure that siblings are up-to-date on vaccinations.
      - □ Provide a diet adequate in proteins and calories.
    - Prevent hemorrhage or injury from bleeding.
      - □ Use a strict aseptic technique for all invasive procedures.
      - □ Use gentle technique when providing mouth care.

□ Clean the perineal area carefully to prevent trauma and avoid obtaining temperatures rectally.

□ Infuse platelets as prescribed.

■ Prevent anemia or injury from anemia.

□ Provide rest periods as needed.

□ Infuse packed red blood cells as prescribed.

o Client Education

■ Reinforce teaching with family members about strategies to recognize complications at home and to prevent damage from infection, hemorrhage, or bleeding.

■ Recommend children avoid activities that can cause injury or bleeding, such as bicycle riding, skateboarding, climbing on playground equipment, and contact sports.

(A) APPLICATION EXERCISES

1. A nurse is caring for a 2-year-old child with Wilms' tumor and is reviewing teaching about chemotherapy with the parent of the child. Which of the following statements by the parent indicates the need for further teaching?

   A. "I should observe my son's mouth for sores."

   B. "Having the PICC line means he won't have to be stuck so often."

   C. "I'm glad he will get all his medications through the PICC."

   D. "He will receive medications to prevent nausea before he has chemotherapy."

2. A nurse is reviewing teaching with an adolescent client on chemotherapy who is receiving epoetin alfa (Procrit). Which of the following statements by the client indicates an understanding of the medication?

   A. "I have to take Procrit so I will manufacture white blood cells."

   B. "My platelet count is low, which is why I need Procrit."

   C. "This medication is an iron supplement."

   D. "Procrit helps build up my bone marrow so I make more red blood cells."

3. A nurse is caring for an adolescent female client experiencing hair loss due to radiation therapy for a brain tumor. How should the nurse assist the client in managing her hair loss?

Scenario: A nurse is caring for a school-age child with leukemia.

4. The nurse is assisting the provider to perform a bone marrow aspiration on the child. Place the following steps of this procedure in the correct order.

   _____ Maintain pressure to the aspiration site for 5 to 10 min.

   _____ Check vital signs frequently.

   _____ Apply EMLA to the biopsy site.

   _____ Apply a pressure dressing.

   _____ Place the child in the fetal position.

   _____ Have the child empty the bladder.

5. The nurse observes that the child has ulcerations of the oral mucosa. Which of the following is an appropriate nursing action to manage the ulcerations? (Select all that apply.)

   _____ Offer lemon glycerin swabs periodically.

   _____ Apply lip balm frequently.

   _____ Use foam-tipped applicators for oral hygiene.

   _____ Encourage soft, bland foods.

   _____ Have the child swish with oral anesthetic solutions.

6. Match the following types of cancer with their anatomic location.

_____	Acute lymphoid leukemia	1. Adrenal gland
_____	Osteosarcoma	2. Kidney or abdomen
_____	Wilms' tumor	3. Bone marrow
_____	Neuroblastoma	4. Long bones
_____	Rhabdomyosarcoma	5. Skeletal muscle

7. A nurse is caring for a school-age child with rhabdomyosarcoma who is undergoing chemotherapy. The child is losing weight, experiencing nausea, and has no appetite. Identify actions the nurse should use to promote adequate nutritional intake.

APPLICATION EXERCISES ANSWER KEY

1. A nurse is caring for a 2-year-old child with Wilms' tumor and is reviewing teaching about chemotherapy with the parent of the child. Which of the following statements by the parent indicates the need for further teaching?

   A. "I should observe my son's mouth for sores."

   B. "Having the PICC line means he won't have to be stuck so often."

   C. "I'm glad he will get all his medications through the PICC."

   D. "He will receive medications to prevent nausea before he has chemotherapy."

   Chemotherapy is administered by various routes – orally, intravenously, or locally. Advise the parent to observe the child's mouth for ulcerations of the oral mucosa Antiemetics are administered orally or intravenously prior to and during chemotherapy. Having a peripherally inserted central catheter (PICC) reduces the frequency of venipunctures.

   NCLEX® Connection: Reduction of Risk Potential, Therapeutic Procedures

2. A nurse is reviewing teaching with an adolescent client on chemotherapy who is receiving epoetin alfa (Procrit). Which of the following statements by the client indicates an understanding of the medication?

   A. "I have to take Procrit so I will manufacture white blood cells."

   B. "My platelet count is low, which is why I need Procrit."

   C. "This medication is an iron supplement."

   D. "Procrit helps build up my bone marrow so I make more red blood cells."

   Procrit is administered to clients with anemia due to bone marrow suppression. Clients with anemia lack red blood cells and Procrit helps to simulate the bone marrow to manufacture red blood cells. Procrit does not stimulate white blood cell or platelet production and is not an iron supplement.

   NCLEX® Connection: Pharmacological Therapies, Expected Actions/Outcomes

3. A nurse is caring for an adolescent female client experiencing hair loss due to radiation therapy for a brain tumor. How should the nurse assist the client in managing her hair loss?

   Talk with the client about her feelings regarding her hair and hair loss. Suggest cutting her hair in an easy-to-manage style and purchasing wigs or colorful scarves and hats. A gentle shampoo and limited brushing reduces the risk of skin injury. The use of hair dryers and curling irons should be avoided. Participation in a support group for adolescents with cancer is another suggestion since members will have comments about dealing with hair loss.

   NCLEX® Connection: Reduction of Risk Potential, Potential for Complications of Diagnostic Tests/Treatments/Procedures

Scenario: A nurse is caring for a school-age child with leukemia.

4. The nurse is assisting the provider to perform a bone marrow aspiration on the child. Place the following steps of this procedure in the correct order.

   __4__   Maintain pressure to the aspiration site for 5 to 10 min.

   __6__   Check vital signs frequently.

   __1__   Apply EMLA to the biopsy site.

   __5__   Apply a pressure dressing.

   __3__   Place the child in the fetal position.

   __2__   Have the child empty the bladder.

   A topical anesthetic, such as EMLA cream, is applied to the biopsy site 45 min to 1 hr prior to the procedure. Have the child empty the bladder before placing the child in the fetal position. Assist the child to remain in that position. Following the aspiration, maintain pressure to the biopsy site for 5 to 10 min and apply a pressure dressing. Check vital signs frequently following the procedure.

   NCLEX® Connection: Reduction of Risk Potential, Diagnostic Tests

5. The nurse observes that the child has ulcerations of the oral mucosa. Which of the following is an appropriate nursing action to manage the ulcerations? (Select all that apply.)

   _____   Offer lemon glycerin swabs periodically.

   __X__   **Apply lip balm frequently.**

   __X__   **Use foam-tipped applicators for oral hygiene.**

   __X__   **Encourage soft, bland foods.**

   __X__   **Have the child swish with oral anesthetic solutions.**

   Management of ulcerations of the oral mucosa focuses on keeping the lips moist by using lip balm to prevent cracking. Frequent oral hygiene is done using soft toothbrushes or disposable foam-tipped applicators. Foods should be soft and bland. Use local anesthetic solutions to minimize pain. Give antifungal and antibacterial agents to prevent mouth infections. Do not use lemon glycerin swabs as they cause tooth decay and tissue erosion.

   NCLEX® Connection: Reduction of Risk Potential, Potential for Complications of Diagnostic Tests/Treatments/Procedures

6. Match the following types of cancer with their anatomic location.

__3__	Acute lymphoid leukemia	1. Adrenal gland
__4__	Osteosarcoma	2. Kidney or abdomen
__2__	Wilms' tumor	3. Bone marrow
__1__	Neuroblastoma	4. Long bones
__5__	Rhabdomyosarcoma	5. Skeletal muscle

(N) **NCLEX® Connection: Physiological Adaptations, Basic Pathophysiology**

7. A nurse is caring for a school-age child with rhabdomyosarcoma who is undergoing chemotherapy. The child is losing weight, experiencing nausea, and has no appetite. Identify actions the nurse should use to promote adequate nutritional intake.

Involve the child in food selection. Do not give the child favorite foods when nauseated. Medicate the child for nausea before meals. Encourage small, frequent meals. Encourage high-protein, high-calorie food choices. Give the child high-protein, high-calorie shakes. Weigh the child daily to monitor weight loss or gain. Make food attractive and unusual, such as cutting a sandwich into a star shape with a cookie cutter. Allow the parents to bring the child's favorite food from home. Involve the parents in order to learn about the child's usual preferences.

(N) **NCLEX® Connection: Basic Care and Comfort, Nutrition and Oral Hydration**

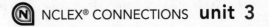

UNIT 3: NURSING CARE OF CHILDREN WITH SPECIAL NEEDS

- Pediatric Emergencies

- Psychosocial Issues of Infants, Children, and Adolescents

NCLEX® CONNECTIONS

When reviewing the chapters in this section, keep in mind the relevant sections of the NCLEX® outline, in particular:

CLIENT NEEDS: HEALTH PROMOTION & MAINTENANCE

Relevant topics/tasks include:
- Data Collection Techniques
  - Collect data for health history.
- Developmental Stages and Transitions
  - Identify and report client deviations from expected growth and development.
- Health Promotion/Disease Prevention
  - Reinforce teaching with client about health risks and health promotion.

CLIENT NEEDS: PSYCHOSOCIAL INTEGRITY

Relevant topics/tasks include:
- Abuse/Neglect
  - Recognize risk factors for domestic, child, and/or elder abuse/neglect, and sexual abuse.
- Crisis Intervention
  - Identify client risk for self injury and/or violence (e.g., suicide or violence precaution).

CLIENT NEEDS: PHYSIOLOGICAL ADAPTATION

Relevant topics/tasks include:
- Alterations in Body Systems
  - Notify primary health care provider of a change in client status.
- Fluid and Electrolyte Imbalances
  - Monitor client response to interventions to correct fluid and/or electrolyte imbalance.
- Medical Emergencies
  - Respond to a client life-threatening situation.

Overview

- Respiratory emergencies

    o   Respiratory failure occurs when there is a diminished ability to maintain adequate oxygenation of the blood. A manifestation of respiratory insufficiency is increased work of breathing.

    o   Airway obstruction prevents adequate air exchange. Obstruction may lead to respiratory failure or arrest if not corrected.

    o   Respiratory arrest occurs when breathing stops completely.

    o   Apnea is the cessation of breathing for more than 20 seconds or for a shorter period of time when associated with hypoxemia or bradycardia.

    o   When respiratory distress is treated or rescue breathing is started in a timely manner, infants and children are less likely than adults to have cardiac arrest.

- Drowning – Asphyxiation while being submerged in fluid

    o   Near-drowning incidents are those in which children have survived for 24 hr after being submerged in fluid.

    o   Drowning may occur in any standing body of water that is at least 1 inch in depth (bathtub, toilet, bucket, pool, pond, lake).

- Sudden infant death syndrome (SIDS)

    o   SIDS is the sudden, unpredictable, and undetectable death of an infant without an identified cause, even after investigation and autopsy.

    o   SIDS is a diagnosis of exclusion that is made only after every other cause of death is discarded. SIDS is not caused by suffocation.

    o   SIDS is a major cause of death in infants from 1 month to 1 year of age, and it occurs frequently in the winter months.

    o   SIDS is not preventable, but risks may be reduced.

    o   Education about reducing the risk of SIDS is increasing.

- Poisoning – Ingestion of or exposure to toxic substances

    o   Most poisonings occur in the child's home or homes of relatives or friends.

    o   Poisonings may also occur in schools or health care facilities.

- o Acetaminophen (Tylenol) is the most common medication poisoning in children (a toxic dose is 150 mg/kg or higher).
- o Toxic substances leading to poisoning are usually ingested, but some may be inhaled.
  - Liquid corrosives cause more damage than granular corrosives.
  - Immediate danger with hydrocarbon ingestion is aspiration.
- o It is vital to use methods to prevent poisoning.

Data Collection

- Risk Factors
  - o Respiratory emergencies (respiratory failure, respiratory arrest)

FUNCTIONAL ALTERATION	POSSIBLE CAUSES
Primary inefficient gas exchange	<ul><li>Cerebral trauma</li><li>Brain tumor</li><li>Overdose of barbiturates, opioids, and/or benzodiazepines</li><li>Asphyxia</li><li>CNS infection (encephalitis)</li></ul>
Obstructive lung disease (increased resistance)	<ul><li>Aspiration</li><li>Infection</li><li>Tumor</li><li>Anaphylaxis</li><li>Laryngospasm</li><li>Asthma</li></ul>
Restrictive lung disease	<ul><li>Cystic fibrosis<ul><li>o Pneumonia</li></ul></li><li>Respiratory distress syndrome</li></ul>

- o Drowning or near-drowning
  - Age of the child
    - □ In children over 12 months of age, drowning is a significant cause of accidental death.
  - Gender
    - □ Males are five times more likely to drown than females.
  - Swimming ability (may be overconfident) or lack of ability
  - Lack of supervision (Children can drown while being supervised.)
  - Boating without life jackets
  - Diving into water

- ○ SIDS
  - Healthy infant
  - Death associated with sleep without signs of suffering
  - Maternal health and behaviors during pregnancy.
    - □ Age less than 20 years
    - □ Alcohol, drug, and/or tobacco use
    - □ Low weight gain during pregnancy
    - □ Anemia
    - □ Placental abnormalities
    - □ Sexually transmitted disease or urinary tract infection
    - □ Inadequate prenatal care
  - Twins
  - Premature birth
  - Small for gestational age
  - Persistent apnea
  - Bronchopulmonary dysplasia
  - Family history of SIDS
  - Environmental risk factors
    - □ Low socioeconomic status
    - □ Crowded living conditions
    - □ Cold weather
    - □ Use of soft items in crib (stuffed animals, blankets)
    - □ Prone sleeping position
    - □ Sleeping with others
- ○ Poisoning
  - Children who are younger than 6 years of age are more likely to ingest toxic substances due to their developmental level. (Infants explore their environment orally, and preschoolers imitate others.)
  - Medications, household chemicals, plants, and heavy metals are potential sources of toxic ingestion.
  - Lead may be ingested or small particles inhaled during renovations of areas with lead-based paint.
  - Common toxic substances ingested by children include acetaminophen, aspirin, iron, hydrocarbons, corrosives, and/or lead.

- Subjective Data

  o Respiratory emergencies

    ■ History of illnesses (chronic or acute)

    ■ History of events leading to respiratory emergency

    ■ Presence of allergies

  o Drowning/Near drowning

    ■ History of event including location and time of submersion

      □ Salt water or nonsalt water drowning

      □ Warm or cold water drowning (bathtub versus cold lake)

  o SIDS

    ■ History of events prior to finding infant

    ■ History of illnesses

    ■ Pregnancy and birth history

    ■ Exposure to tobacco smoke

    ■ Presence of risk factors

    ■ Family coping and support

  o Poisoning

    ■ History of chronic and acute illnesses

- Objective Data

  o Physical Assessment Findings

    ■ Respiratory emergencies

      □ Central or peripheral cyanosis indicates hypoxia

      □ Tachycardia or bradycardia (severe sign of hypoxia)

      □ Tachypnea or bradypnea (severe sign of hypoxia), expiratory grunting, nasal flaring, and presence of retractions and area noted, such as intercostal (between ribs)

      □ Capillary refill greater than 2 seconds indicates decreased perfusion

      □ CNS symptoms ranging from restlessness and lethargy to coma (severe sign)

      □ Diaphoresis

      □ Signs of choking

        ▸ Universal choking sign (clutching neck with thumb and index finger)

        ▸ Inability to speak

        ▸ Weak, ineffective cough

        ▸ High-pitched sounds or no sounds made while inhaling

- ▸ Dyspnea
- ▸ Cyanosis
- ■ Drowning/Near Drowning
  - □ Body temperature for hypothermia
  - □ Bruises, spinal cord injury, or other physical injuries
  - □ Tachypnea or bradypnea (severe sign of hypoxia), expiratory grunting, nasal flaring, and presence of retractions and area noted, such as intercostal (between ribs)
- ■ SIDS
  - □ Blood-tinged fluid is in the mouth.
  - □ The infant was found face down in the bed.
  - □ Fingers may be clenched.
- ■ Poisoning
  - □ List of medications or chemicals that the child may have been exposed to
  - □ Number of pills or amount of liquid ingested
  - □ Time of ingestion
  - □ Physical response
    - ▸ Respiratory rate, rhythm, and effort
    - ▸ Heart rate and rhythm
    - ▸ Level of consciousness
    - ▸ Seizures
    - ▸ Pupil size and response
    - ▸ Swelling of facial area, especially lips and mouth
    - ▸ Color of mucous membranes
    - ▸ Peripheral pulses
    - ▸ Diaphoretic or dry skin
    - ▸ Presence or absence of bowel sounds

SUBSTANCE	CLINICAL MANIFESTATIONS
Acetaminophen	• 2 to 4 hr after ingestion – Nausea, vomiting, sweating, and pallor • 24 to 36 hr after ingestion – Improvement in the child's condition • 36 hr to 7 days or longer (hepatic stage) – Pain in upper right quadrant, confusion, stupor, jaundice, and coagulation disturbances • Final stage – Death or gradual recovery
Acetylsalicylic acid (Aspirin)	• Acute poisoning – Nausea, vomiting, dehydration, disorientation, diaphoresis, hyperpnea, hyperpyrexia, tinnitus, oliguria, lightheadedness, and seizures • Chronic poisoning – Subtle version of acute manifestations, bleeding tendencies, dehydration, and seizures more severe than acute poisoning
Supplemental iron	• Initial period (30 min to 6 hr after ingestion) – Vomiting, hematemesis, diarrhea, gastric pain, and bloody stools • Latency period (2 to 12 hr after ingestion) – Improvement of the child's condition • Systemic toxicity period (4 to 24 hr after ingestion) – Metabolic acidosis, hyperglycemia, bleeding, fever, shock, and possible death • Hepatic injury period (48 to 96 hr after ingestion) – Seizures or coma
Hydrocarbons (gasoline, kerosene, lighter fluid, paint thinner, turpentine, lamp oil)	• Gagging, choking, coughing, nausea, and vomiting • Lethargy, weakness, tachypnea, cyanosis, grunting, and retractions
Corrosives (household cleaners, batteries, denture cleaners, bleach)	• Pain and burning in mouth, throat, and stomach • Edematous lips, tongue, and pharynx with white mucous membranes • Violent vomiting with hemoptysis • Drooling • Anxiety and agitation • Shock
Lead	• Low-dose exposure – Easily distracted, impulsive, hyperactive, hearing impaired, and mild intellectual difficulty • High-dose exposure – Mental retardation, blindness, paralysis, coma, seizures, and death • Other manifestations – Renal impairment, impaired calcium function, and anemia

- ○ Laboratory Tests
  - ▪ Respiratory emergencies
    - ▫ ABGs confirm oxygenation level.
  - ▪ Poisoning
    - ▫ Lead levels in blood or acetaminophen serum levels
    - ▫ CBC with differential to identify anemia
    - ▫ ABGs to assess oxygenation status
    - ▫ Serum iron
- ○ Diagnostic Procedures
  - ▪ Respiratory Emergencies (including near drowning) – Chest radiographs
    - ▫ Chest radiographs determine the status of lungs with respiratory distress in cases of near drowning.
    - ▫ Nursing Actions
      - ‣ Assist with positioning children.
  - ▪ Poisoning – Liver function tests
    - ▫ Liver function tests should be used to identify liver damage.
    - ▫ Nursing Actions
      - ‣ Draw the appropriate amount of serum for laboratory tests.
    - ▫ Client Education
      - ‣ Educate families on the timing of results.

Collaborative Care

- ● Nursing Care
  - ○ Follow the American Heart Association guidelines for CPR for respiratory and cardiac arrest.
    - ▪ Follow the facility's procedure for activating the emergency response team.
    - ▪ Use the current basic life support (BLS) and advanced cardiac life support (ACLS) guidelines for neonates and for pediatric clients.
    - ▪ Maintain current BLS and/or PALS/ACLS skills.
  - ○ Obstructed Airway
    - ▪ Responsive victim
      - ▫ Infants – Use a combination of back blows and chest thrusts.
      - ▫ Children and adolescents – Use abdominal thrusts.

- Remove any obstruction or large debris, but do not reach into the mouth of an infant to prevent pushing the obstruction farther down the throat. No blind finger sweeps.

- Place recovered children (those who resume breathing) into the recovery position (on side with legs bent at knees to stabilize in place).

- Use a calm approach with children and their families.

- Administer oxygen as prescribed.

- Assist with administration of medications, IV fluids, and emergency medications as prescribed.

- Keep the family informed of the child's status.

- ○ SIDS

  - Reduction of risk

    - □ Place infants on back for sleep.

    - □ Prevent exposure to tobacco smoke.

    - □ Prevent overheating.

    - □ Use a firm, tight-fitting mattress in the infant's crib.

    - □ Remove pillows, quilts, and sheepskins from the crib during sleep.

    - □ Ensure that the infant's head is kept uncovered during sleep.

  - Death

    - □ Allow the infant's family an opportunity to express feelings.

    - □ Provide private time for families to be with infants after death.

    - □ Provide support.

    - □ Provide home monitoring for those at high risk, such as a remaining twin.

- ○ Poisoning

  - Assist with intubation if needed, and observe symmetrical movement of the child's chest.

  - Position children with the head of the bed slightly elevated unless contraindicated.

  - Keep emergency equipment (oral airway, suction catheter) at bedside.

  - Apply a cardiac monitor to children.

  - Monitor pulse oximetry for infants.

  - Assist with insertion of an IV and administration of fluids as prescribed.

  - Insert a NG tube as ordered.

  - Insert an indwelling urinary catheter and attach to urine bag.

  - Monitor I&O.

- ▪ Administer the specific antidote as prescribed.
- ▪ Keep the family informed of the child's condition and needs.

INTERVENTIONS FOR SPECIFIC SUBSTANCES	
SUBSTANCE	NURSING INTERVENTIONS
Acetaminophen	• Acetylcysteine (Mucomyst) given orally
Acetylsalicylic acid (Aspirin)	• Activated charcoal • Gastric lavage • Sodium bicarbonate transfusions used to correct metabolic acidosis • Oxygen and ventilation • Vitamin K • Hemodialysis for severe cases
Supplemental iron	• Emesis or lavage • Chelation therapy using deferoxamine mesylate (Desferal)
Hydrocarbons (gasoline, kerosene, lighter fluid, paint thinner, turpentine, lamp oil)	• No induced vomiting • Intubation with cuffed endotracheal tube prior to any gastric decontamination • Treatment of chemical pneumonia
Corrosives (household cleaners, batteries, denture cleaners, bleach)	• Airway maintenance • NPO • No attempt to neutralize • No induced vomiting • Analgesics for pain
Lead	• Chelation therapy using calcium disodium versenate (calcium EDTA)

- • Medications
  - ○ Obstructed airway
    - ▪ Steroids
      - □ Administer for inflammation.
      - □ Nursing Considerations
        - ‣ Administer as prescribed.
        - ‣ Monitor for allergies and effectiveness of the medication.
      - □ Client Education
        - ‣ Reinforce teaching to children and their families how to administer home doses (scheduling).
    - ▪ Bronchodilators – Albuterol (Proventil)

□ Nursing Considerations

‣ Monitor respirations and cardiovascular status.

□ Client Education

‣ Reinforce teaching to children about the importance of using a spacer with the medication if a metered-dose inhaler is prescribed.

- Interdisciplinary Care

  o SIDS

    ▪ Recommend support groups.

    ▪ Recommend counseling.

- Therapeutic Procedures

  o Intubation may be needed with placement on a ventilator.

    ▪ For children with respiratory emergencies, near drowning, and/or poisoning where the airway is unstable and aspiration is likely

    ▪ Nursing Actions

      □ Assist with positioning during intubation to reduce the possibility of injury.

    ▪ Client Education

      □ Reinforce teaching to families about the procedure and what to expect when seeing the child.

- Care After Discharge

  o Client Education

    ▪ Respiratory emergencies

      □ Educate the parents about the risk for obstruction in children. Avoid balloons, small buttons, small candies, hot dogs, and any other foods or objects that may be easily aspirated.

    ▪ Drowning

      □ Encourage the parents of toddlers to lock toilet seats when children are at home.

      □ Do not leave children unattended in the bathtub.

      □ Do not leave children unattended in a swimming pool, even if the children have had swimming lessons.

      □ Make sure private pools have locking gates to prevent the child from wandering into the area.

      □ Have children wear a life jacket while boating.

    ▪ SIDS

      □ Encourage using a home monitoring system for future infants.

      □ Educate or reinforce proper sleeping position, crib environment, smoke-free environment, and the avoidance of overheating.

- Poisoning
  - □ Keep the telephone number for the Poison Control Center (PCC) near the telephone.
  - □ Contact the PCC before taking any action other than maintaining the child's airway.
  - □ Do not give children ipecac.
  - □ Install childproof locks on cabinets containing potentially harmful substances (medications, alcohol, cleaning solutions, mouthwash, outdoor chemicals).
  - □ Supervise children when they are taking medications.
  - □ Do not take medication in front of children.
  - □ Discard unused medications.
  - □ Keep plants out of the reach of children.
  - □ Eliminate lead-based paint in the home.
  - □ Use nonmercury thermometers.
  - □ Reinforce teaching to children about the hazards of ingesting nonfood items.
- Client Outcomes
  - ○ The child will be free of injury.

Complications

- Respiratory arrest
  - ○ Can result from any cause, including drowning, poisoning, and possible SIDS
  - ○ Nursing Actions
    - Initiate CPR.
  - ○ Client Education
    - Encourage families to attend CPR classes.
- Death
  - ○ Nursing Actions
    - Allow private time for the parents to be with the child.
    - Support the parents.

(A) APPLICATION EXERCISES

1. A nurse is reinforcing teaching to a group of parents who have toddlers regarding pool safety. What should the nurse discuss with the parents about pool safety?

2. A nurse is reviewing SIDS prevention with a mother. Which of the following points should the nurse include in the discussion? (Select all that apply.)

    _____ Cover the infant's head with a warm hat when sleeping.

    _____ Do not expose the infant to tobacco smoke.

    _____ Use a space heater in the infant's room.

    _____ Be sure the crib has a firm, tight-fitting mattress.

    _____ Remove pillows and quilts from the crib when the infant is sleeping.

3. Match the following toxic substances ingested by children with the symptoms seen in poisoning caused by the substance.

    _____ Acetaminophen   A. Blindness and seizures

    _____ Iron supplements   B. Lethargy and cyanosis

    _____ Lighter fluid   C. Drooling and white mucous membranes

    _____ Bleach   D. Bleeding and fever

    _____ Lead   E. Confusion and jaundice

4. A nurse is reviewing CPR techniques for an obstructed airway with the parent of an infant. Which of the following statements indicates the parent understands the technique?

    A. "I will use back blows and chest thrusts."

    B. "I need to do a finger sweep of the mouth."

    C. "I will use abdominal thrusts."

    D. "I will place him on his back when he begins breathing."

5. Match the type of poisoning in the first column with the treatment in the second column.

    _____ Hydrocarbons   A. Acetylcysteine (Mucomyst) given orally

    _____ Lead   B. Chelation therapy using deferoxamine mesylate (Desferal)

    _____ Iron supplements   C. Chelation therapy using calcium disodium versenate (calcium EDTA)

    _____ Acetaminophen   D. Intubation with cuffed endotracheal tube prior to any gastric decontamination

Ⓐ APPLICATION EXERCISES ANSWER KEY

1. A nurse is reinforcing teaching to a group of parents who have toddlers regarding pool safety. What should the nurse discuss with the parents about pool safety?

    Locked gates to the pool prevent children from gaining access to the area. Do not permit children in a pool unattended.

Ⓝ NCLEX® Connection: Safety and Infection Control, Accident/Error/Injury Prevention

2. A nurse is reviewing SIDS prevention with a mother. Which of the following points should the nurse include in the discussion? (Select all that apply.)

_____	Cover the infant's head with a warm hat when sleeping.
__X__	**Do not expose the infant to tobacco smoke.**
_____	Use a space heater in the infant's room.
__X__	**Be sure the crib has a firm, tight-fitting mattress.**
__X__	**Remove pillows and quilts from the crib when the infant is sleeping.**

    To reduce the risk of SIDS, tell the parents to avoid exposing the infant to tobacco smoke, have a firm, tight-fitting mattress in the crib, remove pillows and quilts from the crib when the infant is sleeping, keep the infant's head uncovered during sleep, and place the infant on his back while sleeping. A space heater can cause overheating.

Ⓝ NCLEX® Connection: Psychosocial Integrity, End of Life Care

3. Match the following toxic substances ingested by children with the symptoms seen in poisoning caused by the substance.

__E__	Acetaminophen	A. Blindness and seizures
__D__	Iron supplements	B. Lethargy and cyanosis
__B__	Lighter fluid	C. Drooling and white mucous membranes
__C__	Bleach	D. Bleeding and fever
__A__	Lead	E. Confusion and jaundice

Ⓝ NCLEX® Connection: Safety and Infection Control, Accident/Error/Injury Prevention

4. A nurse is reviewing CPR techniques for an obstructed airway with the parent of an infant. Which of the following statements indicates the parent understands the technique?

    A. "I will use back blows and chest thrusts."

    B. "I need to do a finger sweep of the mouth."

    C. "I will use abdominal thrusts."

    D. "I will place him on his back when he begins breathing."

    CPR techniques for an infant who has an obstructed airway include a combination of back blows and chest thrusts. A finger sweep to remove any obstruction is not done to prevent pushing obstructions farther down the throat. Abdominal thrusts are done on children and adolescents. Place the infant who resumes breathing on his side with knees bent, which is the recovery position.

    (N) NCLEX® Connection: Physiological Adaptations, Medical Emergencies

5. Match the type of poisoning in the first column with the treatment in the second column.

__D__	Hydrocarbons	A. Acetylcysteine (Mucomyst) given orally
__C__	Lead	B. Chelation therapy using deferoxamine mesylate (Desferal)
__B__	Iron supplements	C. Chelation therapy using calcium disodium versenate (calcium EDTA)
__A__	Acetaminophen	D. Intubation with cuffed endotracheal tube prior to any gastric decontamination

    (N) NCLEX® Connection: Safety and Infection Control, Accident/Error/Injury Prevention

UNIT 3	NURSING CARE OF CHILDREN WITH SPECIAL NEEDS
Chapter 40	Psychosocial Issues of Infants, Children, and Adolescents

Overview

- Mental health and developmental disorders in children are not always easily diagnosed, and treatment interventions may be delayed or inadequate. This is because:

    o Children do not have the ability or the necessary skills to describe what is happening.

    o Children demonstrate a wide variety of normal behaviors, especially in different developmental stages.

    o It is difficult to determine if the child's behavior indicates an emotional problem.

- A child's behavior is problematic when it interferes with home, school, and interactions with peers.

    o Behaviors become pathologic when they:

        ▪ Are not age appropriate.

        ▪ Deviate from cultural and societal norms.

        ▪ Create deficits or impairments in adaptive functioning.

- Disorders that may appear during childhood and adolescence

    o Childhood depression, including suicide

    o Anxiety disorders

    o Substance abuse – the use of cigarettes, alcohol, illegal drugs, and prescription medications

    o Eating disorders, particularly among females

    o Behavioral disorders, such as attention deficit hyperactivity disorder (ADHD), oppositional defiant disorder, and conduct disorder

    o Pervasive developmental disorders, such as an autistic disorder

- Childhood disorders may have comorbid conditions.

- Characteristics of good mental health for children and adolescents

    o Ability to appropriately interpret reality and have a correct perception of the surrounding environment

    o Positive self-concept

- o Ability to cope with stress and anxiety in a healthy and age-appropriate way
- o Mastery of developmental tasks
- o Ability to express self spontaneously and creatively
- o Ability to develop satisfying relationships

Data Collection

- Risk Factors

  - o Genetics
  - o Biochemical
  - o Social and environmental
  - o Cultural and ethnic
  - o Degree of resiliency
  - o Occurrence of trauma or of experiencing traumatic events in the formative years
  - o Familial tendencies

MOOD DISORDERS

Overview

- Mood (affective) disorders may occur in childhood. Mood disorders that children are at risk for include major depressive and dysthymic disorders.

Data Collection

- Risk factors

  - o Family history of depression
  - o Physical or sexual abuse or neglect
  - o Homelessness
  - o Disputes among parents, conflicts with peers or family, and rejection by peers or family
  - o High-risk behavior
  - o Learning disabilities
  - o Chronic illness

- Subjective and Objective Data

  - o Feelings of sadness
  - o Nonspecific reports related to heath

- o Engaging in solitary play or work
- o Changes in appetite resulting in weight changes
- o Changes in sleeping patterns
- o Irritability
- o Aggression
- o High-risk behavior
- o Poor school performance and/or dropping out of school
- o Difficulty concentrating and/or completing tasks
- o Feelings of hopelessness about the future
- o Sense of helplessness
- o Suicidal thoughts

ANXIETY DISORDERS

Overview

- An anxiety disorder exists when:

    - o Anxiety interferes with normal growth and development.

    - o Anxiety is so serious that the child is unable to function normally in the home, school, and other areas of life.

- Separation anxiety disorder

    - o This disorder is characterized by excessive anxiety when a child is separated from or anticipating separation from home or parents. The anxiety may develop into a school phobia, phobia of being left alone, panic disorder, or another specific phobia. Depression is often a co-occurring disorder.

- Posttraumatic stress disorder (PTSD)

    - o PTSD can be brought on by experiencing or seeing an extremely traumatic event.

    - o Children with PTSD often will respond to the precipitating event in a series of phases. The phases can begin with an arousal that lasts a few minutes to 1 to 2 hr, followed by a period of about 2 weeks in which the child will attempt to deal with the event using defense mechanisms. The last phase, lasting for a period of 2 to 3 months, is when the child may develop psychologic symptoms as attempts are made to cope with the event. Failure to cope can lead to obsession regarding the event.

Data Collection

- Risk Factors

    - o Anxiety may develop after a specific stressor (death of a relative or pet, illness, move, assault).

- Subjective and Objective Data

  - Children with PTSD may have psychologic symptoms of anxiety, depression, phobia, or conversion reactions.

  - If the anxiety resulting from PTSD is displayed externally, it may be manifested as irritability and aggression with family and friends, poor academic performance, somatic reports, belief that life will be short, and difficulty sleeping.

BEHAVIOR DISORDERS

Overview

- ADHD

  - The inability of a person to control behaviors requiring sustained attention.

  - Types of ADHD

    - ADHD combined type (most common)

    - ADHD predominantly inattentive – difficulty paying attention, does not appear to listen, easily distracted

    - ADHD predominantly hyperactive – impulsive, fidgeting, inability to sit still, excessive talking, difficulty waiting for turns, interrupting, disregarding consequences of behavior

  - Behaviors associated with ADHD must have been present prior to age 7 and must be present in more than one setting for the child to be diagnosed with ADHD. Behaviors associated with ADHD may receive negative attention from adults and peers.

  - Inattentive or impulsive behavior may put the child at risk for injury.

- Autism spectrum disorder

  - A complex neurodevelopmental disorder of unknown etiology with a wide spectrum of behaviors affecting an individual's ability to communicate and interact with others. Cognitive and language development are typically delayed. Characteristic behaviors include an inability to maintain eye contact, repetitive actions, and strict observance of routines.

  - The disorder is usually observed before 3 years of age.

  - There is a wide variety of functioning. Abilities may range from poor (inability to perform self-care, inability to communicate and relate to others) to high (ability to function at near-normal levels).

- Mental retardation

  - Below average intellectual functioning indicated by an IQ of less than 70

- Learning disability

  - Group of disorders characterized by difficulty in gaining and using essential skills of listening, speaking, reading, reasoning, performing math, and writing

- Communication disorder
  - May be expressive, receptive, or a combination of both

Data Collection

- Subjective and Objective Data
  - In children with behavior disorders, symptoms generally worsen.
    - Situations that require sustained attention
    - Group situations with less structure, such as playground or classroom activities
  - ADHD
    - Behavioral problems usually occur in school, church, home, and/or recreational activities.
    - Inattention, impulsivity, and hyperactivity are characteristic behaviors of ADHD.

Collaborative Care

- Nursing Care
  - Obtain a complete nursing history.
    - Mother's pregnancy and birth history
    - Sleeping, eating, and elimination patterns and recent weight loss or gain
    - Achievement of developmental milestones
    - Allergies
    - Current medications
    - Peer and family relationships and school performance
    - History of emotional, physical, or sexual abuse
    - Parents' perceptions and reactions to the child's behavior
    - Family history, including current members of the household
    - Substance use/abuse
      - Tobacco products (cigarettes, cigars, snuff, chewing tobacco) and frequency of use
      - Alcohol, frequency of use, driving under the influence, and family history of abuse
      - Drugs (illegal or prescription) used to get high, stay calm, lose weight, or stay awake
    - Safety at home and at school
    - Actual or potential risk for self-injury

- Presence of depression and suicidal ideation, including a plan, the lethality of that plan, and the means to carry out the plan

- Availability of weapons in the home

○ Perform a complete physical assessment, including a mental status examination.

○ Use primary prevention, such as education, peer group discussions, and mentoring to decrease risky behavior and promote healthy behavior and effective coping.

- Work with children to adopt a realistic view of their bodies and to improve overall self-esteem.

- Identify and reinforce the use of positive coping skills.

- Monitor for home safety, including proper storage of medications and weapons.

- Emphasize the use of seat belts when in motor vehicles.

- Encourage the use of protective gear for high-impact sports.

- Provide education on contraceptives and other sexual information, such as transmission and prevention of HIV and other sexually transmitted diseases.

- Encourage abstinence, but keep the lines of communication open to allow adolescents to discuss sexual practices.

- Encourage children and parents to seek professional help if indicated and provide resources.

○ Intervene with children who have engaged in high-risk behaviors.

- Instruct children and families about factors that contribute to substance dependency and tobacco use. Suggest appropriate referrals when indicated.

- Inform children and families about support groups in the community for eating disorders, substance abuse, and general teen support.

- Instruct children regarding individuals within the school environment and community to whom concerns can be voiced about personal safety, (police officers, school nurses, counselors, teachers).

- Involve social services when indicated.

- Discuss the use and availability of support hotlines.

○ Intervene with children who have anxiety disorders.

- Provide emotional support that is accepting of regression and other defense mechanisms.

- Offer protection from panic levels of anxiety.

- Increase self-esteem and feelings of achievement.

- Assist with working through traumatic events or losses and accepting what has happened.

- Suggest group therapy.

- Intervene with children who have behavior disorders.

  - Use a calm, firm, respectful approach with children.

  - Use modeling to demonstrate appropriate behavior.

  - Obtain the child's attention before giving directions. Provide short and clear explanations.

  - Set clear limits on unacceptable behaviors and be consistent.

  - Identify physical activities through which the child can use energy and obtain success.

  - Assist parents to develop a reward system using methods such as a wall chart or tokens. Encourage the child to participate.

  - Focus on the family and child's strengths, not just the problems.

  - Provide a safe environment for the child and others.

  - Provide children with specific positive feedback when expectations are met.

  - Identify issues that result in power struggles.

  - Assist children in developing effective coping mechanisms.

  - Encourage children to participate in a form of either group, individual, or family therapy.

  - Administer medications (antipsychotics, mood stabilizers, anticonvulsants, antidepressants). Monitor for side effects.

- Intervene with children who have an autism spectrum disorder.

  - Request early intervention.

  - Determine emotional and situational triggers.

  - Provide for a structured environment.

  - Carefully monitor the child's behaviors to ensure safety.

  - Consult with the parents to provide consistent and individualized care.

  - Encourage the parents to participate in planning for and giving care to the child.

  - Use short, concise, concrete, and developmentally appropriate communication.

  - Identify desired behaviors and reward them.

  - Role model social skills.

  - Role play situations that involve conflict.

  - Encourage verbal communication.

  - Limit self-stimulating and ritualistic behaviors by providing alternative play activities.

  - Give plenty of notice before changing routines.

  - Carefully monitor the child's behaviors to ensure safety.

- Medications

  o Medications for children and adolescents who have mental health disorders include selective serotonin reuptake inhibitors (fluoxetine [Prozac]), tricyclic antidepressants (amitriptyline [Elavil]), atypical anxiolytics (buspirone [BuSpar]), atypical antidepressants (bupropion [Wellbutrin]), CNS stimulants (methylphenidate [Concerta, Ritalin SR]), and norepinephrine selective reuptake inhibitors (atomoxetine HCl [Strattera]).

- Interdisciplinary Care

  o Learning disabilities

    ■ An individualized approach depends on the disorder and is generally treated within the school setting as an interdisciplinary method (special education, speech therapy, physical therapy, and resource teachers).

  o Communications disorder

    ■ Treated through a variety of modalities (speech and language therapies, adaptive communication devices, hearing aids, sign language)

- Client Outcomes

  o The child achieves a maximum level of physical, cognitive, and social development.

  o The child is able to communicate effectively.

  o The child and family verbalize the need for information and support.

  o The child verbalizes improved mood.

  o The child develops realistic goals for the future.

  o The family identifies strategies for managing long-term care of the child.

  o The family identifies strategies for managing disruptive or inappropriate behavior.

MALTREATMENT OF INFANTS AND CHILDREN

Overview

- Maltreatment of infants and children is attributed to a variety of predisposing factors, which include parental, child, and environmental characteristics. Child maltreatment can occur across all economic and educational backgrounds and racial/ethnic/religious groups.

  o Maltreatment of children is made up of several specific types of behaviors.

    ■ Physical – Any recent act or failure to act that results in imminent risk of serious physical or emotional harm, or death, of a child (less than 18 years of age).

    ■ Sexual – Occurs when sexual contact takes place without consent, whether or not the victim is able to give consent (includes any sexual behavior toward a minor and dating violence among adolescents)

    ■ Emotional – Humiliates, threatens, or intimidates a child (includes behavior that minimizes an individual's feelings of self-worth)

- Neglect – Includes the failure to provide:
  - Physical care (feeding, clothing, shelter, medical or dental care, safety, education)
  - Emotional care and/or stimulation to allow normal development (nurturing, affection, attention)

- Failure to thrive (FTT)
  - FTT is also known as growth failure. It is manifested as inadequate growth resulting from the inability to obtain or use calories required for growth. It is usually described in an infant or child who falls below the fifth percentile for weight (and possibly for height) or has persistent weight loss.
    - FTT can be the result of an organic (physical) cause, the result of a definable psychosocial cause unrelated to disease, or idiopathic, in which the cause is unknown.

Data Collection

- Risk Factors
  - Maltreatment
    - Children under 3 years of age
    - Children that are premature, physically disabled, are the result of an unwanted pregnancy, or have some other trait that makes them particularly vulnerable.
  - FTT
    - Organic causes may include cerebral palsy, chronic renal failure, congenital heart disease, and/or gastroesophageal reflux. However, factors related to nonorganic failure to thrive (NFTT) may include:
      - Parental neglect, lack of parental knowledge, or a disturbed maternal-child attachment
      - Poverty
      - Health or childrearing beliefs
      - Family stress
      - Feeding resistance
      - Insufficient breast milk

- Subjective and Objective Data
  - Inconsistencies between the parent's report and the child's injuries.
  - Maltreatment
    - Inconsistency between nature of injury and developmental level of the child.
    - Repeated injuries requiring emergency treatment.
    - Inappropriate responses from the parents or child.

- Physical signs such as growth failure, bruises, burns, fractures, poor hygiene, and foul odors or discharge from the genital area.
  - Check for unusual bruising on the abdomen, back, and/or buttocks.
  - Identify the mechanism of injury, which may not be congruent with the physical appearance of the injury. Many bruises at different stages of healing may indicate continued beatings. Observe for bruises or welts that have taken on the shape of a belt buckle or other objects.
  - Observe for burns that appear glove- or stocking-like on hands or feet, which may indicate forced immersion into boiling water. Check for an absence of splash marks from water. Small, round burns may be caused by lit cigarettes.
  - Note fractures with unusual features, such as forearm spiral fractures, which could be caused by twisting the extremity forcefully. The presence of multiple fractures and old fractures in various stages of healing are suspicious.
  - Check children for head injuries. Monitor the child's level of consciousness, making sure to note equal and reactive pupils. Also, monitor the child for nausea/vomiting.
- Inappropriate knowledge of or interest in sexual acts
- Seductive behavior
- Avoidance of anything related to sexuality or genitals and the body
- Withdrawn behaviors or excessive aggression towards others
- Fear of a particular person or family member

o Shaken baby syndrome – Shaking may cause intracranial hemorrhage.
  - Observe for:
    - Respiratory distress.
    - Bulging fontanels.
    - Increased head circumference.
    - Retinal hemorrhage.
  - If bruising is present in infants before 6 months of age, it should be deemed as suspicious by nurses.

o Failure to thrive
  - Less than the fifth percentile on the growth chart for weight
  - Malnourished appearance
  - Signs of dehydration
  - Decreased activity level
  - Developmental delays

- Negative interactions between the child and parents (no eye contact, irritability, pushing parents away)
- Difficulty being soothed

○ Laboratory Tests

- CBC, urinalysis, and other tests that assess for sexually transmitted infections or bleeding

○ Diagnostic Procedures

- Diagnostics will depend upon the assessment findings and noted findings or injuries. They may include:
  □ Radiograph
    ▸ CT or MRI scans

Collaborative Care

- Nursing Care

  ○ Maltreatment

  - Report all suspected or actual cases of child abuse. Recognize that mandatory reporting is required of all health care providers.
  - Clearly and objectively document information obtained in the interview and during the physical assessment.
  - Photograph and detail all visible injuries.
  - Conduct the interview about family abuse in private.
  - Be direct, honest, and professional.
  - Use language the child understands.
  - Be understanding and attentive.
  - Inform children and parents if a report must be made to children or adult protective services and explain the process.
  - Check for safety and help reduce danger for the victim.
  - Use questions that are open-ended and require a descriptive response. These questions are less threatening and elicit more relevant information.
  - Provide support for children and families.
  - Demonstrate behaviors for child-rearing techniques with the parents and child.

  ○ FTT

  - Obtain a nutritional history.
  - Observe parent-child interactions.
  - Obtain accurate baseline height and weight. Observe for low weight, malnourished appearance, and signs of dehydration.

- Weigh children daily without clothing or a diaper.
- Perform accurate I&O and calorie counts as prescribed.
- Instruct parents to recognize and respond to the infant's cues of hunger.
- Establish a routine for eating that encourages usual times, duration, and setting.
- Reinforce proper positioning, latching on, and timing for mothers who are breastfeeding.
- Encourage parents to:
  □ Maintain eye contact and face-to-face posture during feedings.
  □ Talk to the infant while feeding.
  □ Burp the infant frequently.
  □ Keep the environment quiet and without distractions.
  □ Be persistent, remaining calm during 10 to 15 min of food refusal.
  □ Introduce new foods slowly.
  □ Never force the infant to eat.
  □ Develop a structured routine.

- Interdisciplinary Care

  ○ A team of health professionals may be involved in the care of the child. These may include a dietician, pediatric feeding specialist, physician, and occupational therapist.

  ○ Coordinate care with community social services.

- Care After Discharge

  ○ Client Education

    - Encourage support groups for parents.
    - Encourage attendance at parenting classes.

  ○ Follow-up

    - Reinforce cooperation with social services and community agencies.
    - Reinforce the need for follow-up care.

Ⓐ APPLICATION EXERCISES

1. A parent suspects her son may have a mood disorder and asks the nurse to describe examples of behaviors than can occur in children. Which of the following behaviors should be discussed? (Select all that apply.)

   _____ Performance in school deteriorates

   _____ Impulsiveness

   _____ Changes in sleeping patterns

   _____ Difficulty paying attention

   _____ Irritability

2. A nurse suspects a case of shaken baby syndrome when she collects which of the following data during the admission process of a 5-month-old infant?

   A. Signs of dehydration

   B. Periorbital bruising

   C. Child avoids eye contact with caregiver

   D. Extensive diaper rash

3. Causes of the organic form of failure to thrive may include _____.

4. Possible causes of the non-organic form of failure to thrive may include _____.

5. A nurse is reviewing methods of home behavior modification that a mother uses for her 7-year-old daughter who has ADHD when she invites other children in the home for group play. Which of the following statements by the mother indicates a need for clarification?

   A. "I will use a calm, firm, respectful manner with my daughter."

   B. "I will plan quiet, low-energy activities such as painting with watercolors."

   C. "I'll let my daughter plan her activities for the day."

   D. "I'll give my daughter positive comments about appropriate behavior."

6. Identify stressful events that can lead to the development of anxiety disorders in children.

7. Which of the following is an example of a central nervous system stimulant that can be prescribed for children who have ADHD?

   A. Fluoxetine (Prozac)

   B. Methylphenidate (Concerta, Ritalin)

   C. Atomoxetine (Strattera)

   D. Amitriptyline (Elavil)

APPLICATION EXERCISES ANSWER KEY

1. A parent suspects her son may have a mood disorder and asks the nurse to describe examples of behaviors than can occur in children. Which of the following behaviors should be discussed? (Select all that apply.)

   __X__ **Performance in school deteriorates**

   _____ Impulsiveness

   __X__ **Changes in sleeping patterns**

   _____ Difficulty paying attention

   __X__ **Irritability**

   Behavioral characteristics of mood disorders include poor school performance and/or dropping out of school, changes in sleep patterns, and irritability. Other typical behaviors can include vague reports of health problems, solitary play or work, loss of appetite and weight, aggression, high-risk behaviors, feelings of hopelessness about the future, and suicidal thoughts. Impulsiveness and difficulty paying attention are more likely to be signs of attention deficit hyperactivity disorder.

    NCLEX® Connection: Psychosocial Integrity, Mental Health Concepts

2. A nurse suspects a case of shaken baby syndrome when she collects which of the following data during the admission process of a 5-month-old infant?

   A. Signs of dehydration

   B. Periorbital bruising

   C. Child avoids eye contact with caregiver

   D. Extensive diaper rash

   Signs of shaken baby syndrome include bruising in the infant before 6 months of age, respiratory distress, bulging fontanels, increased head circumference, and retinal hemorrhage. Signs of dehydration, lack of eye contact, and severe diaper rash may be noted in children who fail to thrive.

    NCLEX® Connection: Psychosocial Integrity, Abuse or Neglect

3. Causes of the organic form of failure to thrive may include **physical conditions such as cerebral palsy, chronic renal failure, congenital heart disease, or GERD.**

   NCLEX® Connection: Reduction of Risk Potential, Potential for Alterations in Body Systems

4. Possible causes of the non-organic form of failure to thrive may include **parental neglect, poverty, ineffective health and childrearing practices, family stress, insufficient breast milk, and the infant resisting feeding.**

   NCLEX® Connection: Psychosocial Integrity, Abuse or Neglect

5. A nurse is reviewing methods of home behavior modification that a mother uses for her 7-year-old daughter who has ADHD when she invites other children in the home for group play. Which of the following statements by the mother indicates a need for clarification?

    A. "I will use a calm, firm, respectful manner with my daughter."

    B. "I will plan quiet, low-energy activities such as painting with watercolors."

    C. "I'll let my daughter plan her activities for the day."

    D. "I'll give my daughter positive comments about appropriate behavior."

    Children with ADHD do better with activities that involve physical exertion and energy expenditure.

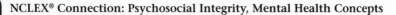 NCLEX® Connection: Psychosocial Integrity, Mental Health Concepts

6. Identify stressful events that can lead to the development of anxiety disorders in children.

    Anxiety may develop after the death of a parent, family member, or pet. Illness can be another cause. A change in family residence or a move to another city and a new school are potential triggers for anxiety. A car accident, physical assault, being bullied, or other violent acts are anxiety-provoking events.

    NCLEX® Connection: Psychosocial Integrity, Mental Health Concepts

7. Which of the following is an example of a central nervous system stimulant that can be prescribed for children who have ADHD?

    A. Fluoxetine (Prozac)

    B. Methylphenidate (Concerta, Ritalin)

    C. Atomoxetine (Strattera)

    D. Amitriptyline (Elavil)

    Methylphenidate is a central nervous system stimulant that can be prescribed for children who have ADHD. Fluoxetine is a SSRI. Atomoxetine is a norepinephrine selective reuptake inhibitor. Amitriptyline is a TCA.

    NCLEX® Connection: Pharmacological Therapies, Expected Actions/Outcomes

References

Centers for Disease Control and Prevention - http://www.cdc.gov

Curren, A. (2008). *Math for meds: Dosages and solutions* (10th ed). Cliften Park, NY: Delmar.

Dudek, S. G. (2010). *Nutrition essentials for nursing practice* (6th ed.). Philadelphia: Lippincott Williams & Wilkins.

Hockenberry, M. J., & Wilson, D. (2009). *Wong's essentials of pediatric nursing* (8th ed.). St. Louis, MO: Mosby.

Lehne, R. A. (2010). *Pharmacology for nursing care* (7th ed.). St. Louis: Saunders.

Perry, S., Hockenberry, M., Lowdermilk, D., Wilson, D. (2010). *Maternal child nursing care.* (4th ed.) Maryland Heights, MO: Mosby.

Pillitteri, A. (2007). *Maternal and child health nursing: Care of the childbearing and childrearing family* (5th ed.). Philadelphia: Lippincott Williams & Wilkins.

Varcarolis, E. M., Halter, M.J., (2010). (2010). *Foundations of psychiatric mental health nursing: A clinical approach* (5th ed.). St. Louis, MO: Saunders.

Wilson, B. A., Shannon, M. T., & Shields, K. M. (2011). *Pearson nurse's drug guide 2011.* Upper Saddle River, NJ: Prentice-Hall.